MIDDLE EAR AND MASTOID SURGERY

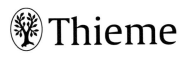

MIDDLE EAR AND MASTOID SURGERY

Edited by

Rex S. Haberman II, M.D.

Assistant Clinical Professor
Department of Otolaryngology
University of Minnesota Medical School
Minneapolis, Minnesota

Consulting Otologist
Department of Otolaryngology
Hennepin County Medical Center
Minneapolis, Minnesota

Department Head of Otolaryngology
Aspen Medical Group
St Paul, Minnesota

Thieme
New York • Stuttgart

Thieme New York
333 Seventh Avenue
New York, NY 10001

Consulting Medical Editor: Esther Gumpert
Associate Editor: Owen Zurhellen
Director, Production and Manufacturing: Anne Vinnicombe
Production Editor: David R. Stewart
Marketing Director: Phyllis Gold
Director of Sales: Ross Lumpkin
Chief Financial Officer: Peter van Woerden
President: Brian D. Scanlan
Medical Illustrator: Anthony M. Pazos
Compositor: Datapage International Limited
Printer: The Maple-Vail Book Manufacturing Group

Library of Congress Cataloging in Publication Data is available from the publisher

Important note: Medical knowledge is ever-changing. As new research and clinical experience broaden our knowledge, changes in treatment and drug therapy may be required. The authors and editors of the material herein have consulted sources believed to be reliable in their efforts to provide information that is complete and in accord with the standards accepted at the time of publication. However, in view of the possibility of human error by the authors, editors, or publisher of the work herein, or changes in medical knowledge, neither the authors, editors, or publisher, nor any other party who has been involved in the preparation of this work, warrants that the information contained herein is in every respect accurate or complete, and they are not responsible for any errors or omissions or for the results obtained from use of such information. Readers are encouraged to confirm the information contained herein with other sources. For example, readers are encouraged to check the product information sheet included in the package of each drug they plan to administer to be certain that the information contained in this publication is accurate and that changes have not been made in the recommended dose or in the contraindications for administration. This recommendation is of particular importance in connection with new or infrequently used drugs.

Some of the product names, patants, and registered designs referred to in this book are in fact registered trademarks or proprietary names even though specific reference to this fact is not always made in the text. Therefore, the appearance of a name without designation as proprietary is not to be construed as a representation by the publisher that it is in the public domain.

Printed in the United States of America

5   4   3   2   1

TNY ISBN 1-58890-173-4
GTV ISBN 3-13-136061-5

To those who strive for excellence and trust their spirit, for without that, enrichment of the mind would serve no purpose

CONTENTS

FOREWORD I

It is indeed a pleasure and honor to be asked to write this foreword to an outstanding textbook on external auditory canal, middle ear, and mastoid surgery. I have truly enjoyed the opportunity to review the outstanding chapters. Having grown up with the many developments in middle ear and mastoid surgery over the past 30 years I have particularly enjoyed the opportunity to review and compare various surgical techniques and approaches that are eloquently described in this text. This textbook addresses solutions to the multitude of problems that present to the otolaryngologist on a daily basis.

Of particular interest is that experts in the field write the chapters. These authors are able to concisely explain and illustrate their techniques. I also found it interesting and exciting to know that many of these authors studied with the great professors of the past and therefore are able to bring a personal perspective to the surgery of the ear. They present the problem, discuss the evaluation of the patient, and describe in detail their surgical technique. It becomes clear that there are many ways to approach the same disease process. This textbook offers the opportunity to compare and contrast these various procedures. Even though I have seen and done most of these techniques, I found reviewing the material

has helped me to understand the differences, advantages, and disadvantages of all these techniques.

By concentrating on the external ear, middle ear, and mastoid, one is able to understand the disease process and surgery that comprise over 90% of the total ear surgery performed today.

This text offers the resident, as well as the practicing physician and the professor, the opportunity to have a basic knowledge and understanding of external ear, middle ear, and mastoid surgery. The textbook is laid out in a well-organized manor, beginning with basic chronic ear surgery and progressing to the more unusual external ear problems and finally the less common labyrinthectomy, middle ear, and cochlear implants.

In summary, the Editor, Dr. Rex Haberman, is to be congratulated on assembling an outstanding group of authors and organizing this well-written and illustrated textbook. This text will be must reading for all those who desire to learn and understand external, middle ear, and mastoid surgery.

John W. House, M.D.
House Ear Clinic
Los Angeles, California

FOREWORD II

Middle ear and mastoid surgical procedures constitute the vast majority of otological procedures utilized by the general otolaryngologist, head and neck surgeon (often 50% of those practice), and especially by the otologist-neurotologist. There are a number of other textbooks that discuss otology as a whole, including information regarding pathogenesis of the many hundreds and even thousands of ear diseases. The recent literature with emphasis on molecular biological studies, including syndromic hearing losses (usually sensorineural), with particular relevance and frequency of studies enhancing our understanding of nonsyndromic hearing losses, represent a new wave of important information regarding etiology and pathogenesis. Other texts also emphasize medical management of otological diseases as well as information regarding intracranial diseases and related surgical procedures. The above serve as an essential background to this practical text, which focuses on the most common surgical procedures (middle ear and mastoid) that will provide information, reference, and assistance to residents, fellows, general otolaryngologists, and otologists-neurotologists, as well as others in associated fields with an interest in otological surgery.

In this text, *Middle Ear and Mastoid Surgery*, Dr. Rex Haberman (Editor) has most of the common surgical procedures covered, with a nicely balanced selection of authors for the various chapters. Each chapter necessarily stresses the authors' point of view and the reader will benefit from this information relative to his/her personal experience and database of otological surgery. The authors also blend new and slightly older "blood," so that on the whole this book incorporates current innovative procedures with more experienced time-proven surgical procedures.

Once more, this text will prove to be of interest and useful to all involved in these common otological surgical procedures, which represent the majority of surgical otology.

Michael M. Paparella, M.D.
Minnesota Ear, Head & Neck Clinic
Clinical Professor and Chairman Emeritus
Department of Otolaryngology
University of Minnesota
International Hearing Foundation

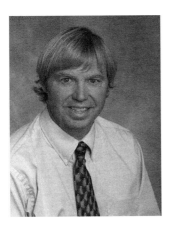

PREFACE

On a day prior to September 11, 2001, at the American Academy of Otolaryngology–Head and Neck Surgery annual meeting in Denver, Colorado, I had dinner with Esther Gumpert, consulting editor from Thieme Medical Publishers for otolaryngology, ophthalmology, and orthopaedics titles. She told me that she had some ideas about a new otologic textbook and wanted to know if I had any thoughts regarding the same. She asked if I would be interested in editing and authoring this new text. The task seemed daunting. After a long discussion, however, it became clear to me that otolaryngology needed a book that was applicable to the general otolaryngologist and otolaryngology resident, and was defined, chapter by chapter, by operative procedure and not by anatomy or disease state. We thought that the book should be a frequently used addition to the libraries of otolaryngologists and not one to sit on the shelf. With that in mind, we set off to recruit the best otologic surgeons in the world to contribute to the project. We asked them to write in a way that is easily understood and can be quickly referenced. Our intent is for practitioners and residents to open the book regularly to review and prepare for upcoming otologic surgeries.

The table of contents clearly demonstrates our idea. At first, simple otologic procedures, such as myringoplasty and tympanoplasty, are presented. Tympanoplasty is presented in its many forms, with both medial and lateral techniques discussed. If an ear surgeon needs to make a decision regarding whether it would be better to do a lateral graft versus a cartilage graft, all that is necessary is to compare Chapter 4 and Chapter 6. The surgeon should be able to assimilate the different techniques and determine which best fits the patient. A variety of mastoid techniques are presented next, including wall up, wall down, intact bridge, revision, recon-

structive, and pediatric mastoidectomy. Virtually all chronic ear diseases can be handled by having a thorough knowledge of those techniques. Some otologists believe that general otolaryngologists should not perform stapedectomy, an opinion I do not agree with. If an otolaryngologist is performing at least five stapedectomies per year and has predictably excellent results, I see no reason to limit that activity. Therefore, three chapters are devoted to the operation, including a chapter on endoscopic procedures relating to otosclerosis. Our intent is to present stapedectomy as a procedure that the surgeon may relatively quickly review prior to performing it to enhance operator poise and surety. We present two chapters on ossiculoplasty, each written by internationally renowned otologists, with the idea that the reader should be given more choice when it comes to reconstructing the ossicular chain. There are many ways to get a satisfactory result and those options should be readily available.

Later on, the text presents some procedures that may require additional training or expertise, but nevertheless remain true otolaryngologic procedures. Canaloplasty for atresia can be one of the most demanding of all otologic procedures. Our chapter makes each step seem clear as possible, and is an excellent review for those about to take that operation on. Surgery for Meniere's disease has had its controversy over the decades, but many otologists, including me, believe that endolymphatic sac surgery has its place and should be part of the surgeon's armamentarium. Labyrinthectomy and basic neurotologic procedures present more options on how to treat recalcitrant Meniere's and other diseases. Finally, the book presents the newest technology and information regarding cochlear implants and implantable hearing aids. The future may indeed lie in those areas, particularly in implantable hearing aids, once costs are held to reasonable levels so that the general public can afford such operations or third-party payers decide it is good policy to cover implantation.

I am confident that once the general otolaryngologist and otolaryngology resident becomes familiar with this text, it will be used often. The future will determine the course of the next edition. I am convinced that our approach, presenting each chapter as a procedure, is an excellent way to present this information. I hope you, the reader, will enjoy the book as much as we enjoyed preparing it.

Rex S. Haberman II, M.D.

ACKNOWLEDGMENTS

Many hours have been spent reading, editing, writing, and reviewing documents related to this project. My authors were given guidelines, but I allowed significant latitude to allow opportunities to express their styles and present their expertise. It pays off in the final product. Each chapter represents a skillfully written dissertation, armed with exacting illustrations that make understanding easier than ever.

There are many people I wish to thank. Esther Gumpert, consulting medical editor at Thieme Medical Publishers, has been very supportive of the project since day one. Also, J. Owen Zurhellen, associate editor at Thieme, has been enormously helpful in getting information to and from the authors and has helped me make decisions regarding important issues related to the book. I'd like to thank my many contributors, for without their knowledge there could be no book. Anthony M. Pazos, our medical illustrator, has done a magnificent job of preparing the drawings in a way that is accurate and complete. I'd like to thank my family for their understanding of how many hours are required to prepare such a manuscript. My office staff, both academic and private, has also been very supportive. Finally, I'd like to thank the surgeons before me who paved the way for us in modern medicine. Without their ingenuity and courage, we would never have come this far.

Rex S. Haberman II, M.D.

CONTRIBUTORS

Patrick J. Antonelli, M.D., M.S.
Professor and Vice Chair
Department of Otolaryngology
University of Florida
Gainesville, Florida

Seilesh C. Babu, M.D.
Fellow
Department of Otology/Skull Base Surgery
Providence Hospital/Michigan Ear Institute
Southfield, Michigan

Robert A. Battista, M.D.
Northwestern University Medical School
Hinsdale, Illinois

Dennis I. Bojrab, B.S., M.D.
Associate Professor of Otolaryngology
Wayne State University
Detroit, Michigan;
Michigan Ear Institute
Farmington Hills, Michigan;
Chief of Otolaryngology–Head and Neck Surgery
William Beaumont Hospital
Royal Oak, Michigan;
Chief of Skull Base Surgery
Providence Hospital
Southfield, Michigan

Larry K. Burton, Jr., M.D.
Ear, Nose, and Throat Department
Mayo Clinic
Rochester, Minnesota

John L. Dornhoffer, M.D.
Associate Professor
Department of Otolaryngology–Head and Neck
  Surgery
University of Arkansas for Medical Sciences
Little Rock, Arkansas

Karen J. Doyle, M.D.
Department of Otolaryngology–Head and Neck
  Surgery
University of California Davis Medical Center
Sacramento, California

Colin L.W. Driscoll, M.D.
Ear, Nose, and Throat Department
Mayo Clinic
Rochester, Minnesota

Carlos R. Esquivel, M.D.
Assistant Professor
Department of Surgery
Madigan Army Medical Center
Uniform Services University Health Sciences Center
Tacoma, Washington

Jay B. Farrior, M.D.
Farrior Ear Clinic
Tampa, Florida

Jill B. Firszt, Ph.D.
Associate Professor
Department of Otolaryngology and Communication
  Sciences
Medical College of Wisconsin
Milwaukee, Wisconsin

Rick A. Friedman, M.D., Ph.D.
Associate, House Ear Clinic;
St. Vincent's Medical Center/Los Angeles County–
  USC Medical Center
Los Angeles, California

Oleg Froymovich, M.D.
Assistant Professor
Department of Otolaryngology–Head and Neck
  Surgery
University of Minnesota;
Minnesota Ear, Head, and Neck Clinic
Minneapolis, Minnesota

Edward K. Gardner, M.D.
Fellow
The Otology Group
Baptist Hospital
Nashville, Tennessee

Gary E. Garvis, M.D., F.A.C.S.
Assistant Clinical Professor of Otolaryngology
University of Minnesota Medical School;
Ear, Nose, and Throat Specialty Care of Minnesota
Minneapolis, Minnesota

William J. Garvis, M.D.
Ear, Nose, and Throat Specialty Care of Minnesota
Minneapolis, Minnesota

Norman N. Ge, M.D.
Department of Otolaryngology–Head and Neck
  Surgery
University of California Davis Medical Center
Sacramento, California

Rex S. Haberman II, M.D.
Assistant Clinical Professor
Department of Otolaryngology
University of Minnesota Medical School
Minneapolis, Minnesota;
Consulting Otologist
Department of Otolaryngology
Hennepin County Medical Center
Minneapolis, Minnesota;
Department Head of Otolaryngology
Aspen Medical Group
St Paul, Minnesota

Marlan R. Hansen, M.D.
House Ear Clinic
Los Angeles, California

Tina C. Huang, M.D.
University of Minnesota Medical School
Minneapolis, Minnesota

Gordon B. Hughes, M.D., F.A.C.S.
Professor and Head, Otology and Neurotology
Department of Otolaryngology and Communicative
  Disorders

Cleveland Clinic Foundation
Cleveland, Ohio

Raleigh O. Jones, M.D., F.A.C.S.
Associate Professor
Department of Surgery
University of Kentucky Medical Center
Lexington, Kentucky

Andrew N. Karpenko, M.D.
Wayne State University
Detroit, Michigan

John F. Kveton, M.D.
Clinical Assistant
Department of Surgery/Otolaryngology
Yale University School of Medicine
New Haven, Connecticut

Joseph L. Leach, M.D.
Department of Otolaryngology
University of Texas Southwestern Medical Center
Dallas, Texas

Samuel C. Levine, M.D.
Department of Otolaryngology
University of Minnesota
Minneapolis, Minnesota

Pramit S. Malhotra, M.D.
Department of Otolaryngology
University of Minnesota
Minneapolis, Minnesota

Thomas J. McDonald, M.D.
Professor of Otolaryngology
Mayo Medical School;
Department of Otorhinolaryngology–Head and
  Neck Surgery
Mayo Clinic
Rochester, Minnesota

Edwin M. Monsell, M.D., Ph.D.
Professor
Department of Otolaryngology–Head and Neck
  Surgery
Wayne State University School of Medicine
Detroit, Michigan

Tam Q. Nguyen, M.D.
Department of Otolaryngology–Head and Neck
  Surgery
Wayne State University School of Medicine
Detroit, Michigan

Sarah L. Pertzborn, M.D.
Resident Physician
Department of Otolaryngology–Head and Neck
 Surgery
University of Florida
Gainesville, Florida

Dennis S. Poe, M.D.
Harvard Medical School
Boston, Massachesetts

G. Mark Pyle, M.D.
Associate Professor
Department of Surgery
Division of Otolaryngology–Head and Neck Surgery
University of Wisconsin Hospitals and Clinics
Madison, Wisconsin

Frank Rimell, M.D.
Associate Professor
Department of Otolaryngology–Head and Neck
 Surgery
University of Minnesota
Minneapolis, Minnesota

Franklin M. Rizer, M.D. [deceased]
Department of Otolaryngology and Communication
 Science
Ohio State University
Warren, Ohio

Peter S. Roland, M.D.
Department of Otolaryngology
University of Texas Southwestern Medical Center
Dallas, Texas

Seth I. Rosenberg, M.D., F.A.C.S.
Clinical Assistant Professor
Department of Otorhinolaryngology
University of Pennsylvania
Philadelphia;
Florida Ear and Sinus Center
Sarasota, Florida

Bassem M. Said, M.D.
Private Practice
Otolaryngology–Head and Neck Surgery
Brentwood, California

Hamed Sajjadi, M.D., F.A.C.S.
Clinical Associate Professor
Department of Otology/Neurotology
Stanford University Medical Center
San Jose, California

Weiru Shao, M.D.
Fellow
Department of Otolaryngology–Head and Neck
 Surgery
University of Minnesota;
Minnesota Ear, Head, and Neck Clinic
Minneapolis, Minnesota

Michele St. Martin, M.D.
Department of Otolaryngology
University of Minnesota
Minneapolis, Minnesota

John Stewart, D.O.
Private Practice
Minnesota Ear, Head, and Neck Clinic;
Fairview-University Medical Center
Minneapolis, Minnesota

Trang Vo-Nuygen, M.D.
Resident
Department of Otolaryngology–Head and Neck
 Surgery
University of Minnesota
Minneapolis, Minnesota

Phillip A. Wackym, M.D., F.A.C.S.
John C. Koss Professor and Chairman
Department of Otolaryngology and Communication
 Sciences
Medical College of Wisconsin
Milwaukee, Wisconsin

Chapter 1

An Overview of Middle Ear and Mastoid Surgery

Rex S. Haberman II

There are many indications for middle ear and mastoid surgery. Traumatic and nontraumatic perforations of the eardrum need repair, accomplished through a variety of ways. For a small defect, a myringoplasty or repair of the eardrum without lifting a tympanomeatal flap might suffice; for larger perforations, tympanoplasty becomes necessary. Techniques of tympanoplasty vary according to the size of the perforation and underlying disease. A transcanal approach may be all that is required, but frequently that does not give the surgeon sufficient exposure, so a postauricular approach becomes necessary. Medial and lateral grafting techniques all have their place, depending on the nature of the primary problem and training and preference of the surgeon. Both techniques have excellent results, as the take rate exceeds 90%.

Chronic otitis media with and without cholesteatoma is the major disease that leads the otologic surgeon to perform a mastoid operation. There are different approaches to mastoid surgery. Many believe that the logical approach to mastoidectomy is to leave the posterior ear canal intact and perform a canal-wall-up mastoidectomy. Others believe that leaving the posterior ear canal intact leaves the patient with too high a risk for recurrence of disease and that it is necessary to take the posterior canal wall down or perform a canal-wall-down mastoidectomy. There are modifications of those two basic mastoid surgeries, such as leaving the incus bridge intact, limiting the amount of bone removed, or even bypassing the mastoid completely if the disease is limited to the epitympanum.

In the middle ear, an assortment of conditions exist that call for surgical intervention. Erosion of the incus is a familiar condition that the ear surgeon encounters. There are many ossiculoplasty techniques that address that problem, including the insertion of various prostheses. Other ossicles may be involved in disease, either destroyed or fixed by fibrous tissue or tympanosclerosis, at times requiring complete replacement of the ossicular chain. Since the advent of stapedectomy almost 50 years ago, refinement of that technique has led to predictable and excellent results. There are many prostheses available to the general market, and most have led to the expected good result. Some new innovative prostheses are on the horizon, based on novel ideas regarding connection between the inner ear vestibule and incus.

Surgical treatment for Meniere's disease and other vertiginous conditions, such as benign paroxysmal positional vertigo, typically involves performing mastoidectomy. At a minimum, simple mastoidectomy provides the basic entry to the labyrinth and endolymphatic sac. A thorough knowledge of the mastoid becomes a prerequisite for performing more complex temporal bone operations. From the mastoid, entry into the membranous labyrinth and internal auditory canal is possible, as is exposure of the posterior fossa dura, endolymphatic sac, and retrolabyrinthine area. Control of vertigo is the primary reason to perform inner ear surgery, although other symptoms such as hearing loss or tinnitus are often affected.

In the last few years, implantable hearing aids appeared, and implanting them may be a commonly performed procedure in the future. The technology continues to be refined, and as a result there is high expectation. Cochlear implants are relatively commonplace today. They have helped many patients who previously may have required sign language or lip reading. In the future, we can expect changes that could fulfill the desired objectives of otologists and otolaryngologists, that is, serving the needs of the hearing impaired to the greatest degree.

This book provides general otolaryngologists and residents of otolaryngology with a comprehensive presentation of the current status of middle ear and mastoid surgery. A chapter is assigned to each procedure, allowing easy reference to a specific operation in which the otolaryngologist may be interested. Each chapter describes in detail patient preparation and surgical technique. There is less focus placed on disease depiction, as other texts already provide that. After reviewing a chapter, the physician may then proceed to perform the selected surgery with added confidence and understanding of appropriate elements of the procedure.

PATIENT SELECTION AND INFORMED CONSENT

Virtually all patients who require middle ear or mastoid surgery have endured chronic symptoms. Patients with cholesteatoma typically present with purulent otorrhea that has plagued them for years. Otosclerotic patients often complain that their hearing has diminished gradually over many years. It is not uncommon for Meniere's disease patients to have received treatment by a primary care physician for a long period before finally seeing the specialist, enduring many episodes of vertigo that may even have elicited trips to the emergency room. Thus, by the time the otolaryngologist sees the patients, expectations are high to find a cure and improve their lifestyle. Patients may exhibit unrealistic expectations about their condition and believe that a quick turnaround is imminent once treated by the otolaryngologist.

The initial consultation is usually a time to become familiar with the patient's condition. This consultation may not be the appropriate time to schedule surgery. Instead, a second appointment becomes the logical time to present surgical options, especially if diagnostic tests such as computed tomography (CT) need to be done before contemplating an operation.

A second, third, and fourth appointment, as necessary, allow for the development of rapport and trust, which are required if the surgeon is to perform complicated otologic procedures. There are times, however, when a patient arrives at the appointment, audiograms and CT scans in hand, ready to be scheduled. Those patients, typically referred from an otolaryngologist to an otologist, can be scheduled for surgery, as the patient and the referring otolaryngologist expect as much and may be dissatisfied if those needs are not met.

It is important to present a reasonable prognosis based on a variety of information. First, otolaryngologists must review their own results and make determinations of outcome based on that data. In addition, presentation of results published in the current literature informs the patient about regional and national outcomes. If an insufficient number of cases exist to make reasonable predictions, reliance on published data is acceptable as long as this is clearly explained to the patient. Intraoperative and postoperative risks and complications must be presented to the patient, including risks of hearing loss, both sensorineural and conductive, vertigo, altered taste, and facial nerve injury, both temporary and permanent. Other complications and postoperative expectations should also be explained depending on the type of surgery performed. A consent form, specific to a particular doctor or office, may be utilized, but that form would not replace the hospital or surgery center's document. It would only serve to document within the practitioner's own medical record that informed consent has been obtained. In addition to discussing risks and complications of the operation, the surgeon must also present risks and complications of refusal to comply with the recommended treatment. If a mastoidectomy is indicated but the patient refuses to have the procedure, he must be told about the suppurative complications of chronic otitis media such as meningitis and temporal lobe abscess. The point is not to overwhelm the patient. Instead, care must be taken to educate patients about the serious and complex nature of their disease. Important decisions require information; if maximal information is available, a better choice is made.

SCHEDULING AND PERIOPERATIVE MANAGEMENT

After the patient agrees to comply with recommendations of surgery, the operation is scheduled. It is important to schedule an appropriate amount of time for the otologic procedure, including adequate turnover. That will depend on many factors, such as determination of facility, experience of the support staff, anesthesia, and proficiency of the surgeon. A canal-wall-up tympanomastoidectomy with complete exposure and opening of the facial recess will require at least 2 hours for an expert team, including operating room turnover; the same procedure may require 3½ hours for a less experienced crew. Ample time is a prerequisite for a successful outcome. Earnest consideration should be given to schedule these surgeries on days when no other obligation is needed, especially if a full-day block is available. Otherwise, a cushion of extra time will allow for unsuspected findings that may prolong the operation. As an example of a perilous scenario, a surgeon finds he will be late for office hours because he is operating near a dehiscent facial nerve that is covered by cholesteatoma. Rather than facing that situation, allocate more time than expected.

The otologic surgeon must take a multifaceted approach to preparing the patient and the operating room for commencement of the surgery. After anesthesia induction, the surgeon should be in the operating room, making sure the microscope assembly and organization are correct and that the patient's position is appropriate. That effort, not left to the operating room staff, is the responsibility of the operating surgeon. Ultimately, the surgeon is accountable for making sure that the instrumentation is as it should be and the otologic drill is suitable. A case scheduled at a facility that is new or infrequently attended requires that the surgeon coordinate his plans with the nursing supervisor for otolaryngology. If possible, document the procedure with photographs, obtainable from a standard printer or via digital capture. With photographs, the medical record reflects permanent verification of the operation. In addition, the surgeon can distribute a copy to the patient, which supplements patient understanding and education about the disease. Coordination with anesthesia is crucial. During surgery, the patient must not be moving and the patient must not be paralyzed, two goals that can be difficult to achieve at times. If there is unwanted repositioning because of the patient's awakening prematurely from anesthesia, the operating field may be altered adversely, requiring stoppage of the procedure to realign the patient. Waking from anesthesia should be smooth and without bucking to minimize labyrinthine stimulation and prevent dislodging a prosthesis. Once fully recovered from anesthesia, the patient can be discharged unless an underlying medical condition dictates admission.

Follow-up after surgery can be in a week or as long as 6 weeks, depending on the operation and the experience of the surgeon. After sufficient time has passed, cleaning of the ear under the microscope takes place without risking dislodging a graft or prosthesis. If granulations are present, treatment topically with gentian violet, antibiotic drops, or combination powders allows adequate healing. Obtain postoperative audiograms after 6 to 12 weeks but not before unless indicated. Otherwise, misleading results will cause undue stress and prevent appropriate presentation of the prognosis. Following assessment of the initial postoperative audiogram

and otomicroscopic exam of the ear, the surgeon may present the prognosis, making sure that a realistic picture is presented. If an unexpected poor hearing result occurs in the face of an excellent medical result, as may occur in tympanomastoid surgery, one should wait 6 months and repeat the audiogram. Sometimes, resolution of edema of middle ear mucosa and graft tissue will lead to improvement of the hearing over time. If an excellent hearing result is present after 6 weeks, the patient needs counseling regarding potential diminution of the hearing over time, as recurrent disease or other situations that are out of the surgeon's control may occur. If they do, the patient must understand that no one is at fault, Instead, the natural course of the disease may dictate the eventual outcome.

COMPLICATIONS

If a surgeon operates enough times, complications will be encountered—it is unavoidable. That is not to say that care should not always be taken to avoid them, but rather sometimes circumstances are out of our control. Other times, a surgical mishap leaves the patient with an obvious complication such as facial nerve injury or vertigo due to a lateral canal fistula. In those cases, it is most important to recognize the problem intraoperatively and treat it at that time rather than later. If the facial nerve is injured during surgery, specific treatment should take place at that time. If the labyrinth is inadvertently entered, repair is necessary at that time. Once the complication occurs and is treated, the surgeon must explain the condition to the patient and the family. That discussion can be as difficult as any conversation in medicine. The surgeon must present the facts without assigning blame, which can be delicate as well as challenging. The best way to present the case is to be straightforward and discuss what is current and relevant, not to circumvent the situation or try to deflect responsibility. On the other hand, it is paramount not to apologize or admit to a surgical error. Situations arise that happen in an instant, and before you know it the damage is done. Surgeons are not perfect technicians. If a surgeon experiences repeated complications, then an assessment of some kind must be done to ensure patient safety. Ideally, the surgeon will realize that limitations in practice are not a sign of ineptitude, but instead are an honest appraisal of personal strengths and weaknesses. If a surgeon refuses to evaluate results, lawsuits or complaints may render the final answer on what a surgeon does or does not do.

With experience, most surgeons identify what operative procedures make sense in their practices.

For some, chronic ear disease becomes their forte. Others may become proficient in otosclerosis surgery. Some may find that skull base surgery and treating complicated tumors of the temporal bone is their calling. With neurotology fellowships now 2 years in length and often oriented toward steering fellows into academic careers, opportunities exist and will continue to be available for otolaryngologists to develop strong otologic private practices. In fact, otolaryngologists will necessarily perform many of the otologic cases in the future. Thus, it is important to identify surgical strengths and incorporate them into your practice. In large groups, neurotologists may be hired. There may be situations where one or two of the associates have an interest in otology and eventually become otologists for the group by default.

OBJECTIVES

This book provides the reader with written descriptions and visual presentations of otologic surgical procedures and presents detailed information regarding how the procedures are performed, so that practicing otolaryngologists and otolaryngology residents may be better prepared for surgery. Nearly all otologic procedures are presented, with the exception of skull base and neurotology surgeries that are beyond this book's scope. Practitioners and residents can utilize the text on a regular basis, both for review and for preparing to perform an otologic procedure.

Recognized experts in otology, whose time and effort are greatly appreciated, have written the chapters. They present standard techniques in ear surgery as well as new and innovative techniques that are on the cutting edge of surgery. After reviewing a specific chapter, the practitioner should be able to comfortably proceed with the intended operation with an understanding of the technique and an awareness of operative variables. Optimistically, over time and with the experience gained with performing otologic surgeries repeatedly, practitioners can routinely expect to achieve predictable, outstanding results. With regular review of surgical procedures and standard temporal bone dissection, otolaryngologists can become unquestionably proficient in performing otologic surgery.

Chapter 2

MYRINGOPLASTY

Raleigh O. Jones

Confusion has existed for many years regarding the nomenclature used to describe surgery on the tympanic membrane (TM), middle ear, and ossicular chain. Wullstein's classic classification system (types I–V) was based on the relative position of the TM to the other middle ear structures including the ossicles and inner ear membranes.[1] This description was developed prior to the introduction of many of the procedures and prostheses that are used so commonly today in middle ear surgery, so its ability to adequately describe current surgical techniques is limited. Consequently, the term *tympanoplasty* by itself is not adequately descriptive, simply indicating some sort of reconstructive surgery on the TM or middle ear. It is therefore necessary for the surgeon to use further descriptive terms in addition to the term *tympanoplasty* to communicate effectively which procedures are being described.

The term *myringoplasty* refers to reconstructive surgery that is limited to the TM. It was actually introduced by Berthold, who successfully closed a TM perforation using a full thickness skin graft in 1878.[2,3] He was the first to report the use of autologous tissue in an effort to repair the TM; prior to that, several different artificial or animal-based materials were used dating back to as early as 1640.[4] By definition, any manipulation of the ossicular chain is beyond the scope of a pure myringoplasty. Because the term *tympanoplasty* includes surgery on both the TM and middle ear, however, many cases of myringoplasty are labeled tympanoplasty by surgeons, further adding to the confusion. The terms *myringoplasty* and *tympanoplasty without ossicular reconstruction* are synonyms unless other manipulation of the middle ear such as removal of cholesteatoma is included in the tympanoplasty procedure. Within the more limited surgery of the TM, many different approaches to myringoplasty have been described.

PATIENT PRESENTATION

Patients with perforations of the TM may present acutely or with symptoms suggestive of a chronic perforation. Acute perforations are usually the result of acute otitis media with rupture of the TM due to increased pressure in the middle ear, trauma to the ear canal or temporal bone, or sudden pressure changes transmitted to the TM.

The majority of cases of acute otitis media resolve spontaneously with or without medical treatment and without any significant injury to the TM. Certain infections, however, build up sufficient pressure within the middle ear space, which is effectively closed due to eustachian tube blockage, that the flexible TM ruptures, thereby relieving this pressure. This acute event is associated with sudden drainage from the ear that is often both bloody and purulent, and also with an increase in pain followed by a marked diminution of pain. This rupture of the TM effectively releases the infection from out of the skull and away from other fragile and vital structures such as the central nervous system (CNS) and the inner ear. Most cases of acute TM perforations due to infection will heal without surgical treatment over a period from a few days to a few weeks. Resolution of the infection is an important consideration as to whether this healing will occur because a perforation is more likely to remain open if the drainage persists. Treatment of such infections with both systemic antibiotics and aural antibiotic drops is highly recommended. Although not proven, it is believed that thin, atelectatic TMs are more likely to rupture and less likely to heal without surgery than normal membranes.

Trauma can produce a tear in the TM either directly, such as a penetrating injury, or indirectly, such as from a shearing movement in bone as seen in a temporal bone fracture. Although any small object could produce a penetrating injury, the cotton-tipped swab is a particularly common offender, because it is used in an attempt to clean or scratch the ear canal and too often finds its way through the TM. These perforations are typically central in location and can be quite large. A discussion of the possible trauma to the ossicles and inner ear is beyond the scope of this chapter, but the perforation will be accompanied by a moderate amount of self-limited bleeding and sudden pain. Temporal bone fractures may present with hemotympanum when the TM is intact or with a perforation and bleeding when the annulus or TM is torn. Longitudinal fractures are particularly prone to tearing the TM, but mixed or transverse fractures may also present in this manner.

Significant changes in pressure in the outer ear may also produce ruptures of the TM. This can be negative pressure, as is seen in injuries that occur while flying in which the cabin pressure is not maintained adequately, or positive pressure such as a slap with a cupped hand to the ear canal, resulting in pushing on the TM. Again, a sudden onset of pain and bleeding accompanied by some degree of hearing loss are usually present. The pain and bleeding usually resolve quickly without treatment, and unless infection develops, no otorrhea occurs and the patient is asymptomatic with the exception of a hearing loss.

Patients with a chronic perforation of the TM usually present with a conductive hearing loss, otorrhea, or both. Nearly all patients with a chronic perforation of their TM have otorrhea to some degree. There is a wide spectrum of the severity of this symptom. Some patients are not able to recall ever having an episode of drainage, whereas other patients have constant drainage of malodorous, discolored material that drains into their conchal bowl, onto their ear lobe, and even onto their upper neck on a daily basis. Between these two extremes, most patients have intermittent drainage that may occur spontaneously or be brought on by getting water in the ear or suffering from an upper respiratory infection. These infections are typically caused by multiple microorganisms, particularly *Pseudomonas*, *Staphylococcus*, *Proteus*, and various anaerobic bacteria. They are frequently resistant to most orally administered antibiotics presumably due to the repeated courses of antibiotics that have been used

to treat this condition over the period of the existence of the perforation.

Audiologic Considerations

Patients with a chronic TM perforation generally present with a conductive hearing loss. The degree of hearing loss varies significantly among patients, from no detectable loss up to a moderate conductive loss. Among the factors influencing the degree of hearing loss present are the size and location of the perforation, the presence of otorrhea, and the status of the ossicular chain. Other chapters of this book address details of ossicular absence, erosion, or fixation, but with an intact ossicular chain the conductive hearing loss associated with a TM perforation rarely exceeds 35 dB, regardless of the size or location of the hole.

Small perforations may be associated with no significant impairment of hearing. Generally speaking, the larger the perforation, the greater the degree of hearing loss. Initially the conductive hearing impairment affects only the very low frequencies, but as the size of the perforation increases, the hearing loss increases and involves more of the middle frequencies.[5] Anterior perforations tend to produce smaller hearing losses than their posterior counterparts, presumably due to the exposure of the round window to the effect of sound waves penetrating directly through the perforation and striking the round directly setting up a competing fluid wave within the inner ear. Even large anterior perforations rarely produce greater than 15 dB of conductive hearing loss in the absence of infection or ossicular involvement. In addition to the effect of the exposing the round window directly to the sound waves, perforations also produce hearing loss by diminishing the surface area of the TM available to collect the energy in the form of sound waves and then transmit that energy onto the inner ear via the ossicular chain. It is therefore understandable that larger perforations produce a greater degree of hearing impairment.

Preoperative Assessment

For a patient presenting with a perforation of the TM, the physician should take a thorough history and perform a physical examination. The history should attempt to determine if the perforation is acute or chronic and what if any event precipitated the perforation. Because most acute perforations heal spontaneously with proper medical treatment, determining when the perforation developed is a prime consideration. Ears with acute perforations should be cleaned and examined carefully under a microscope. If edges of the perforation can be seen to be deflected medially into the middle ear, it is desirable to elevate them gently with a suction to prevent squamous epithelium from growing in the middle ear. It is neither necessary nor desirable to treat these acute perforations with antibiotic eardrops, as many of the currently available drops contain materials that may be ototoxic when exposed to the round window. It is indeed desirable to prevent infection, so these patients are advised to keep all water out of their ears and watch for any signs or symptoms that would suggest infection. When infection does occur, treating it aggressively will increase the likelihood that spontaneous healing will occur.

Patients with chronic infection rarely recall when their perforation first developed. Their history should focus on the presence of other factors that may influence eustachian tube function and healing after surgery, as well as on what other attempts have been made to treat this condition. Eustachian tube function is a major factor in determining the ultimate success of tympanoplasty or myringoplasty surgery. Patients with poor eustachian tube function may heal their perforations successfully after surgery, only to be left with a conductive hearing loss equal to or even greater than the loss they had prior to surgery if serous otitis media should develop. Indeed, small perforations may act in a manner similar to a PE tube placed by an otolaryngologist in an ear with poor eustachian tube function and at times should be viewed positively by both patient and surgeon. This is particularly true in children, among whom eustachian tube dysfunction is a common problem. Unfortunately, there are no tests that can predict with a high degree of success the status of the eustachian tube function prior to surgery to close a perforation.[6] In fact, there is evidence that merely closing a perforation may have a beneficial effect on the function of the eustachian tube.[7–9] The status of the eustachian tube in the other ear gives some indication of the function in the involved ear, but this is not a universally effective predictor either. Though opinions vary, many surgeons prefer not to repair dry perforations associated with minimal hearing loss in children's ears until the child is 6 or 7 years old, hoping that eustachian tube function will be adequate at that point to yield an air-containing middle ear space with normal hearing after the procedure. Even if the procedure is successful in closing the perforation, recurrence of the perforation is a particular concern in children. Reperforation rates of 10

to 20% have been reported,[8] although Tos and Lau[9] reported reperforation rates in children as low as 4%, although approximately 6% developed serous otitis media significant enough to require PE tube placement after successful closure.

Preoperative planning also includes a careful inspection for evidence of cholesteatoma that would require a more extensive surgery to eradicate. Routine imaging of patients with TM perforations is not required, nor justifiable, but circumstances may exist that would make a computed tomography (CT) scan appropriate to evaluate the extent of infection. Among the reasons for preoperative scanning are dizziness, unusual pain, or a suspected intracranial complication. It is important to realize, however, that the presence of infection does not mean that a procedure other than a myringoplasty will be needed to close a perforation.

A serious effort to resolve all active drainage from an ear prior to an operation is an important adjunct to the surgery. Pignataro et al[10] have confirmed a commonly held belief among ear surgeons that dry perforations are more likely to heal following myringoplasty or tympanoplasty than those with persistent infection. This is particularly true when a myringoplasty is considered because any infection in the middle ear is not addressed by this procedure. Most ears with active drainage can be improved with proper treatment to the point where the drainage stops or is significantly decreased. Careful microscopic cleaning is the first step in this process. Repeated cleaning alone without any other treatment often produces dramatic results, and when combined with appropriate antibiotic treatment usually leaves the patient with a dry perforation ready for surgery. Antibiotic cultures are not routinely obtained, but when the patient does not respond to treatment, these cultures can be helpful in directing further therapy. It is important to remember the possibility of unusual infections, such as with *Mycobacterium*, in patients who are immunocompromised or who do not respond as expected to treatment. In addition, many of these patients have been treated extensively with antibiotics, and fungal infections are frequently seen. Cultures may help direct therapy successfully when the usual improvement is not seen with local cleaning and antibiotic drops.

Successful medical treatment of otorrhea has benefits beyond that of improving the success rate of the surgery. Landmarks are more readily visible and the surgery is often accomplished in a shorter period than in ears with active infection. In addition, polypoid, chronically infected, and thickened mucosa with or without granulation tissue make the surgery more difficult and increase the possibility of a surgical complication. Still, the presence of active drainage in an ear does not mean that a perforation cannot be successfully closed with a good surgical procedure, although the procedure may need to address more than the perforation itself, including removal of infection from the middle ear and/or mastoid.

Every patient who is a potential candidate for surgery on the TM should have a current audiogram to document for legal purposes any presurgical hearing deficit, but also to provide a valuable piece of information regarding the status of the ossicular chain prior to the operation. This information helps determine whether the patient is a candidate for a myringoplasty or needs formal tympanoplasty.

OPERATIVE PROCEDURES

Many different techniques have been developed over the past 50 years in an attempt to close perforations and several materials have been used for grafting material. Initially, split or full-thickness skin grafts were employed. The material was readily available near the operative site and was inexpensive, autologous, and readily shaped. However, many cases of improper growth of squamous epithelium either within the TM or in the middle ear occurred with this technique, leading to the search for other materials. Vein grafts, perichondrium, cartilage, fat, and homologous dura or fascia have been used,[11–14] although the most common material used today is temporalis muscle fascia harvested from a small incision behind and slightly above the patient's ear within the operative field. This fascia is semitransparent and flexible like a TM, and has roughly the same thickness as a TM when properly prepared. In addition, other synthetic materials such as rice paper and dissolvable synthetic collagen (Gelfilm) have been utilized in certain specific situations discussed below.

How and where these materials are placed relative to the remaining perforation also varies from one technique to another. Two of the most common methods for myringoplasty include the underlay and overlay methods discussed in detail in Chapters 3 and 4. These procedures are named according to the position of the graft relative to the remaining anterior TM, although both techniques place the graft medial to the handle of the malleus when the perforation involves the superior half of the TM. The underlay technique also allows good exposure to the middle ear required for tympanoplasty, but for myringoplasty alone this is not needed.

Although the surgical repair of acute perforations is not required to yield good results for closure, it is thought that certain perforations may benefit from surgical manipulation in a limited manner. The desirability of elevating depressed remnants of TM out of the middle ear has already been mentioned. In addition, many surgeons attempt to put a temporary covering over these perforations to aid healing, serving as a scaffold for the TM to grow beneath and also as a barrier to keep infection from migrating into the middle ear from the external ear. A special instance frequently encountered is the acute perforation created surgically when retained PE tubes are removed. It is known that patients who have PE tubes removed that have been in place for 3 years or longer are at significantly greater risk for nonhealing following removal. Patching these perforations acutely at the time of tube removal has been done in an effort to reduce this rate of permanent perforation, although two studies have called the efficacy of this procedure into question.[15,16] Rice paper has been used and described most extensively for this procedure.

This procedure is generally done in the clinic without any anesthesia. An operating microscope is utilized and the external canal is cleaned. The edges of the perforation are elevated gently with a small suction; then a circular patch approximately 3 mm larger than the perforation is cut from cigarette paper that has been previously sterilized with steam. It is desirable to leave the paper dry when placing it directly on top of the remaining TM, ensuring that the perforation is completely covered. The patch needs to sit directly on the TM. If it is bent slightly and therefore not in direct contact, a small drop of saline can be placed on the paper patch allowing it to conform to the contour of the TM. The patient is then instructed to keep all water out of the ear and to notify you if any discharge occurs. The procedure is nearly painless and should take 5 minutes or less. The patient returns to the office in approximately 2 weeks and the patch is removed under the microscope. The success rate for closure of acute perforations is quite high, with smaller perforations having a nearly 100% success rate and even larger perforations close at a rate of approximately 90%. Gold and Chaffoo[17] created acute perforations in guinea pigs and randomized them to treatment with fat myringoplasty, paper patch, or control. They demonstrated healing in 88, 56, and 75% of these groups, respectively. Although statistical significance was not reached in this study, it does demonstrate the expected high rate of spontaneous healing and the safety of these minor procedures in the guinea pig model. Imamoglu et al[18] did a similar study in rats where the success rates for small perforations using fat, paper, and control were 95, 94, and 67%, but in larger perforations were 53, 56, and 27% respectively. Subsequent series in humans have confirmed these results. It remains unclear which acute perforations would benefit from patching, although it seems as if larger perforations at higher risk for nonhealing may be considered good candidates for this procedure.

Gelfilm has been used in a similar manner as the paper patch. It has the added advantage of being self-dissolving and therefore does not need to be removed later, a particular advantage in children who may not tolerate this manipulation in the clinic without anesthesia.

Chronic perforations can also be closed through a simple myringoplasty technique without the flaps and extensive exposure required for an underlay or overlay tympanoplasty. Many different substances have been used, but the fat myringoplasty has been utilized and studied extensively for 40 years. It has also been used for bilateral TM perforation repair in children with a 91% success rate reported.[19] Although some variations in the technique exist, it is important to manipulate the TM to create a fresh surface to which the fat graft adheres. This requires anesthesia of some sort. Although various local anesthetics have been used, a brief general anesthetic is preferred in most cases. The ear canal is thoroughly cleaned under the microscope and then the edges of the perforation are "freshened." This is an extremely important part of the procedure and is accomplished by using a sharp instrument or needle to puncture the TM just lateral to the edge of the perforation removing approximately 1 mm of tissue circumferentially around the perforation. This enlarges the perforation somewhat, so it is desirable to remove the minimal amount of tissue necessary to get back to a fresh edge. Numerous studies have shown that the smaller the perforation, the greater the success of this technique, so it is important not to remove any more TM than necessary. The fat is harvested from any site, but generally the ear lobe is readily accessible to the field and fat is readily available. A single piece of Gelfoam (Upjohn Laboratories, Kalamazoo, MI) is placed in the middle ear. A piece of fat just larger than the freshened perforation is harvested and then placed in the perforation in an hourglass shape, with a small amount of the fat protruding through the perforation into the middle ear and a small amount extending just lateral to the TM.[20] It is important that the fat is lodged in the perforation and stays firmly in that position (Fig. 2–1). Generally, a small amount of Gelfoam is placed lateral to the graft in the medial ear canal, although this is not absolutely essential.

The patient is instructed to keep all water out of the ear until seen back in the office in approximately 2 to 3 weeks. The success rate for small perforations is quite good ranging from 76 to 92%,[21–23] but the success rate for larger perforations (> 4 mm) is poor, approximately 30%. Even at this low success rate the procedure is so quick, safe, well tolerated, and relatively inexpensive that it is often desirable to try this approach first, with the patient's understanding that if it is not successful, it will be followed with a formal tympanoplasty later, which should accomplish a greater than 90% success rate for closure. It needs to be emphasized that this procedure is appropriate only for completely dry perforations where there is no concern for cholesteatoma and where preoperative audiometry reveals no suggestion of an ossicular problem. Studies have shown that attempts at closing perforations with active or recent drainage carry a very low success rate, so this procedure is not recommended in those circumstances.

AlloDerm (LifeCell Corporation, Branchburg, NJ) has also been used in a similar fashion to close small perforations in adults under local anesthesia in the office with good success. The graft should be 1.5 times as large as the perforation, because it is placed onto the TM covering after it is rimmed and a small amount of the outer squamous epithelium around the perforation is removed, leaving a denuded segment of TM adjacent to the perforation. The AlloDerm is then gently pressed onto the perforation, and is then covered with Gelfoam soaked in antibiotic drops (Fig. 2–2A,B). The ear is kept clean and dry for 6 weeks. Healing has been reported in 86% of cases when small perforations that are dry and stable are treated.

RESULTS

Simple myringoplasty techniques as described in this chapter are highly successful when utilized in the correct circumstance. One- and 2-year follow-up success rates of 80 to 90% have been reported, although some recidivism is reported in children with longer follow-up. Gross et al[24] nicely summarized the benefits of myringoplasty (over formal tympanoplasty) when utilized in the proper setting:

1. Minimal manipulation of the middle ear minimizing the risk of operative injury.
2. Relative simplicity of the procedure.
3. Decreased operative and postoperative morbidity.

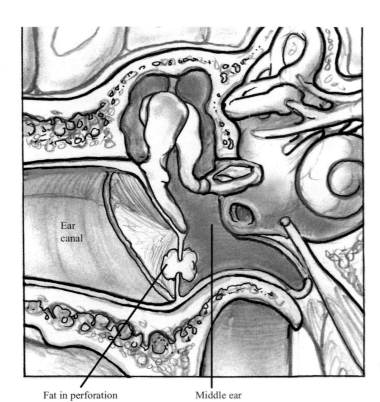

Ear canal

Fat in perforation

Middle ear

FIGURE 2–1 Fat myringoplasty.

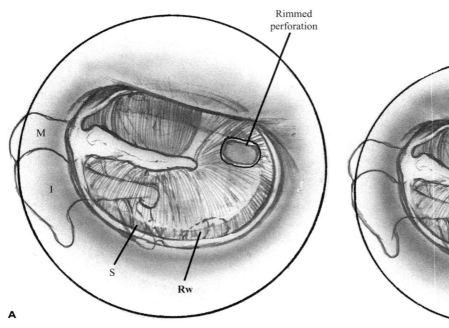

Rimmed perforation

M

I

S

Rw

A

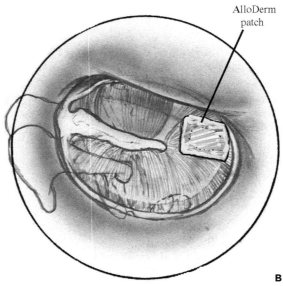

AlloDerm patch

B

FIGURE 2–2 (A,B) AlloDerm myringoplasty.

4. Little postoperative care or manipulation is needed, which is particularly important in children.
5. Decreased operative and recovery time, resulting in decreased cost.
6. Bilateral procedures are possible at the same sitting.

Because of these real benefits, this procedure should be considered in all patients who present with a small, dry perforation without concern about cholesteatoma or ossicular problems.

REFERENCES

1. Wullstein H. Theory and practice of tympanoplasty. *Laryngoscope* 1956;66:1076–1093.
2. Berthold E. Uber myringoplastik. *Medicinisch-Chuurgisches Central-Blatt* 1879;14:195–207.
3. Guthrie D. The history of otology. *J Laryngol* 1940;55:473–494.
4. Banzer M. *Disputatio de Audiotione Laesa.* Wittebergae, 1640. Cited by House H. XVIII Wherry Memorial Lecture: otology in orbit. *Trans Am Acad Ophthalmol Otolaryngol* 1963;67:233–259.
5. Tonndorf J, McCardle F, Kruger B. Middle ear transmission losses caused by tympanic membrane perforations in cats. *Acta Otolaryngol* 1976;81:330–336.
6. Todd NW. There are no accurate tests of eustachian tube function. *Arch Otolaryngol Head Neck Surg* 2000;126:1041–1042.
7. Tos M. Tubal function and tympanoplasty. *J Laryngol Otol* 1974;88:1113–1124.
8. Kessler A, Potsic WP, Marsh RP. Type 1 tympanoplasty in children. *Arch Otolaryngol Head Neck Surg* 1994;120:487–490.
9. Tos M, Lau T. Stability of tympanoplasty in children. *Otolaryngol Clin North Am* 1989;22:15–28.
10. Pignataro L, Grillo Della Berta L, Capaccio P, Zaghis A. Myringoplasty in children: anatomic and functional results. *J Laryngol Otol* 2001;115:694–698.
11. Goodhill V. Articulated polyethylene prosthesis with perichondrial graft in stapedectomy. *Rev Laryngol (Bordeaux)* 1951;82:305–320.
12. Tabb HG. Closure of perforations of the tympanic membrane by vein grafts: a preliminary report of 20 cases. *Laryngoscope* 1960;70:271–286.
13. Storrs L. Myringoplasty with the use of Fascia Grafts. *Arch Otolaryngol* 1961;74:45–49.
14. Yetiser S, Tosun F, Satar B. Revision myringoplasty with solvent-dehydrated human dura mater (Tutoplast). *Otolaryngol Head Neck Surg* 2001;124:518–521.
15. Nichols PT, Ramadan HH, Wax MK, Santrock RD. Relationship between tympanic membrane perforation and retained ventilation tubes. *Arch Otolaryngol Head Neck Surg* 1998;124:417–419.
16. Pribitkin EA, Handler SR, Tom LW, Potsic WP, Wetmore RF. Ventilation tube removal: indications for paper patch myringoplasty. *Arch Otolaryngol Head Neck Surg* 1992;118:495–497.
17. Gold SR, Chaffoo RAK. Fat myringoplasty in the guinea pig. *Laryngoscope* 1991;101:1–5.
18. Imamoglu M, Isik AU, Acuner O, Harova G, Bahadir O. Fat-plug and paper-patch myringoplasty in rats. *J Otolaryngol* 1998;27:318–321.
19. Mitchell RB, Pereira KD, Younis RT, Lazar RH. Bilateral fat graft myringoplasty in children. *Ear Nose Throat J* 1996;75:655–656.
20. Mitchell RB, Pereira KD, Lazar RH. Fat graft myringoplasty in children: a safe and successful day-stay procedure. *J Laryngol Otol* 1997;111:106–108.
21. Terry R, Belline M, Clayton M, Gandhi A. Fat graft myringoplasty: a prospective trial. *Clin Otolaryngol* 1998;13:227–229.
22. Ringenberg J. Closure of tympanic membrane perforations by the use of fat. *Laryngoscope* 1978;88:982–983.
23. Althaus S. "Fat plug" myringoplasty: a new technique for repairing small tympanic membrane perforations. In: Brackman DE, ed. *Otologic Surgery.* Philadelphia: WB Saunders; 1994:112–119.
24. Gross CW, Bassila M, Lazar RH, Long TE, Stagner S. Adipose plug myringoplasty: an alternative to formal myringoplasty techniques in children. *Otolaryngol Head Neck Surg* 1989;101:617–620.

Chapter 3

UNDERLAY TYMPANOPLASTY

Edwin M. Monsell and Tam Q. Nguyen

DEFINITIONS

The current era of tympanoplasty began in 1952 with Wullstein and Zollner.[1] Shea,[2,3] Hough,[4] Storrs,[5] Herrmann,[6] Austin,[2,7,8] Sheehy,[9,10] Glasscock,[11,12] Tos,[13–15] and others have since made important contributions. Today tympanoplasty is a highly developed set of techniques. Most tympanic membrane perforations can be closed with underlay or overlay techniques regardless of location or size.[11,16–18] This chapter presents the technique of tympanic membrane repair with underlay grafting. In the underlay technique the graft material is placed medial to the tympanic membrane remnant and medial to the manubrium of the malleus. Other strategies and techniques for grafting are described elsewhere in this book.

The overall goals of treatment of chronic otitis media in order of priority are (1) to make the ear safe; (2) to make the ear clean, dry, comfortable, and relatively free of maintenance; and (3) to restore hearing. Otologists pursue these goals with medical and surgical treatment. Tympanoplasty is defined as a procedure to remove disease from the middle ear and to reconstruct with or without tympanic membrane grafting. Tympanic membrane grafting is a component of tympanoplasty when the disease involves the tympanic membrane; for example, in cases of perforation or atelectasis. Tympanoplasty often includes reconstruction of the ossicular chain for hearing. Sometimes mastoidectomy is also performed either to remove disease or to provide exposure through a posterior tympanotomy approach.

EVALUATION

A careful evaluation of diseased ears is necessary for planning treatment. Important points of history include the patient's age, history of prior otologic surgery, general health, and the frequency and character of drainage, pain, hearing loss, and vestibular symptoms. It is important to understand what symptoms are most bothersome and most important to the patient.

The physical examination should include an examination of the tympanic membranes and the outer ears for incisional scars from previous otologic surgery. The nasopharynx should be examined, if possible, for evidence of potential causes of eustachian tube dysfunction. The size and location of the perforation or retraction of the tympanic membrane, the presence of middle ear polyps, cholesteatoma, tumors, masses, atelectasis, tympanosclerosis, and erosion of the ossicular chain should be noted.

In appropriate instances, high-resolution computed tomography of the temporal bones or microbial cultures should be considered.[19,20] Audiometric testing is indicated. We have not found routine tests of eustachian tube function to be useful guides to therapy.

Patients should be evaluated holistically, with due consideration given to the status of the opposite ear and the ability to maintain middle ear aeration, and to estimate the long-term prospects for helping with the patient's needs and goals. In some cases, medical treatment and debridement will be needed to control active infection prior to consideration for surgical repair. The assessment guides the treatment recommendations and counseling. The elective nature of most cases of tympanoplasty should be kept in mind. Surgery in the only hearing ear should be reserved for dangerous ear conditions, such as progressive cholesteatoma, and should be carried out by experienced surgeons.[15,21]

CONSIDERATIONS IN GRAFT HEALING

The normal tympanic membrane has a complex layered structure consisting of thin stratified squamous epithelium on the lateral surface, flat respiratory epithelium on the medial surface, and two fibrous layers, one radial and one longitudinal, between the two epithelial layers. The fibrous layers also contain vascular elements. Successful, functional repair of the tympanic membrane requires reconstitution of the epithelial layers and enough of a fibrous middle layer to provide satisfactory mechanical support.

When a tympanic membrane heals spontaneously without grafting, the perforation is often closed by the squamous epithelium before fibrous elements develop. The fibrous layer may be attenuated or even lacking. The resultant tympanic membrane has an area that lacks the tensile strength, elasticity, blood supply, and resistance to future perforation of a fully reconstructed tympanic membrane. Such areas are referred to as "dimeric" because the squamous epithelium lies against the mucous membrane without intermediate fibrous elements.

The healing process after grafting appears to be initiated by angiogenesis within the tympanic membrane remnant, especially at the margin of the perforation. During healing the fascia is a scaffold for epithelialization. The margins of the freshened edges of the perforation (see below) are the sources for the migrating epithelia. Fascia is composed of fibroblasts in a collagen matrix. Its low metabolic rate and its extracellular matrix permit it to persist until it becomes vascularized.

A critical problem early in the development of tympanoplasty was finding a suitable material for tympanic membrane grafting. Since the 1950s, several tissues have been proposed for donor graft materials, including split-thickness skin, full-thickness skin, vein, allograft tympanic membranes, and prepared collagen materials.

This chapter describes the use of temporalis fascia, which is now the most widely used material.[5,6] Temporalis fascia results in rapid, reliable healing of an appropriately thin tympanic membrane. It can be obtained from the same operative field, often from the same incision used for access to the ear (Fig. 3–1). Epidermal growth factors have been used to enhance healing experimentally.[22]

Medial grafting techniques take advantage of the ability of respiratory epithelium (unlike squamous epithelium) to incorporate the graft material when the graft is placed against it. The squamous and respiratory epithelial layers and the fibrous layer are in contact with the rest of the tympanic membrane after healing.[23,24]

TECHNIQUE

A graft of temporalis fascia is harvested early in the procedure to allow time for the graft to dry (Fig. 3–1). Any muscle tissue adherent to the fascia is removed. We prefer to use the true temporalis fascia, rather than the areolar fascia. The areolar fascia has more of a trabecular structure, which occasionally results in the formation of small perforations. These small perforations sometimes appear months after primary healing.

The *transcanal approach* is appropriate for small posterior perforations where the entire margin can be seen through the ear canal (Fig. 3–2). Either local anesthesia (adults) or general anesthesia can be used. After sterile preparation and draping of the ear, local anesthetic with epinephrine is injected to supplement the general anesthetic and aid in hemostasis. The graft is harvested and allowed to dry on a smooth, hard surface. The size of the fascial graft depends on the size of the perforation. The trimmed perforation should overlap the graft by at least 1 mm, and preferably by 2 mm or more, in all directions. Once harvested, the fascia is allowed to dry on a block of dense fluoroplastic.

Tympanic membrane perforations are fistulas between the ear canal and the middle ear space. They are stable because contact inhibition between the squamous epithelium of the lateral surface of the tympanic membrane and the mucous membrane of the medial surface prevents active growth of either epithelium. Consequently, it is necessary to disrupt the junction between the squamous and respiratory epithelia.[23] The authors prefer to accomplish this step by removing a 1-mm rim of the perforation circumferentially (Fig. 3–2). This step is sometimes referred to as "freshening" the edges of the perforation.

Plaques of tympanosclerosis are patches of hyalinized (calcified) scar that replace portions of the fibrous layers of the tympanic membrane following periods of inflammation from chronic otitis media. They probably interfere with healing by blocking vascularization of the graft. Tympanosclerosis can be removed from the medial surface of the tympanic membrane with an angled pick. It is also useful to score the medial surface of the tympanic membrane remnant to stimulate the respiratory epithelium to incorporate the graft.

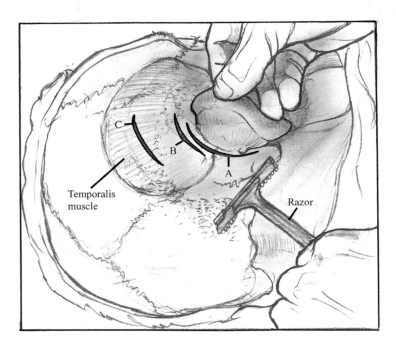

FIGURE 3–1 Temporalis fascia may be harvested from the same postauricular incision used for exposure to the middle ear (incision A). If a transcanal approach is used, a smaller incision over the fascia may be used to obtain the graft (incision B). If fascia has already been harvested during a previous operation, it may be necessary to harvest fascia from a more superior position using a supplemental incision (incision C). Use of incision C requires shaving and sterile preparation of a larger area before starting the operation. It is important to be aware of the location of the temporalis muscle, because the true temporalis fascia makes a more suitable graft material than areolar fascia or the periosteum of the skull.

A simple myringoplasty can be accomplished for small perforations without a tympanomeatal flap. In most cases, however, a tympanomeatal flap is raised to provide exposure to remove disease, reconstruct the ossicular chain, or facilitate placement of the graft.

The flap should be planned to expose at least the posterior half of the middle ear space. The flap should be folded anteriorly at the manubrium. Thus, incisions are made laterally from the annulus at the 6 and 12 o'clock positions, and directed posteriorly. The inferior incision may be placed more anteriorly if more anterior exposure is needed.

Three canal incisions are made to create the medially based flap (Fig. 3–3A). The two radial incisions are made first. Then they are connected by a third incision placed laterally. The flap should be long enough to accommodate curettage of the

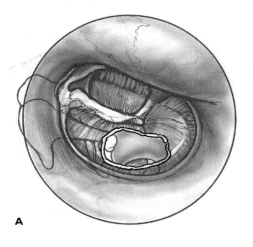

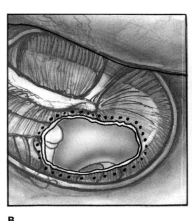

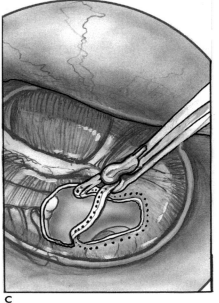

FIGURE 3–2 The transcanal approach is suitable for repair of a small posterior tympanic membrane perforation (A). A series of full-thickness punctures is made 1 mm from the edge of the perforation circumferentially using a sharp curved needle (B). The margin of the perforation is then stripped off using a cup forceps (C).

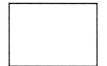 **SINGLE Tu** **I**

Customer:
Dana Freese

Middle Ear and Mastoid Surgery

Rex S. Haberman

6C-20-04-D1

P1-CBS-340

No CD

Used - Very Good

9781588901736

Picker Notes:
M _____ 2 _____
WT _____ 2 _____
CC _____

55439336

1 Item

1053926645

Reno International Tuesday Singles

Ship. Created: 11/27/2017 11:40:00 AM

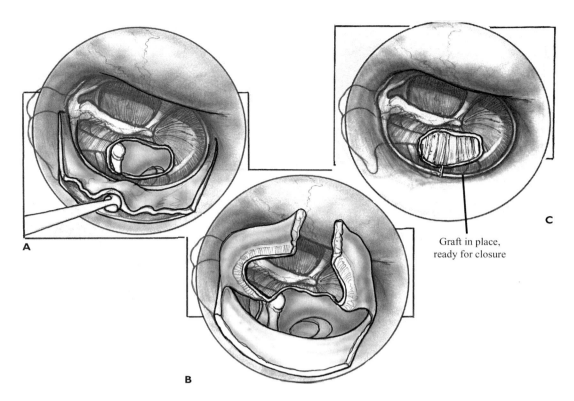

FIGURE 3–3 A tympanomeatal flap is raised to the annulus (A). Dividing the flap through the fibrous annulus to the perforation provides additional exposure (B). The graft is placed under the perforation allowing for generous overlapping of the tympanic membrane, and the tympanomeatal flap is returned to its normal position (C) prior to placement of absorbable packing lateral to the tympanic membrane.

posterior scutum if needed for exposure. To avoid troublesome bleeding, the flap should not be extended more than necessary into the thicker posterosuperior canal skin (the "vascular strip"). Also, a large flap can obstruct exposure to the middle ear. In general the flap should extend two thirds of the distance from the annulus to the bony–cartilaginous junction of the external auditory canal, or about 7 mm from the annulus (Fig. 3–3A).

The flap is elevated until the fibrous annulus is identified. To avoid unnecessary trauma to the flap it should be elevated by gently scraping the skin from the bone, hugging the bone, advancing along a broad front. As much as possible the suction tip is applied only to the back of the elevator, not directly to the flap. Spherical pledgets of nonlinting, nonabsorbable sponge material (4-mm diameter) soaked in 1:5000 epinephrine solution are applied to the subcutaneous surface of the flap for several minutes to achieve hemostasis. Sometimes a speculum holder is brought into use while the epinephrine is applied.

After the epinephrine pledgets are removed, elevation of the tympanomeatal flap continues by elevation of the fibrous annulus from the sulcus of the bony annulus. An effort is made to keep the

fibrous annulus intact. Care is taken not to injure the chorda tympani nerve, or to tear the flap off the annulus.

We usually make a fourth incision from the posterior midpoint of the flap medially through the flap, the annulus, and the tympanic membrane to the middle of the perforation (Fig. 3–3B). This incision creates two "wings" that can be separated, greatly enhancing exposure of the middle ear.

With maximum exposure thus achieved, we now lyse adhesions in the middle ear and remove inflammatory tissue. Care is taken to avoid trauma to any viable middle ear mucosa. If the promontory has been traumatized, it is important to retard the formation of adhesions to the newly grafted tympanic membrane. Either nonabsorbable (silicone sheeting of 0.16-mm thickness) or slowly absorbable sheeting may be used at the discretion of the surgeon.

If necessary, a postauricular incision is made and a mastoidectomy is performed. The ossicles are inspected for mobility and continuity. Ossicular chain reconstruction is performed as indicated.[25]

Pledgets of gelatin sponge are thoroughly moistened in normal saline, balanced salt solution, or an antibiotic solution, squeezed dry in a lint-free microwipe, and placed in the middle ear to support the graft. If the ossicles are absent, the epitympanum should also be packed so the packing will be stable. Enough packing material should be placed to fill the space but not to extend lateral to the tympanic membrane. If the packing starts to swell after it is placed, the surgeon can remove the excess packing or apply suction indirectly through a nonabsorbable 4-mm sponge to remove excess fluid and compress the packing material.

The temporalis fascia graft is trimmed so that the tympanic membrane remnant will overlap it by 2 mm or more circumferentially. The graft is grasped at the leading edge with a cup forceps and pushed under the remnant and lateral to the middle ear packing. It is spread out under the remnant so it is flat between the medial surface of the tympanic membrane and the gelatin sponge. The graft is extended posteriorly onto the bony portion of the external auditory canal to provide additional stability during healing (Fig. 3–3C).

After the graft is placed the external auditory canal is packed with absorbable gelatin sponges. The first few pieces are placed very carefully onto the grafted surface, beginning with the anterior sulcus of the external auditory canal, so the graft is not pulled out of position. A cotton ball saturated with bacitracin ointment is placed in the ear canal. The incision for the graft donor site is closed with buried stitches of absorbable suture material.

Although there is little more than anecdotal supporting evidence, clinical experience teaches that anterior and large tympanic membrane perforations are less likely to heal than small or posterior perforations when underlay grafting techniques are used. Consequently, it is author Monsell's preference to use underlay grafting techniques only for small posterior tympanic membrane perforations.

Some authors have described techniques to supplement underlay techniques to improve results (Figs. 3–4 and 3–5). These include a postauricular skin incision and canal skin incisions to access the middle ear from a posterior approach for better exposure. When a postauricular approach is used, the fascia can be harvested from the same incision (Fig. 3–1). During closure the ear canal is packed with absorbable gel sponges. The postauricular incision is closed with absorbable suture. The remainder of the ear canal is packed with absorbable gel sponges, and a mastoid dressing is applied.

An anterior canaloplasty also enhances exposure (Fig. 3–4B). This can be performed through either the transcanal or the postauricular approach, though it is easier to accomplish through a postauricular approach. A medially based flap of anterior canal skin is elevated to the annulus. A graded series of diamond burs is used on the surgical drill with continuous suction-irrigation. A piece of metal foil from a suture package may be fitted over the canal skin flap to prevent the flap from catching in the bur during drilling. The anatomic goal is to be able to see the entire circumference of the annulus from a single position.

If adhesions form between the graft and the promontory, a conductive hearing loss will result. Adhesions can usually be prevented by placing silicone sheeting material in the middle ear whether or not the operation is staged.[26,27]

Oral analgesics are prescribed for postoperative pain. We do not routinely prescribe prophylactic antibiotics. The mastoid dressing can be removed 1 to 2 days after surgery. Dry ear precautions are maintained until the ear is healed, usually after 4 to 8 weeks, depending on the size of the perforation. Antibiotic eardrops are applied three times per day after surgery until healing is complete. The patient is advised not to blow forcefully through the nose, to avoid contact sports, and to avoid air travel for at least 2 weeks.

RESULTS

Caution is advised in reading the literature on tympanic membrane repair because of uncontrolled variations in patient selection, and reporting methods (Table 3–1). Prospective, randomized, controlled clinical trials comparing groups undergoing underlay versus overlay tympanic membrane grafting do not exist. In author Monsell's experience, the socioeconomic status of the patient is an important factor in success with chronic ear surgery generally.

In 1995, the American Academy of Otolaryngology–Head and Neck Surgery (AAO-HNS) Committee on Hearing and Equilibrium recommended uniform reporting methods.[28] Under the reporting guidelines, the pure tone average (PTA) is evaluated at 500, 1000, 2000, and 3000 Hz for air and bone conduction postoperatively. The 4000-Hz threshold can replace the 3000-Hz threshold in the calculation of the PTA. The postoperative air–bone gap (ABG) is determined by subtracting the postoperative bone PTA from postoperative air PTA. Sensorineural hearing loss as a complication of the procedure is defined as changes in the bone conduction PTA at 1000, 2000, and 4000 Hz.[28] Patients should be followed for at least 12 months.

Postoperative reperforation of the tympanic membrane occurs in some cases. The postoperative interval chosen to assess successful graft closure

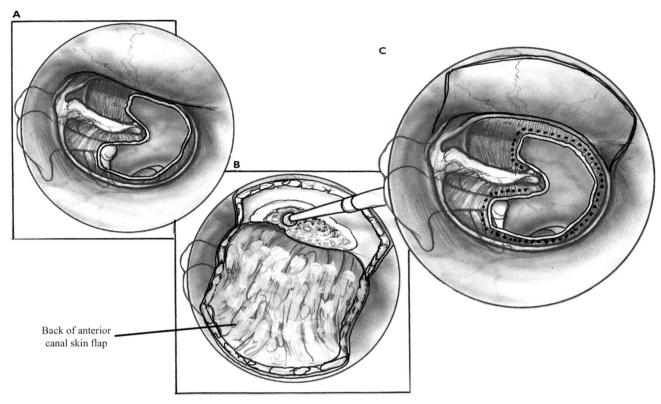

FIGURE 3–4   To facilitate exposure for repairing larger and anterior perforations, a postauricular incision is made and a tympanoplasty retractor is placed (not shown). No additional exposure is needed if the anterior tympanic sulcus can be seen (A). If additional exposure is needed, an anterior canaloplasty can be performed by drilling the anterior canal wall bone with a diamond bur behind a medially based flap of anterior canal wall skin (B). The skin flap is returned to its original position after the canal bulge has been removed (C).

varied among published studies. Thus, the same case might be reported as a success, a failure, or a complication depending on the postoperative interval chosen for assessment. Many published studies predated the AAO-HNS guidelines, or the guidelines were not consistently followed. Most reports have included the postoperative ABG and complications.

Most cases in the series listed in Table 3–1 involved tympanoplasty without ossicular repair or mastoidectomy. Rates of complete closure of the tympanic membrane are generally greater than 90% in most series. In centers that use overlay grafting techniques predominantly, the rate of closure for overlay grafts tends to be higher, about 97%, than with underlay grafting techniques, 93 to 95%. Patients were followed for at least 6 months postoperatively in most series reported here. Most graft failures occurred 6 to 12 months postoperatively.

Some reports of personal series cannot be generalized to compare the merits of underlay versus overlay techniques except as used by those authors. For example, one study compared the results of underlay tympanoplasty on 79 ears versus overlay

techniques in 52 ears.[17] The authors reported a lower failure rate and better postoperative hearing result (closure of ABG) with the underlay technique. However, they exclusively employed the endaural approach for both underlay and overlay techniques. Exposure of the anterior tympanic sulcus, which is important to the success of lateral grafting techniques, is restricted with the endaural approach. Also, the operations were often performed by residents, who may not have been experienced with the more technically demanding overlay grafting technique. Another prevalent source of bias in published personal series is that surgeons may use underlay techniques for healthier ears and smaller perforations (selection bias).

Hough[4] reported a series of 208 cases with medial grafting and the transcanal approach. Perforations were closed in more than 99%, with 81% ABG closure to within 10 dB. The cause of perforation and middle ear pathology did not influence the result. Lee and Schuknecht[29] reported similar hearing results in their series. They also noted slightly less success with vein and split-thickness skin grafts in comparison with fascia grafts. They reported

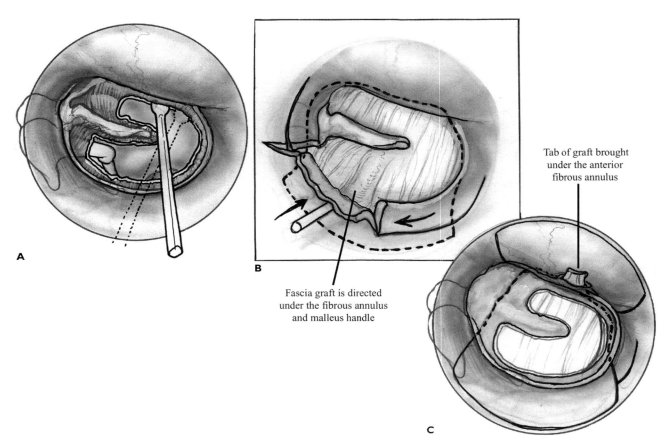

Tab of graft brought
under the anterior
fibrous annulus

Fascia graft is directed
under the fibrous annulus
and malleus handle

FIGURE 3-5 Supplemental techniques may improve the success rate in large and anterior perforations. To create a larger surface of raw tissue for graft healing, elevate the annulus and up to 1 mm of medial canal wall skin (A).[34] The graft can then be placed between the fibrous and bony annulus. For large perforations the graft can be placed lateral to the malleus and superior scutum (B).[35] The superior and inferior flaps of canal wall skin are placed over the fascia graft. A 4 × 4 mm tab of fascia can be placed through a tunnel under the anterior canal wall skin to help ensure adequate coverage of the perforation and retention of the graft in the desired position (C).

significantly different success rates between attending surgeons and residents (89% vs. 68%).

Glasscock[11] reported the results of 180 ears with underlay techniques versus 57 ears with overlay techniques. The areolar fascia was used instead of true temporalis fascia. All procedures employed a postauricular approach. The graft take rate was better with the underlay technique (96%) versus with the overlay technique (91%). Glasscock et al[12] later reported an overall graft success rate of over 93% in his series of 1556 ears, all performed with postauricular incisions and underlay techniques. There were 19 cases of early graft failure and 91 cases of graft failure noted 3 months after surgery. Success with cholesteatomatous ears was slightly less (92%) compared with those without cholesteatoma (93.2%). There was no difference in the rate of graft healing between draining and dry ears. The graft closure rate for children under age 12 was 91.5%, and 93.3% for those 12 and older.[12] Various graft materials were used, including aerolar temporalis tissue, true temporalis fascia, perichondrium, and cartilage. In general, the postauricular approach was associated with a slightly better success rate than transcanal techniques. In contrast, Sheehy[10,27] reported better success rate, 97%, with overlay techniques.

Rizer[16] addressed the question of whether differences in success rates in comparative studies may reflect the surgeon's preference for a particular technique. He reported results of 551 procedures with underlay techniques versus 158 ears with overlay techniques. The location and size of the perforations, the middle ear status, and the causes of perforation (infection or trauma) were evenly distributed in both groups. All operations were performed by the same surgeons, who were experienced with both techniques. Rizer concluded that both techniques have high success rates, although drum healing was more successful with overlay grafting (95.6%) versus underlay techniques (88.8%), $p = 0.050$.[16] There were no statistically sig-

TABLE 3–1   ILLUSTRATIVE RESULTS

Author	Technique	Closure of Perforation (%)	Postoperative Air–Bone Gap	Comments	Complications: Reperforation, Retraction, SNHL
Lee 1971[29]	Underlay n = 235	81	< 10 dB: 78%	Included various graft materials	3% (estimated)
Hough 1970[4]	Underlay n = 208	99.63	< 10 dB: 81% < 40 dB: 92.3%	Transcanal Myringoplasty only from a larger series of 644 Children included	2%
Austin 1976[8]	Underlay n = 52	94	< 10 dB: 59% < 20 dB: 76% < 30 dB: 96%	Transcanal	Less than 1%
Sheehy 1980[10]	Overlay n = 153	97.4	< 10 dB: 88% < 20 dB: 97%		Loss of BC of more than 10 dB at 2 kHz and 4 kHz = 3%
Shelton and Sheehy 1990[27]	Overlay n = 39	97	< 10 dB: 31 to 45% < 20 dB: 68 to 80% < 30 dB: 79 to 85% Tested after second stage	Myringoplasty only from a larger series of 400	As SNHL, including cases with mastoidectomy: < 2%, mostly from cholesteatomatous ears with mastoidectomies
Doyle 1972[17]	Underlay n = 79 Overlay n = 52	86 64	< 15 dB: 62% < 15 dB: 27%	Mostly endaural approaches with both techniques	10% 38%
Glasscock 1982[12]	Underlay, postauricular n = 1556	93	Not reported	Aerolar fascia, true fascia, allograft, perichondrium, and cartilage used Children included	6–8%
Koch 1990[30]	Underlay, endaural mostly n = 64	73	< 10 dB: 42% < 20 dB: 50% < 30 dB: 72%	Children only; mostly fascia with perichondrium	Estimated to 12%: infection, cholesteatoma, atelectasis
Shih 1991[36]	Overlay n = 59	78	< 10 dB: 17% < 30 dB: 68%	Children from 6 to 16 years of age	Not reported
Rizer 1997[16]	Underlay n = 554 Overlay n = 158	89 96	< 15 dB: 90% < 15 dB: 89%	Overall results	8%

BC, bone conduction threshold; SNHL, sensorineural hearing loss.

nificant relationships between the hearing results or complications with techniques used.

Special considerations may apply to tympanoplasty in children. Recommended ages for pediatric tympanoplasty and success rates vary widely. Some authors have proposed that tympanoplasty in children should be deferred until eustachian tube maturation is achieved and the risk of infection is lessened, typically age 8 to 10. Others have argued that closing the perforations would better protect the middle ear from further infections and minimize delay in speech development from hearing loss.

Koch et al[30] reported complete healing of 73% in one series of 64 pediatric cases. Graft failures were more common in children under 8 years of age. The middle ear status, the condition of the contralateral ear, and the size and location of the perforation did not influence results. In contrast, Raine and Singh[31] noted a statistically lower success rate with bilateral perforations. They also reported better success with children older than 8 years of age in their 114 cases.

In 170 pediatric cases (124 underlay, 46 overlay), Rizer[16] found no correlation between age and success rate; however, 75% of patients were older than 9 years of age in his series. The success rate for 35 patients under age 9 was 100% for overlay grafts and 89% for underlay grafts. Lau and Tos[13] concluded that long-term success, which was 92% in their series, depended on whether the ear remained dry, rather than on the age at surgery.

COMPLICATIONS AND MANAGEMENT

Failure of graft healing is usually due to improper placement of the graft (due to technical error or inadequate exposure) or infection. Office myringoplasty or revision surgery may be considered.[32] Failure to achieve the desired improvement in hearing may occur because of failure of the graft to heal (persistent perforation), recrudescence of disease, adhesions between the tympanic membrane and the promontory, or ossicular problems. An inclusion keratoma may form if a piece of viable squamous epithelium is trapped under the tympanic membrane. Most keratomas can be unroofed in a minor office procedure.

Sensorineural hearing loss is rare. The probable causes include ossicular trauma from drilling, dissection, or the persistence of active disease. Facial paralysis is also rare. If it occurs immediately, early exploration is usually needed. Mild facial paralysis of delayed onset can be managed expectantly, and usually will recover to normal without surgical intervention.[33]

Tympanoplasty has many variations, but is essentially a mature set of procedures. Future progress will require research to achieve more successful control of chronic otitis media and to manage the processes of wound healing in the middle ear. The advantages and disadvantages of the underlay technique are listed in Table 3–2.

TABLE 3–2 ADVANTAGES AND DISADVANTAGES OF UNDERLAY TECHNIQUES

Advantages

   Potentially less invasive

   Shorter healing time

   Less technically challenging

   Lateralization and blunting are avoided

   Failures are easier to repair

   Local anesthesia and a transcanal approach are possible

Disadvantages

   Less exposure than lateral grafting techniques

   Less suitable for difficult cases, e.g., anterior or recurrent perforation

   Diseased portions of the remnant cannot be removed as readily as with overlay techniques

   Lower rates of success for closure of the perforation

   More prone to adhesions to the promontory

REFERENCES

1. Wullstein H. Funktionelle Operations in Muttelohr mit Hilfe des fresen Spalthappen-Transplantes. *Arch Ohr Nas Hehlkopfheilkunde* 1952;161:22–427.

2. Austin D, Shea J. A new system of tympanoplasty using vein graft. *Laryngoscope* 1961;71:596–602.

3. Shea JJ. Vein graft closure of eardrum perforations. *J Laryngol Otol* 1960;74:358–362.

4. Hough JVD. Tympanoplasty with the interior fascial graft technique and ossicular reconstruction. *Laryngoscope* 1970;80:1385–1413.

5. Storrs LA. Myringoplasty with the use of fascia grafts. *Arch Otolaryngol Head Neck Surg* 1961;74:45–49.

6. Herrmann H. Trommelfellplastic mit Fasciengewebe von Musculus Temporalis nach Begradigung der vorderen Gehorganswand. *HNO* 1961;9:136–137.

7. Austin D. Reporting results in tympanoplasty. *Am J Otol* 1985;6:85–89.

8. Austin D. Transcanal tympanoplasty: a 15-year report. *Trans Am Acad Ophthalmol Otol* 1976;82:30–38.

9. Sheehy JL, Glasscock ME. Tympanic membrane grafting with temporalis fascia. *Arch Otolaryngol* 1967;86:391–402.

10. Sheehy JL, Anderson RG. Myringoplasty: a review of 472 cases. *Ann Otol Rhinol Laryngol* 1980;89:331–334.

11. Glasscock ME. Tympanic membrane grafting with fascia: overlay vs underlay technique. *Laryngoscope* 1973;5:754–770.

12. Glasscock ME, Jackson CJ, Nissen AJ, Schwaber MK. Postauricular undersurface tympanic membrane grafting: a follow up report. *Laryngoscope* 1982;92:718–727.

13. Lau T, Tos M. Tympanoplasty in children: an analysis of late results. *Am J Otol* 1986;7:55–59.

14. Tos M. Stability of myringoplasty based on late results. *Otorhinolaryngology* 1980;42:171–181.

15. Tos M, Falbe-Hansen J Jr. Tympanoplasty in only hearing ears. *J Laryngol Otol* 1975;89:1057–1064.

16. Rizer FM. Overlay versus underlay tympanoplasty. Part II: the study. *Laryngoscope* 1997;107(suppl 84):26–36.

17. Doyle JP, Schleuning AJ, Echevarria J. Tympanoplasty: should grafts be placed medial or lateral to the tympanic membrane? *Laryngoscope* 1972;82:1425–1430.

18. Rizer FM. Overlay versus underlay tympanoplasty. Part I: historical review of the literature. *Laryngoscope* 1997;107(suppl 84):1–25.

19. Leighton SE, Robson AK, Anslow P, Milford CA. The role of CT imaging in the management of chronic suppurative otitis media. *Otolaryngol Clin North Am* 1993;18:23–29.

20. Garber LZ, Dort JC. Cholesteatoma: diagnosis and staging by CT scan. *J Otolaryngol* 1994;23:121–124.

21. Perez de Tagle JRV, Fenton JE, Fagan PA. Mastoid surgery in the only hearing ear. *Laryngoscope* 1996;106:67–70.

22. Clymer MA, Schwaber MK, Davidson JM. The effects of keratinocyte growth factor on healing of tympanic membrane perforation. *Laryngoscope* 1996;106:280–285.

23. Spandow O, Hellstrom S, Dahlstrom M. Structural characterization of persistent tympanic membrane perforations in man. *Laryngoscope* 1996;106:346–352.

24. Gladstone HB, Jackler RK, Varav K. Tympanic membrane wound healing: an overview. *Otolaryngol Clin North Am* 1995;28:913–932.

25. Monsell E. Ossiculoplasty. In: English G, ed. *Otolaryngology: Head and Neck Surgery*. Philadelphia: Lippincott Williams & Wilkins; 1998.

26. Sheehy JL. Plastic sheeting in tympanoplasty. *Laryngoscope* 1973;83:1144–1159.

27. Shelton C, Sheehy JL. Tympanoplasty: review of 400 staged cases. *Laryngoscope* 1990;100:679–681.

28. Committee on Hearing and Equilibrium. Committee on Hearing and Equilibrium guidelines for the evaluation of results of treatment of conductive hearing loss. *Otolaryngol Head Neck Surg* 1995;113:186–187.

29. Lee KJ, Schuknecht HF. Results of tympanoplasty and mastoidectomy at the Massachusetts Eye and Ear Infirmary. *Laryngoscope* 1971;81:529–543.

30. Koch WM, Friedman EM, McGill TJ, Healy GB. Tympanoplasty in children: the Boston Children's Hospital experience. *Arch Otolaryngol Head Neck Surg* 1990;116:35–40.

31. Raine CH, Singh SD. Tympanoplasty in children: a review of 114 cases. *J Laryngol Otol* 1983;97:217–221.

32. Derlacki E. Residual perforations after tympanoplasty: office technique. *Otolaryngol Clin North Am* 1982;15:861–867.

33. Monsell E. Iatrogenic facial nerve injury: prevention and management. In: Jackler RK, Brackmann DE, eds. *Neurotology*. St. Louis: Mosby; 1994:1333–1343.

34. Shea MC. Tympanoplasty: the undersurface graft technique: transcanal approach. In: Brackmann D, Shelton C, Arriaga A, eds. *Otologic Surgery*. Philadelphia: WB Saunders; 2001:106–112.

35. Jackson C, Glasscock M, Strasnick B. Tympanoplasty: the undersurface grafting technique—postauricular approach. In: Brackmann D, Shelton C, Arriaga A, eds. *Otologic Surgery*. Philadelphia: WB Saunders; 2001:113–124.

36. Shih L, Thomas DT, Crabtree JA. Myringoplasty in children. *Otolaryngol Head Neck Surg* 1991;105:74–77.

Chapter 4

Overlay Tympanoplasty

Rick A. Friedman and Marlan R. Hansen

The modern era of tympanoplasty began in the 1950s with the work of Zollner[1] and Wullstein[2] using full- and split-thickness skin grafts to repair the tympanic membrane (TM). Subsequent innovations included the use of other grafting material including canal skin, vein, perichondrium, and temporalis fascia.[3–5] Modern approaches to tympanoplasty differ in whether the graft is placed lateral or medial to the TM remnant.[6–10] This chapter describes lateral grafting or overlay tympanoplasty techniques. The advantages of lateral grafting techniques are:

1. High success rate. There was a 97% success rate in closure of the perforation in a review of the experience at the House Ear Clinic of over 1700 cases of overlay tympanoplasty.[11]
2. Excellent intraoperative and postoperative visualization of the anterior meatal angle. This is especially helpful in cases of anterior perforation with a large anterior canal wall bony overhang.
3. Preservation of the middle ear space. Because the graft is placed lateral to the drum remnant, the middle ear space is less likely to be reduced by overlay tympanoplasty.

The disadvantages of lateral grafting are:

1. The potential for lateralization of the graft or blunting of the anterior meatal recess if proper surgical techniques are not carefully applied. This occurs more commonly in cases where the surgeon is inexperienced with the procedure.
2. Squamous epidermal inclusion cysts may develop if the TM epithelium is not completely removed prior to grafting. These cysts may also occur along the external auditory canal. In either

case, they are generally easily treated with simple unroofing and marsupialization in the office.
3. Relative to underlay tympanoplasty, healing from overlay techniques takes longer, lasting up to 4 to 6 weeks.

Patient Presentation

Patients with chronic otitis media usually present with recurrent or persistent otorrhea or with hearing impairment. Patients with a central perforation of the TM without cholesteatoma usually describe recurrent episodes of otorrhea that resolve promptly with topical treatment. Persistent malodorous discharge most commonly reflects advanced middle ear and mastoid disease, often in association with a cholesteatoma. The degree of hearing impairment depends on several factors including the size and location of the perforation, the extent and duration of middle ear mucosal disease, and the status of the ossicles. Rarely, a patient with advanced disease including cholesteatoma may present with pain, vertigo, facial paralysis, or central nervous system (CNS) complications of otitis media.

Indications for Surgery

The goals of surgery in chronic otitis media are to produce a dry, safe ear; to restore hearing; and to preserve normal anatomic structures and contours when possible. Careful evaluation of the patient is necessary to determine the necessity and urgency of surgery. In patients with a unilateral dry, central perforation and minimal hearing loss, the main indication for surgery is to prevent further episodes of otorrhea, and surgery is elective. Patients with advanced mucosal disease or cholesteatoma usually require surgical intervention to eradicate infection and produce a safe ear.

PREOPERATIVE EVALUATION

Successful and safe tympanoplasty demands careful preoperative examination of the patient. The preoperative examination alerts the surgeon to potential complications of the disease process that may be encountered in surgery and to predict the outcome of surgery. This is helpful, not only in planning the surgical procedure, but also in advising patients about realistic postoperative expectations and alerting them to potential complications.

Examination of the TM is best performed with a microscope. Cleaning of any debris or discharge in the external canal allows visualization of the entire TM. Specific notes are made regarding the type of perforation, the character of the discharge, and the status of the middle ear mucosa and ossicles.

EXAMINATION

PERFORATION

In general, perforations can be divided into central or marginal. Central perforations maintain a margin of drum remnant around the circumference of the perforation. Typically, these perforations only intermittently drain and are not associated with cholesteatoma. Marginal perforations involve the periphery of the TM. They are most often located in the posterior-superior quadrant or in the pars flaccida; present with persistent, malodorous discharge; and frequently involve cholesteatoma.

RETRACTION POCKETS/CHOLESTEATOMA

Deep retraction pockets and cholesteatoma usually involve the pars flaccida or the posterior-superior quadrant of the pars tensa. Occasionally a polyp or granulation tissue may prevent inspection of the retraction pocket or cholesteatoma. Not infrequently deep retractions in the pars flaccida extend into the attic and even the mastoid without significant ossicular involvement. These patients may have a normal-appearing pars tensa, minimal hearing loss, and no otorrhea, highlighting the importance of careful inspection of the entire TM with an operating microscope prior to tympanoplasty.

MIDDLE EAR/OSSICULAR STATUS

Often the status of the middle ear mucosa and ossicular chain can be evaluated by careful examination through the perforation. A normal or near-normal mucosa predicts a favorable outcome. Likewise, an intact ossicular chain improves the prognosis for hearing improvement. Tympanosclerosis, a hyaline degeneration in the middle ear, is frequently seen in ears with chronic otitis media. Although tympanosclerosis rarely affects the success of the TM graft, it may contribute to ossicular fixation. Stapedial fixation by tympanosclerosis, although rare, requires a second operation. Ossicular erosion or necrosis usually involves the incus. The status of the stapes can often be determined and is the most important ossicular variable in hearing improvement.

PNEUMATIC OTOSCOPY/FISTULA

A pneumatic otoscope is used to compress and rarefy the air of the external ear canal. When a labyrinthine fistula is present, the patient often complains of vertigo, and nystagmus is present. A negative fistula test, however, does not exclude a fistula, a point that should be kept in mind during surgery. Pneumatic otoscopy also helps determine the mobility of the remnant of the par tensa or the presence of a perforation that is difficult to see.

AUDIOLOGY

Preoperative air and bone pure tone thresholds and speech discrimination scores should be performed on every patient undergoing tympanoplasty. This information not only helps the surgeon predict the potential for hearing improvement, but also may alert the surgeon to potential complications of chronic otitis media such as labyrinthine fistula. Audiometric results are confirmed with tuning fork testing.

EUSTACHIAN TUBE FUNCTION TESTING

We do not routinely test the function of the eustachian tube prior to tympanoplasty. A careful history and physical examination predict outcome more accurately than any test of the eustachian tube.

RADIOLOGY

Likewise, we do not routinely order radiographic studies in patients with chronic otitis media. If a patient has a complication of the disease such as labyrinthine fistula or facial nerve weakness, or in selected revision cases, the temporal bone is imaged with high-resolution computed tomography.

OPERATING ROOM SETUP AND PATIENT POSITION

Attention to operating room setup and patient positioning greatly facilitates the ease with which tympanoplasty is performed. The anesthesiologist is positioned at the foot of the patient and therefore needs an extra-long ventilation tubing. It is helpful to have the blood pressure cuff on the arm opposite to the ear to be operated on; therefore, the intravenous (IV) is best placed in the forearm of the side to be operated on. As the head may need to be repositioned frequently during surgery, it is important that the endotracheal tube be adequately taped and secured prior to placement of sterile drapes and that there is some laxity in the ventilation tubing. The scrub nurse is positioned directly across from the surgeon.

Proper patient positioning improves intraoperative exposure and allows the surgeon to operate in a relaxed and comfortable position. The patient is positioned so that his head and shoulders are as near to the surgeon as possible. The patient is then adequately padded and secured to the table with wide adhesive tape or Velcro straps. The patient's head is turned away and flexed onto the opposite shoulder. The table is placed in a few degrees of the Trendelenburg position and rolled slightly toward the surgeon. The surgeon sits on a chair with his back against a rest and his arm and back muscles completely relaxed.

SPECIFIC TECHNIQUE

The main objectives of tympanoplasty are to eliminate disease and restore hearing. Achievement of these goals requires an intact TM; an air-containing, mucosally lined middle ear space; and a secure connection from the TM to the inner ear. Lateral graft tympanoplasty accomplishes these objectives in a high percentage of patients. Presented here are the specific steps taken in lateral graft tympanoplasty and suggestions to avoid the common potential complications.

TRANSMEATAL CANAL INCISIONS

Incisions along the tympanomastoid and tympanosquamous suture line demarcate the vascular strip, which is the area of skin in the superior and posterior-superior external ear canal. It is important to carry these incisions laterally into the cartilage of the concha to permit greater mobility of the vascular strip and improve the ultimate postauricular exposure. These incisions are connected with a medial incision made 1 to 2 mm lateral to the annulus and drum remnant, and the vascular strip is elevated from medial to lateral. A beaver knife with a No. 64 blade is then used to make a lateral semilunar incision in the outer third of the ear canal that connects the two vascular strip incisions (Fig. 4–1). This cut is beveled toward the bony canal, which thins the 1 to 2 mm of membranous canal included.

POSTAURICULAR EXPOSURE AND HARVESTING OF TEMPORALIS FASCIA

The skin incision begins at the anterior extent of and 1 cm above the postauricular fold. It is carried forward inferiorly, either in or just posterior to the postauricular crease, to the level of the floor of the external auditory canal. This allows adequate exposure of the bony external canal when the ear is retracted forward. A large piece (2 × 3 cm) of temporalis fascia is harvested, cleaned of any adherent muscle or fat, and pressed for 5 minutes. It is then dried under a heating lamp. The periosteum overlying the mastoid cortex is incised horizontally at the level of the linea temporalis posteriorly to the level of the skin incision. The periosteal incision is then carried inferiorly to the full extent of the skin incision. The auricle with the periosteal flap and the vascular strip are retracted forward with self-retaining retractors, exposing the mastoid cortex and bony external canal.

REMOVAL OF CANAL SKIN AND DE-EPITHELIALIZATION OF THE TYMPANIC MEMBRANE REMNANT

The skin and periosteum are dissected from the bony canal from lateral to medial along a broad front until the fibrous annulus is reached (Fig. 4–2). Removal of the canal skin medial to the anterior canal bulge may require blind dissection because the bulge often obscures vision of the anterior meatal recess. Tears in the skin are avoided by keeping the dissecting knife firmly against the bone and by not suctioning on the skin. Once the skin is elevated to the level of the annulus, a plane is developed between the skin of the canal and TM remnant, and the annulus and fibrous layer of the TM. Working in a plane parallel to the annulus, the skin of the canal and TM remnant

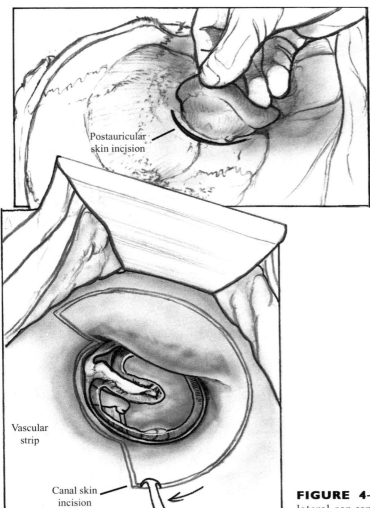

Postauricular skin incision

Vascular strip

Canal skin incision

FIGURE 4–1 Transmeatal incisions of vascular strip and lateral ear canal.

are removed. Beginning superiorly and anteriorly, the skin of the canal and TM remnant can often be removed in continuity by using a small cup forceps. To prevent epithelial pearls from developing in the reconstructed drum, it is important that all remaining squamous epithelial components be completely removed from the drum remnant.

DRILLING OF EAR CANAL

Drilling of the bony canal is routine in all lateral graft procedures, as it enlarges the field of surgery and allows satisfactory graft placement. Under continuous irrigation, drilling begins laterally and posteriorly with removal of the spine of Henle and the tympanosquamous suture line. Care is taken not to enter the mastoid air cells. Next, the anterior and inferior canal bulges are removed (Fig. 4–3). The posterior wall of the temporal mandibular joint

represents the anterior wall of the bony canal. It is most prominent in the midportion of the bony canal in both the superior to inferior and medial to lateral planes. It is important not to violate the joint when drilling the bony canal, and therefore superior and inferior troughs are drilled first, followed by thinning of the midportion of the canal wall over the joint. Final medial dissection just lateral to the annulus completely exposes the anterior sulcus and converts the acute anterior meatal angle into an obtuse angle. This is critical to prevent postoperative blunting.

INSPECTION OF THE OSSICLES AND MIDDLE EAR

Once the bony canal is drilled and the diseased TM remnant removed, the surgeon has a maximal view of the middle ear cleft. This allows thorough inspec-

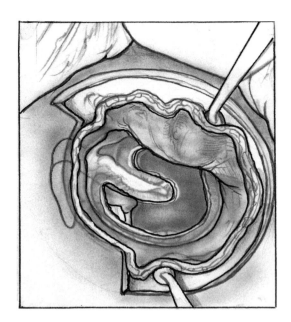

FIGURE 4–2   Removal of canal skin.

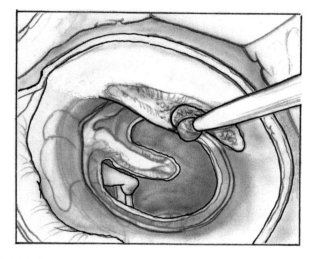

FIGURE 4–3   Drilling to enlarge ear canal.

tion of the middle ear and ossicles. Any disease (e.g., tympanosclerosis, cholesteatoma) is appropriately removed. Canal-wall-intact mastoidectomy and the facial recess approach are performed as necessary. Ossicular reconstruction, if indicated, is performed following placement of the temporalis graft.

GRAFTING

Prior to grafting, the middle ear space is packed with Gelfoam. The Gelfoam supports the graft as well as any ossicular prosthesis that is to be placed. It is important to adequately pack the protympanum at the eustachian tube orifice; however, the packing should not extend lateral to the handle of the malleus. The now-dried temporalis fascia is trimmed to a 1.3 × 1.6 cm oval shape, and a superior slit is cut in the fascia. This slit allows placement under the manubrium. If the manubrium is absent, two small 2 × 2 mm tabs are cut in the anterior and superior aspects of the graft. These tabs are tucked medial to the anterior canal wall and the lateral wall of the epitympanum. This is critical to prevent lateralization of the graft in the absence of the malleus handle.

The fascia is gently rehydrated by immersion for a few seconds in physiologic solution such as Tis-U-Sol. It is placed over the perforation and TM remnant and the two free edges of the slit are slipped under and around the manubrium (Fig. 4–4). The apex of the slit should contact the tensor tympani tendon. The graft is then positioned over the perforation. It is important that the graft does not extend onto the anterior canal wall to reduce postoperative blunting. The free edges of the slit are positioned in an overlapping fashion to cover the manubrium. This two-layered repair gives added strength to the pars flaccida region and helps avoid retraction pockets in this area.

REPLACEMENT OF CANAL SKIN

The canal skin is trimmed of any irregular edges and is replaced over the bony canal (Fig. 4–5). Medially it is positioned to overlap the fascia graft by 1 to 2 mm, which helps promote epithelialization of the drum and prevent anterior blunting. It is important to ensure that no edges of the skin remain rolled under, because small epithelial cysts may develop. The canal is now packed firmly with Gelfoam. The first piece of packing is a cigar-shaped, tightly rolled piece of Gelfoam that is placed in the anterior sulcus to give definition to the angle. The posterior aspect of the canal is not fully packed to leave room for the vascular strip.

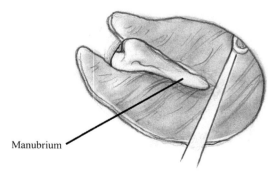

Manubrium

FIGURE 4–4   Rehydrated fascia is placed under the malleus handle and on outer surface of remnant.

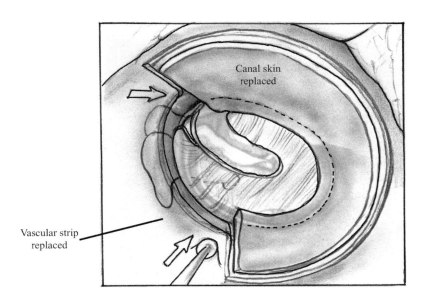

Canal skin
replaced

Vascular strip
replaced

FIGURE 4–5 Replacement of canal skin.

POSTAURICULAR CLOSURE AND PLACEMENT OF VASCULAR STRIP

The retractors are removed and the vascular strip is replaced anteriorly in the bony canal. The periosteal layer is closed over the mastoid cortex or the mastoidectomy defect. Transmeatally, the vascular strip is elevated and pulled forward to uncurl it to its full length. It is then replaced along the posterior canal wall and the remainder of the canal is packed with Gelfoam. The postauricular incision is closed subcutaneously followed by Steri-Strips, and a standard mastoid dressing is applied.

POSTOPERATIVE CARE

The patient or the patient's family removes the mastoid dressing the day following surgery. One week postoperative the patient is seen in the office, the ear is inspected, and the postauricular Steri-Strips are removed. To loosen the packing, the patient begins using antibiotic eardrops twice a day 3 weeks following surgery. The drops may be started sooner if drainage occurs. The second postoperative visit occurs 6 to 8 weeks following surgery, by which time the ear should be well healed.

COMPLICATIONS: AVOIDANCE AND MANAGEMENT

Although there are many advantages to outer surface grafting, there are several potential healing problems that may occur including lateralization of the graft, anterior blunting, and epithelial cysts.

Careful adherence to proper surgical technique avoids most of these complications; nevertheless, in certain individuals the potential complications may outweigh the advantages of lateral grafting.

LATERALIZATION

Lateralization of the TM was one of the first problems encountered in lateral grafting and resulted from placement of the fascia graft lateral to the malleus handle when the technique was first developed. Placement of the graft underneath the malleus handle has greatly reduced the incidence of this complication. When the manubrium is missing, small tabs in the graft are placed under the lateral wall of the epitympanum and the anterior canal wall to avoid lateralization. Lateralization usually becomes apparent 6 to 12 months following tympanoplasty and is recognized by a small, mobile eardrum with poor landmarks that lies at a right angle to the line of vision. The patient's hearing is often reduced. Correction of this problem requires revision tympanoplasty with placement of the graft medial to the malleus handle.

ANTERIOR BLUNTING

Blunting of the anterior sulcus is the complication most often encountered by the inexperienced surgeon. It results from excess fibrous tissue formation, especially anterior-superiorly, and when significant enough to involve the malleus handle, can reduce hearing. With severe blunting, the anterior half of the membrane assumes a concave appearance with no clear junction with the skin of the anterior canal wall and is often immobile. The manubrium is often indistinguishable. If blunting persists for 6 months and hearing is impaired, revision tympanoplasty is required to correct it.

There are several specific steps that are taken to avoid anterior blunting. First, the entire anterior canal wall bulge is removed and the anterior angle is opened from an acute to an obtuse angle. Second, whenever possible the anterior fibrous annulus should be preserved and the fascia graft should not be placed onto the anterior canal wall bone. Third, the replaced canal wall skin should overlap the fascia graft anteriorly by 1 to 2 mm. Finally, placement of a tightly rolled, cigar-shaped piece of Gelfoam packing in the anterior sulcus to re-create the anterior angle helps prevent blunting.

EPITHELIAL CYSTS

It is not unusual for epithelial cysts to develop as small pearls on the TM or ear canal. They result from the turning under of the skin edges when the canal skin is replaced and are easily managed by simple unroofing in the office. Much less frequently, an epithelial cyst may develop between the TM remnant and the fascia graft anterior-inferiorly adjacent to the canal wall bone where a small nerve and artery enter the ear canal just lateral to the annulus. This results from inadequate de-epithelialization of the canal bone and TM remnant next to the bone in this area. It is managed by incision and evacuation of the cyst.

SUMMARY

Lateral graft tympanoplasty provides a reliable technique for reconstruction of the middle ear and TM in chronic otitis media. Appropriate patient selection and counseling mandates a thorough understanding of the disease processes of chronic otitis media and detailed preoperative evaluation. Lateral graft techniques provide maximal exposure of the ear canal and middle ear space and have a very high graft success rate. Most of the potential complications can be avoided by strict adherence to proper surgical technique. Once mastered, it provides the otologic surgeon with a technique that can be reliably used to treat nearly all cases of chronic otitis media and restore middle ear function.

REFERENCES

1. Zollner F. The principles of plastic surgery of the sound-conducting apparatus. *J Laryngol Otol* 1955;69:637–652.
2. Wullstein H. Theory and practice of tympanoplasty. *Laryngoscope* 1956;66:1076–1093.
3. House WF, Sheehy JL. Myringoplasty: use of ear canal skin compared with other techniques. *Arch Otolaryngol Head Neck Surg* 1961;73:407–415.
4. Storrs LA. Myringoplasty with use of fascia graft. *Arch Otolaryngol Head Neck Surg* 1961;74:45–49.
5. Sheehy JL, Glasscock ME III. Tympanic membrane grafting with temporalis fascia. *Arch Otolaryngol* 1967;86:391–402.
6. Glasscock ME III. Tympanic membrane grafting with fascia: overlay vs. undersurface technique. *Laryngoscope* 1973;83:754–770.
7. Glasscock ME III, Jackson CG, Nissen AJ, Schwaber MK. Postauricular undersurface tympanic membrane grafting: a follow-up report. *Laryngoscope* 1982;92:718–727.
8. Sheehy JL, Anderson RG. Myringoplasty: a review of 472 cases. *Ann Otol Rhinol Laryngol* 1980;89:331–334.
9. Rizer FM. Overlay versus underlay tympanoplasty. Part I: historical review of the literature. *Laryngoscope* 1997;107:1–25.
10. Rizer FM. Overlay versus underlay tympanoplasty. Part II: the study. *Laryngoscope.* 1997;107:26–36.
11. Sheehy JL. Tympanic membrane grafting: early and long-term results. *Laryngoscope* 1964;74:985–988.

Chapter 5

OVER-UNDER TYMPANOPLASTY: INDICATIONS AND TECHNIQUE

Dennis I. Bojrab and Andrew N. Karpenko

Today the goal of successful tympanoplasty is to create a mobile tympanic membrane or graft with an aerated mucosal-lined middle ear space and a sound-conducting mechanism between the mobile membrane and the inner ear fluids. A review of the literature reveals that many techniques have been developed and employed successfully; there is a rich history of the evolution of techniques to produce this end. This chapter gives a brief history of the evolution of the over-under tympanoplasty, and discusses the indications and technical aspects of the technique.

NORMAL TYMPANIC MEMBRANE

Embryologically, the tympanic membrane is derived from the fusion of the ectodermal meatal plugs from the first branchial cleft and the endodermally derived first branchial pouch (tubotympanic recess). The tympanic membrane and middle ear cavity is the area of contact between these two structures. The tympanic membrane separates the delicate middle and inner ear structures from the external environment. It measures approximately 10 mm in diameter, and is conically shaped with the apex of the cone at the umbo.

Histologically, the tympanic membrane has three layers. This structure contains an outer ectodermal layer composed of keratinizing squamous epithelium, a middle mesodermal fibrous layer, and an inner endodermal mucosal layer. The outer epidermal layer is composed of stratum corneum, granulosum, spinosum, and basale. This layer has cell growth and migratory properties responsible for the self-cleaning and replacement function of the tympanic membrane.[1,2] Studies have demonstrated the presence of epidermal growth factor and fibroblast growth factor, which are thought to promote healing of membrane perforations and contribute to the success of tympanoplasty procedures.[3]

The mesodermal fibrous layer is the intermediate layer or the lamina propria. There are different compositions depending on the location along the tympanic membrane.[4] In the pars tensa, the lamina propria has a subepidermal loose connective tissue layer containing the internal blood vessels and nerves and a fibrous layer made of outer radial and inner circular fibers. These fibers are made of collagen. This should contribute to the vibratory functions of the tympanic membrane.[5,6] The pars flaccida or Shrapnell's membrane has elastic fibers and accounts for the flaccidity of this variably sized area.[4]

There are two major blood supplies of the tympanic membrane. An external plexus from the tympanic branch of the deep auricular artery sends large manubrial branches along Shrapnell's membrane and the manubrium and numerous radial branches into the tympanic membrane from along its circumference.[7] The malleal artery is the major blood supply of the posterior half of the tympanic membrane, which is better perfused than the anterior half.[8] The anterior half is supplied from smaller radial branches that enter around the annulus derived from the internal plexus from the stylomastoid branch of the postauricular artery.[9]

HISTORICAL REVIEW

The tympanoplasty operation is a surgical procedure to eradicate disease in the middle ear and to reconstruct the hearing mechanism, with or without mastoid surgery and with or without tympanic membrane grafting. This procedure was defined by the American Academy of Ophthalmology and Otolaryngology's Committee on Conservation of Hearing in 1964.[10] Hippocrates[11] himself recognized that "acute pain of the ear, with continued strong fevers, is to be dreaded, for there is danger that the man may become delirious and die." Early surgery for the draining ear was basically a mastoid operation and was lifesaving. The first attempt of repairing a tympanic membrane was performed in 1640 when Banzer[12] used a pig's bladder stretched across an ivory tube and placed in the ear and obtained hearing improvement temporarily. In 1853 Toynbee[13] placed a rubber disk attached to a silver wire over a perforation, resulting in hearing improvement. In 1877 Blake[14] placed a paper patch over a perforation, and in many patients a hearing improvement was noted.

Berthold[15] is credited with performing the first true tympanoplasty, in 1878. His technique involved de-epithelializing the tympanic membrane by applying plaster against the membrane for 3 days, removing the epithelium, and then placing a skin graft over the defect. The modern era of tympanoplasty began in the 1950s due to many developments, including antibiotics, instrumentation, and the operating microscope.

Following the introduction of tympanoplasty in the early 1950s by Wullstein[16] and Zollner,[17] all surgeries used an overlay graft. Wullstein's article, "Tympanoplasty as an Operation to Improve Hearing in Chronic Otitis Media and Its Results," set the stage for this operation to improve hearing and protect the middle ear from the outside environment. At that time, this operation consisted of full-thickness and split-thickness skin grafts. By the end of the decade, graft eczema, desquamation, and a poor long-term take rate had prompted many surgeons to seed alternate grafting materials and techniques.[18] In 1956 Sooy[19] had reported the use of canal skin pedicle graft to close marginal perforations. In 1958 House and Plester, working independently, began using canal skin as a free overlay graft.[20,21] In 1959 Shea, Austin, and Tabb, working independently, employed vein as an undersurface graft to repair tympanic membrane perforations.[22–24] The vein graft tended to atrophy over a few months and occasionally reperforated.

In 1961 Storrs[25] described the first undersurface fascia technique to be used in the United States. With the use of connective tissue, most of the problems incurred with free skin grafts were eliminated. The first successful use of homograft tympanic membrane in the United States was by Ned Chalat[26] in 1964. His experience was reported in the Harper Hospital Bulletin and went unnoticed for several years. Many authors reported promising results with this technique starting in 1968 with House and Glasscock, and soon to be followed by Perkins, Smith, and Wehrs.[27–30] With this technique, procurement and sterilization of the donor material have been problematic. Over the years surgeons have used various living or homograft grafting materials mentioned above including loose areolar connective tissue, perichondrium, cartilage, fat, and periostium.[31,32]

Fascia has been the preferred material because of the internal structure of this material and because of the plentiful amount in the operative field. The high success rate of this material probably resides in the internal structure of collagen and mucopolysaccharides. It is interesting to note that both collagen and mucopolysaccharides have been implicated as playing a critical role in wound healing. Collagen is believed to contribute to wound tensile strength, and there is evidence that the chemically and biologically complex mucopolysaccharides play a positive role in the healing process, attracting fibroblasts into the wound area through chemotaxis.[33]

EVOLUTION OF TECHNIQUES

The over-under tympanoplasty is an evolution of technique that combines benefits of the earlier described techniques. A review of the literature reveals that many techniques have been developed and employed successfully. Tympanoplasty techniques have employed approaches such as transcanal, endaural, or postauricular. The grafts have been placed over and under the tympanic membrane or the malleus, and the biologic material used has been full-thickness skin, partial-thickness skin, fascia, perichondrium, cartilage, and periosteum. We will describe the various techniques and approaches commonly used in the past with the evolution of the presented technique of the over-under tympanoplasty.

Previous authors have demonstrated the technique of placing a graft lateral to the malleus but medial to the remnant of tympanic membrane. As early as 1972, Austin[35] stated that the graft may be secured either over or under the malleus tip, depending on the ease of positioning, and then some of the skin covering the malleus is dissected and replaced on the graft surface. Other authors such as Glasscock,[36] Wehrs,[37] and Hough[38] have also made similar inferences when describing underlay grafting in particular situations, usually with significant retraction of the malleus, large perforations, or anterior middle ear disease.

In 2002 Kartush et al[34] presented their results with this technique as an article dedicated to the technique with excellent long-term results for closure of perforations, hearing improvement or stabilization, and low incidence of complications. The authors used this technique with and without mastoidectomy and with and without ossicular reconstruction.

UNDERLAY (UNDERSURFACE) TECHNIQUE

The underlay or undersurface technique employed grafting material medial to or under the remnant tympanic membrane, typically under the malleus when the perforation extended to that area. The free edges of the perforation are prepared using a right-angled hook. The intent is to separate the outer cutaneous layer from the inner mucosal layer. This develops a fresh edge for healing. This technique originally described by Shea in 1957, was used initially for iatrogenic tympanic membrane perforations caused at the time of middle ear surgery.[29] Austin and Shea[23] in 1961 published their combined experience with this technique, stating that vein was an ideal material because it did not substitute for the missing squamous layer of the drum, but as a replacement for the fibrous layer across which normal epithelium will grow. The great hardiness of the vein as a free graft was also thought to be desirable. Their approach began as a transcanal or transmeatal procedure. The postauricular approach was used as a surgeon's decision at the time of surgery. Long-term results with vein proved to be fraught with atrophy over a few months, and the veins occasionally reperforated. These results were improved with the use of fascia, loose areolar connective tissue, or perichondrial tissue, and have been the preferred material over the past 30 years.

OVERLAY TECHNIQUE

The overlay technique as practiced in the 1960s consisted of accessing the drum head through the surgeon's preferred incision. The epithelium of the surface of the drum was removed and a fascia graft was placed on the perforation[39] and the ear packed with various material. Sheehy and Glasscock[40] replaced the pedicled canal skin grafts earlier described by authors with temporalis fascia overlay grafts. After comparing cases of canal skin and fascia grafts the following conclusions were made:

1. Fascia grafts (97.5% take rate) are generally superior to canal skin grafts (91.8% take rate).
2. Fascia grafts are also superior (91%) to canal skin grafts (70%) in closing total perforations.
3. Fascia is an excellent material to close ears that are draining at the time of surgery as evidenced by higher success rate (98%) than dry perforations using canal skin.

This technique was to be performed from the postauricular approach. Once the vascular strip incision is dissected out of the ear canal, it is held anteriorly with the retractor. The medial superior, anterior, and inferior canal wall skin is incised near the bony cartilaginous junctional site and then carefully elevated medially to the annulus. The entire cuff of skin is then cut free, leaving the annulus in its physiologic position. This skin is then removed from the operative site and placed into saline for the duration of the procedure.

Canal-wall widening is performed with a small drill as needed to visualize the anterior portion of the annulus. The squamous layer of the tympanic membrane remnant fascia is placed in the physiologic position of the drum, and then the ear canal skin is replaced over the fascia. The vascular strip is replaced, and the ear canal is packed with pledgets of absorbable gelatin sponge moistened in an antibiotic solution. With this technique, there is obvious marked dissection necessary and eardrum blunting is common.

INDICATIONS FOR OVER-UNDER TYMPANOPLASTY

By combining the benefits of both techniques, the over-under tympanoplasty has become the preferred technique for various approaches to tympanoplasty.[41–43] This technique places the tympanic membrane fascia graft lateral to the malleus, but medial to the remnant of tympanic membrane or fibrous annulus. This allows excellent exposure to the anterior middle ear space and prevents medialization of the graft to the promontory, and ossicular reconstruction may be placed directly to the underside of the malleus. Over-under tympanoplasty has become the authors' preferred technique for perforations that abut the malleus in both anterior and posterior perforations and for large or near-total perforations, when there is significant malleus retraction (making the classic underlay technique impractical), significant anterior tympanosclerosis, or anterior middle ear cholesteatoma.

SURGICAL TECHNIQUE OF OVER-UNDER TYMPANOPLASTY

Postauricular over-under tympanoplasty technique is begun with appropriate preoperative decisions common in all tympanoplasty surgery previously described in the literature.

SURGICAL PREPARATION

Most patients undergo general anesthesia with endotracheal intubation for this type of surgery. After the general anesthesia with endotracheal intubation is secured, the patient is then turned 180 degrees, and the surgeon sits at the surgical side of the patient with the scrub nurse across the patient from the surgeon. An area of hair is removed from around the ear for approximately 2 cm above and behind the auricle. The natural oils of the skin are removed with alcohol solution or acetone, adherence material is placed on the edges of the prepped area, and plastic drapes are placed on the shaved area to hold the hair out of the field. The ear is injected with lidocaine HCl 1% with 1:100,000 epinephrine, in a subdermal plane at the postauricular incision site and a four-quadrant external ear location. A cotton ball is placed in the ear canal (to keep the scrub solution from the middle ear space), and the ear is then washed with an iodine solution, with the solution kept in contact with the ear for about 6 minutes. The ear is then dried from the solution by the scrub nurse, the ear is folded forward, and a plastic drape (attached to a waterproof barrier) is applied.

Drill cord, irrigation and suction tubes, and cautery lines are wrapped in a towel and placed and secured to the top of the drape over the patient. A second pouch is made to hold the drill hand piece, suction tips, and cautery devices. This prevents the lines from tangling or falling off of the surgical field.

The surgeon then cuts the drape directly over the surgical site. A wet sponge is used to clean the external ear from any dried iodine solution and then the ear is dried. The ear canal is then suctioned free from any ear canal debris or iodine solution. The vascular strip area is examined and then injected with the same lidocaine-epinephrine solution at the bony–cartilaginous junction site. The surgeon is to observe blanching of the skin of the vascular strip skin. The ear is then irrigated with sterile saline solution to further debride and clean the ear canal and examine the tympanic membrane pathology.

INCISIONS

The auricle is then held with the left hand (by right-handed surgeons), pulling the ear forward and laterally. The incision is made with a No. 15 blade approximately 5 mm behind the postauricular fold. Once the area of the loose areolar tissue overlying the temporalis fascia is seen, this bloodless plane is carried to the mastoid tip inferiorly. The nurse holds the auricle, and bleeding points are controlled with an electrocautery. A self-retaining retractor is then placed.

HARVESTING FASCIA

The scrub nurse holds the superior edge of the wound laterally with a small retractor to help visualize the fascia. We attempt to harvest true fascia for the reasons previously mentioned. Fascia of the temporalis muscle posteriorly is ideal, as anteriorly the fascia thickens and occasionally splits with adipose tissue interposed. An incision is made in the fascia superior and parallel to the linea temporalis, and then a delicate iris scissors is used to harvest simply the fascia without areolar tissue laterally or muscle tissue medially. For a subtotal perforation the graft is about 10 × 15 mm, and for larger perforations a 15 × 20 mm graft is harvested. The graft is then placed on a Teflon block, cleaned of any areolar or muscle tissue, and then straightened on the block. The block is then placed onto the scrub nurse's back table where a lamp is placed near the graft to dehydrate the graft. Once the graft is dehydrated, the lamp is turned off to prevent excessive drying of the graft.

EXPOSING THE EAR CANAL AND MIDDLE EAR

The area of the linea temporalis is palpated and then an incision is made along this line, between the temporalis muscle and the ear canal. A T incision is made through the tissue overlying the mastoid to the mastoid tip. A Lempert periosteal elevator is used to expose the mastoid bone, and the spine of Henle is visualized.

The self-retaining retractor is placed in this deeper plane. Now with the use of the operating microscope, a smaller periosteal elevator in the surgeon's right hand and a fine 20-gauge needle suction in the left hand are used to elevate the soft tissue of the bony external ear canal. Care is taken not to tear the delicate skin of the medial portion of the ear canal skin. The tympanomastoid suture line and the tympanosquamous suture line are visualized. The surgeon then utilizes a No. 6400 Beaver

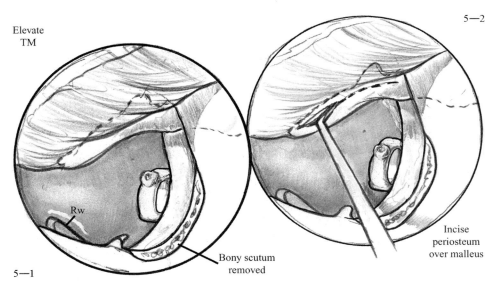

FIGURE 5–1 Elevate tympanomeatal flap.

FIGURE 5–2 Incise periosteum on malleus.

blade to make the superior and inferior incisions of the vascular strip, and a No. 7200 Beaver blade to make a parallel to annulus cut about 4 to 5 mm lateral to the annular rim. The vascular strip is then held anteriorly in the self-retaining retractor. This exposure now allows the surgeon to visualize the pathology of the tympanic membrane more clearly.

Now with the 20-gauge needle suction in the surgeon's left hand and a small round dissector in the right hand, the cuff of medial ear canal skin is elevated to the annulus. Generally a relaxing incision is made on the medial ear canal wall skin of the tympanic bone, 4 to 5 mm lateral and parallel to the inferior annulus. The middle ear is entered by elevating the cuff of skin until the fibrous annulus is visualized inferior to the chordae tympani nerve and then elevating the annulus inferiorly and anteriorly. At the point, the middle ear may be well visualized (Fig. 5–1).

CONTROL OF DISEASE

These initial steps are carried out in all cases. Once the middle ear is well exposed, the decision about which type of tympanoplasty technique to use (over-under, underlay, or overlay) is made. Indications for the over-under tympanoplasty technique are outlined in Table 5–1.

Middle ear cholesteatoma, granulation tissue, diseased mucosa, and so forth are dealt with at this time. If a mastoidectomy is required to remove tissue safely from the middle ear or if there is disease in the mastoid, then an intact canal mastoidectomy with facial recess approach is employed. Further

TABLE 5–1 INDICATIONS FOR OVER-UNDER TYMPANOPLASTY

Perforations or retractions that abut the malleus
Large or near total perforations
Severe malleus retraction
Significant anterior tympanosclerosis
Anterior middle ear cholesteatoma
To assist in ossicular reconstruction

treatment decisions are made, as described in subsequent chapters of this book.

PREPARATION OF TYMPANIC MEMBRANE REMNANT

When the disease process is under control, the tympanic membrane remnant is prepared for grafting. A rim of tissue is removed from the perforation edge to remove diseased tissue or mucosal thickening and encourage migration of healthy epithelium and the mucosal layer. For those patients where an over-under tympanoplasty is to be employed, the malleus is clearly visualized by elevating the tympanic membrane. The periosteum of the malleus is incised with a fine sharp needle (Fig. 5–2). This periosteal cuff is then used to elevate the tympanic membrane off the short process of the malleus, neck of the malleus, and then the long process of the malleus to the fibrous umbo area (Fig. 5–3). At this point either a microalligator-type scissors or the laser

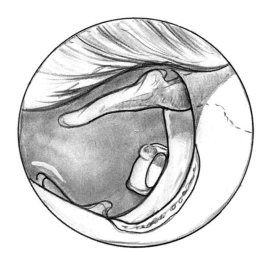

FIGURE 5–3 Drum lifted off malleus.

is used to totally remove the remnant from the malleus.

Internal Packing

When there is significant middle ear mucosal disease or severely retracted malleus, a fitted sheet of Silastic is placed on the entire promontory area (0.25 mm thickness). Generally the sheeting is fashioned to about 10 to 12 mm in diameter, with a small cutout where the stapes is located. Gelfoam (Pharmacia, Peapack, NJ) is used to pack the eustachian tube. An 8-mm Gelfoam disk is placed on the Silastic sheet medial to the malleus. The middle ear space up to the annulus is filled with one-half of 8-mm disk pledgets of Gelfoam.

Placement of Graft

The parchment-like fascia graft is now removed from the Teflon block and trimmed to the appropriate

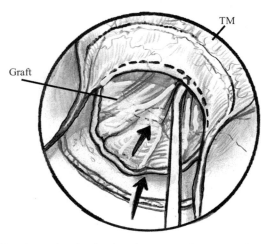

FIGURE 5–4 Graft placed on top of malleus (lateral).

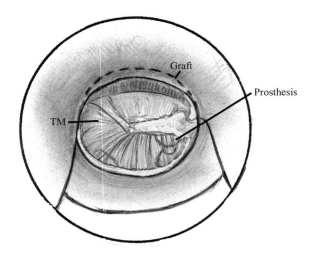

FIGURE 5–5 Same view with graft visible through a tympanic defect.

size. Generally for near-total perforations, the fascia is trimmed to a tongue shape with the anterior edge about 10 mm in diameter; the graft is then made about 15 mm in length. This allows the graft to be tucked under the anterior, inferior, and superior bony annulus, over the malleus and then onto the posterior bony canal wall (Fig. 5–4). The remnant of tympanic membrane is then placed onto the lateral surface of the graft and the remainder of the ear canal skin flaps are replaced into their normal position (Fig. 5–5). A disk of EpiFilm (Medtronic Xomed, Inc., Jacksonville, FL), a bioactive lamina composed of an ester of hyaluronic acid, is placed onto the lateral surface of the tympanic membrane. A Gelfoam 8-mm disk is placed lateral to the EpiFilm, and then antibiotic ointment is applied through a 14-gauge soft catheter on a 5-cc syringe placed onto the Gelfoam, filling the anterior sulcus of the ear canal.

The self-retaining retractors are removed, hemostasis is secured, and then the T incision is closed with an absorbable suture. The postauricular incision is sutured with an absorbable suture in a subcuticular manner. No skin sutures are necessary.

The ear canal is then visualized under the operating microscope and evacuated from blood, making sure not to suction onto the graft, but placing the vascular strip skin onto the fascia graft. This is held

Table 5–2 Over-Under Tympanoplasty High Points

Fascia

Periosteum incised and elevated

Fibrous tissue removed from umbo

Graft placement

into position with a nonabsorbable sponge moistened with an antibiotic steroid suspension. A mastoid dressing is placed. Table 5–2 summarizes the high points of the technique.

POSTOPERATIVE CARE

The mastoid dressing is removed the first postoperative day. The ear canal sponge is moistened with the antibiotic steroid suspension a couple of times each day. The pack is removed on the first postoperative appointment in about a week.

CONCLUSION

Over-under tympanoplasty is the preferred method of tympanoplasty for the indications previously noted. Flexibility of technique is ensured by the experience of the surgeon, and with any technique the surgeon should review long-term results for successful take rate, hearing improvement, and low complication rate. This technique should be included in the repertoire of the otologic surgeon.

REFERENCES

1. Litton W. Epithelial migration over the tympanic membrane and external canal. *Arch Otolaryngol* 1963;77:254–257.
2. Boxall JD, Proops DW, Michaels L. The specific locomotive activity of tympanic membrane and cholesteatoma epithelium in tissue culture. *J Otolaryngol* 1988;17:140–144.
3. Mondain M, Ryan A. Epidermal growth factor and basic fibroblast growth factor are induced in guinea-pig tympanic membrane following traumatic perforation. *Acta Otolaryngol (Stockh)* 1995;115:50–54.
4. Shimada T, Lim DJ. The fiber arrangement of the human tympanic membrane: a scanning electron microscopic observation. *Ann Otol Rhinol Laryngol* 1971;80:210–217.
5. Decraemer WF, Dirckx JJ, Funnel WR. Shape and derived geometrical parameters of the adult, human tympanic membrane measured with a phase-shift moiré interferometer. *Hear Res* 1991;51:107–121.
6. Hussl B, Timpl R, Lim D, Ginsel M, Wick GG. Immunohistochemical analysis of connective tissue components in tympanosclerosis. In: Lim DJ, Bluestone CD, Klein JO, Nelson JD, eds. *Recent Advances in Otitis Media: Proceedings of the Fourth International Symposium.* New York: BC Decker; 1988:402–406.
7. Wilson JG. Nerves and nerve endings in the membrana tympani of man. *Am J Anat* 1911;11:101–115.
8. Applebaum EL, Deutsch EC. Fluorescein angiography of the tympanic membrane. *Laryngoscope* 1985;95:1054–1058.
9. Wilson JG. Nerves and nerve endings in the membrana tympani of man. *Am J Anat* 1911;11:101–115.
10. Committee on Conservation of Hearing of the American Academy of Ophthalmology and Otolaryngology. Standard classification for surgery of chronic ear disease. *Arch Otolaryngol* 1964;81:204–205.
11. Hippocrates. *De Carnibus* [in German and Greek]. Teubner BB, trans. Leipzig, Berlin; 1935.
12. Banzer M. *Disputatio de Audiotone Laesa.* Wittenbergae: Johannis Rohrerei; 1651.
13. Toynbee J. *On the Use of an Artificial Membrane Tympani in Cases of Deafness Dependent Upon Perforations or Destruction of the Natural Organ.* London: J Churchill & Sons; 1853.
14. Blake CJ. *Transactions of the First Congress of the International Otological Society.* New York: D Appleton; 1887.
15. Berthold E. Ueber myringoplastik. *Wier Med Bull* 1878;1:627.
16. Wullstein H. The restoration of the function of the middle ear in chronic otitis media. *Ann Otol Rhinol Laryngol* 1971;80:210–217.
17. Zollner F. The principles of plastic surgery of the sound conducting apparatus. *J Laryngol Otol* 1955;69:637–652.
18. Plester D. Myringoplasty methods. *Arch Otolaryngol* 1963;78:310–316.
19. Sooy FA. A method of repairing a large marginal tympanic perforation. *Ann Otol Rhinol Laryngol* 1956;65:911–914.
20. House WF, Sheehy JL. Myringoplasty: use of ear canal skin compared with other techniques. *Arch Otolaryngol* 1961;73:407.
21. Plester D. Myringoplasty methods. *Arch Otolaryngol* 1963;78:310–316.
22. Shea JJ. Fenestration of the oval window. *Ann Otol Rhinol Laryngol* 1958;67:932–951.
23. Austin DF, Shea JJ Jr. A new system of tympanoplasty using vein graft. *Laryngoscope* 1961;71:596–611.
24. Tabb HG. Closure of perforations of the tympanic membrane by vein grafts: a preliminary report of 20 cases. *Laryngoscope* 1960;70:271–286.
25. Storrs LA. Myringoplasty with the use of fascia grafts. *Arch Otolaryngol* 1961;74:65–69.
26. Chalat NI. Tympanic membrane transplant. *Harper Hosp Bull* 1964;22:27–34.
27. Glasscock ME III, House WF. Homograft reconstruction of the middle ear: a preliminary report. *Laryngoscope* 1968;78:1219–1225.
28. Perkins R. Human homograft otologic tissue transplantation: buffered formaldehyde preparation. *Trans Am Acad Ophthalmol Otolaryngol* 1970;74:278–282.
29. Smith MF. Viable homograft reconstruction of the middle ear transformer mechanism and posterior osseous external canal. *Trans Pac Coast Otoophthalmol Soc Annu Meet* 1972;53:63–69.
30. Wehrs RE. Homograft tympanic membrane in tympanoplasty. *Arch Otolaryngol* 1971;93:132–139.
31. Goodman WS. Tympanoplasty: areolar tissue graft. *Laryngoscope* 1971;81:1819–1825.
32. Goodhill V. Tragal perichondrium and cartilage in tympanoplasty. *Arch Otolaryngol* 1967;85:480–491.

33. Patterson ME, Lockwood RW, Sheehy JL. Temporalis fascia in tympanic membrane grafting: tissue culture and animal studies. *Arch Otolaryngol* 1967;85:73–77.

34. Kartush JM, Michaledes EM, Becvarovski Z, LaRouere MJ. Over-under tympanoplasty. *Laryngoscope* 2002;112:802–807.

35. Austin DF. Transcanal tympanoplasty. *Otolaryngol Clin North Am* 1972;5:127–143.

36. Glasscock ME. Tympanic membrane grafting with fascia: overlay versus underlay technique. *Laryngoscope* 1973;5:754–770.

37. Wehrs RE. Grafting techniques. *Otolaryngol Clin North Am* 1999;32:443–455.

38. Hough JV. Tympanoplasty with the interior fascial graft technique and ossicular reconstruction. *Laryngoscope* 1970;80:1385–1413.

39. Patterson ME, Lockwood RW, Sheehy JL. Temporalis fascia in tympanic membrane grafting. *Arch Otolaryngol* 1967;74:65–69.

40. Sheehy JL, Glasscock ME. Tympanic membrane grafting with temporalis fascia. *Arch Otolaryngol* 1967;86:57–68.

41. Bojrab DI, Causse JB, Battista RA, Vincent R, Gratacap B, Vandeventer G. Ossiculoplasty with composite prostheses: overview and analysis. *Otolaryngol Clin North Am* 1994;27:759–776.

42. McFeely WJ Jr, Bojrab DI, Kartush JM. Tympanic membrane perforation repair using AlloDerm. *Otolaryngol Head Neck Surg* 2000;123:17–21.

43. Jackson CG, Glasscock ME III, Nissen AJ, Schwaber MK, Bojrab DI. Open mastoid procedures: contemporary indications and surgical technique. *Laryngoscope* 1985;95:1037–1043.

Chapter 6

CARTILAGE TYMPANOPLASTY

John Dornhoffer and Edward Gardner

Generally speaking, there are two distinct techniques utilized for cartilage reconstruction of the tympanic membrane (TM): the perichondrium/cartilage island flap, which uses tragal cartilage, and the palisade technique, which uses cartilage from the tragus or cymba, depending on the surgical approach. Either technique can be used to reconstruct the TM; however, the choice of technique is typically dictated by the specific middle ear pathology or, in cases where the TM reconstruction is in conjunction with ossiculoplasty, the status of the ossicular chain. The palisade technique is preferred in cases of cholesteatoma and when ossicular reconstruction is needed in the malleus-present situation. The perichondrium/cartilage island flap is preferred for management of the atelectatic ear and the high-risk perforation. This chapter describes the two techniques in detail, followed by descriptions of the modifications that should be taken in response to specific surgical indications.

Tympanoplasty, or repair of the TM, was first introduced by Zoellner[1] and Wullstein[2] in 1952. Since that time, numerous graft materials and methods of placement have been described to reconstruct the TM. Skin, fascia, vein, and dura mater have all been described as grafting materials for the TM.[3-9] Temporalis fascia and perichondrium remain the most commonly employed materials for closure of TM perforations, and successful reconstruction is anticipated in approximately 90% of primary tympanoplasties.[10]

In certain situations, such as the atelectatic ear, cholesteatoma, and revision tympanoplasty, however, the results have not been as gratifying. In these situations, fascia and perichondrium have been shown to undergo atrophy and subsequent failure in the postoperative period, regardless of placement technique.[11] The recurrent perforation and discharging ear are likewise associated with less than optimal results.[12-14] These observations have led to the use of less compliant, more rigid grafting materials for TM reconstruction, such as the cartilage graft. Although one might anticipate a significant conductive hearing loss with cartilage, due to its rigidity, it is this quality that tends to resist resorption and retraction, even in the milieu of continuous eustachian tube dysfunction. It has been shown in both experimental and clinical studies that cartilage is well-tolerated by the middle ear, and long-term survival is the norm.[15-18] It appears that cartilage grafts are nourished largely by diffusion and become well-incorporated in the TM.[19] Human and animal studies[20,21] have shown that although some softening occurs with time, the matrix of the cartilage remains intact, but with empty lacunae, demonstrating degeneration of the chondrocytes.

The use of cartilage in middle ear surgery is not a new concept, but the last decade has shown a renewed interest in this material as an alternative to more traditional grafting materials for TM reconstruction. Cartilage has been recommended on a limited basis to manage retraction pockets by advocates such as Sheehy,[22] Glasscock and Hart,[23] Levinson,[19] Eviatar,[24] and Adkins,[25] all of whom have reported excellent anatomic results. Cartilage also has been described for use in cases of recurrent perforation and revision tympanoplasty with encouraging results.[14,26,27]

Given the good anatomic results, more attention also has been given to the acoustic properties of cartilage compared with more traditional grafting materials. In a retrospective comparison between perichondrium and cartilage in type I tympanoplasties, we reported no significant difference in hearing between groups.[28] Graft take was 100% in the cartilage group and 85% in the perichondrium group. These results were supported by other researchers who have shown excellent closure of the air–bone gap with cartilage tympanoplasty techniques.[14,26,27,29]

TECHNIQUES FOR RECONSTRUCTION

HARVEST OF THE CARTILAGE GRAFT

Cartilage for TM reconstruction is typically harvested from two areas, the tragus and the cymba, depending on the type of reconstruction to be performed. The perichondrium/cartilage island flap is nearly always constructed with cartilage harvested from the tragus. This cartilage is ideal because it is thin, flat, and in sufficient quantities to permit reconstruction of the entire TM. The cartilage is used as a full-thickness graft and is typically slightly less than 1 mm thick in most cases. Although Zahnert et al[30] suggested a slight acoustical benefit could be obtained by thinning the cartilage to 0.5 mm, this advantage is offset by the unacceptable curling of the graft that occurs when the cartilage is thinned and perichondrium is left attached to one side.

When the palisade technique is used for reconstruction of the TM, cartilage can be harvested from either the tragus or the cymba. Cartilage from the cymba area of the conchal bowl is used if the surgical approach involves a postauricular incision. Tragal cartilage is used if the approach is transcanal or endaural. The cartilage of the cymba is similar to the tragus in that it has an acceptable thickness of about 1 mm compared to other areas of the concha, which are thicker and irregular. It is different, however, in that it is curved, making it difficult to create a perichondrium/cartilage island flap suitable for reconstruction of the entire TM.

PERICHONDRIUM/CARTILAGE ISLAND FLAP

The general technique of reconstruction using the perichondrium/cartilage island flap begins with harvest of the cartilage from the tragal area.[28] An initial cut through skin and cartilage is made on the medial side of the tragus, leaving a 2-mm strip of cartilage in the dome of the tragus for cosmesis (Fig. 6–1). The cartilage, with attached perichondrium, is dissected medially from the overlying skin and soft tissue by spreading a pair of sharp scissors in a plane that is easily developed superficial to the perichondrium on both sides. At this point, it is necessary to make an inferior cut as low as possible to maximize the length of harvested cartilage. The cartilage is then grasped and retracted inferiorly, which delivers the superior portion from the incisura area. The superior portion is then dissected out while retracting, which produces a piece of cartilage typically measuring 15 × 10 mm in children and somewhat larger in adults.

The perichondrium from the side of the cartilage furthest from the ear canal is dissected off, leaving the thinner perichondrium on the reverse side. A perichondrium/cartilage island flap is constructed as described previously.[28] Using a round knife, cartilage is removed to produce an eccentrically located disk of cartilage about 7 to 9 mm in diameter for total TM reconstruction. A flap of perichondrium is produced posteriorly that will eventually drape over the posterior canal wall. A complete strip of cartilage 2 mm in width is then removed vertically from the center of the cartilage to accommodate the

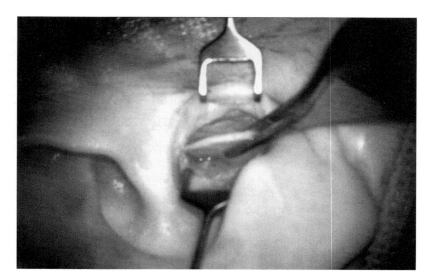

FIGURE 6–1 Harvest of cartilage, leaving small rim of cartilage in dome for cosmesis (right ear).

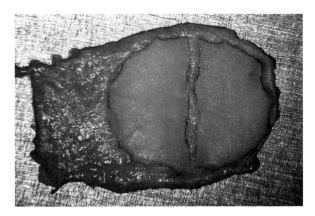

FIGURE 6–2 Prepared perichondrium/cartilage island graft, showing strip of cartilage removed to facilitate malleus.

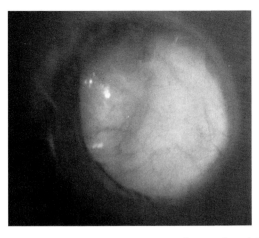

FIGURE 6–4 Postoperative ear with perichondrium/cartilage island graft (left ear).

entire malleus handle (Fig. 6–2). The creation of two cartilage islands in this manner is essential to enable the reconstructed TM to bend and conform to the normal conical shape of the TM. When the ossicular chain is intact, an additional triangular piece of cartilage is removed from the posterior-superior quadrant to accommodate the incus. This excision prevents the lateral displacement of the posterior portion of the cartilage graft that sometimes occurs because of insufficient space between the malleus and incus.

The entire graft is placed in an underlay fashion, with the malleus fitting in the groove and actually pressing down into and conforming to the perichondrium, as shown in Figure 6–3. The cartilage is placed toward the promontory, with the perichondrium immediately adjacent to the TM remnant, both of which are medial to the malleus. Failure to remove enough cartilage from the center strip will cause the graft to fold up at the center instead of lying flat in the desired position. Likewise, if the strip is insufficient, the cartilage may be displaced

medially instead of assuming a more lateral position in the same plane as the malleus.

Gelfoam (Upjohn Laboratories, Kalamazoo, MI) is packed in the middle ear space underneath the anterior annulus to support the graft in this area, and the posterior flap of perichondrium is draped over the posterior canal wall. Middle ear packing is avoided on the promontory and in the vicinity of the ossicular chain. One piece of Gelfoam is placed lateral to the reconstructed TM, and antibiotic ointment is placed in the ear canal (Fig. 6–4).

THE PALISADE TECHNIQUE

In the palisade technique, the cartilage is cut into several slices that are subsequently pieced together, like the pieces of a jigsaw puzzle, to reconstruct the TM (Fig. 6–5). Because of the nature of the reconstruction, it is not necessary to have one large, flat piece of cartilage, and the more curved cymba cartilage, which is harvested from the postauricular incision, is suitable (Fig. 6–6). A large area of conchal eminence can be exposed by elevating the subcutaneous tissue and postauricular muscle from the conchal perichondrium. The cymba cartilage is the prominent bulge at the superior aspect of the concha (Fig. 6–7). A circumferential cut the size of the anticipated graft is made through the perichondrium and cartilage, but not through the anterior skin. The perichondrium is removed from the postauricular side, and the cartilage, with the perichondrium on the anterior aspect, is dissected from the skin. This technique is also used for harvesting cartilage for canal wall reconstruction when the retrograde mastoidectomy technique is used for cholesteatoma surgery.

The technique described here differs somewhat from the palisade tympanoplasty of Heermann et

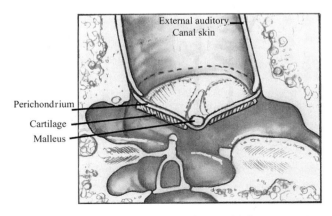

FIGURE 6–3 Lateral line drawing demonstrating proper placement of graft.

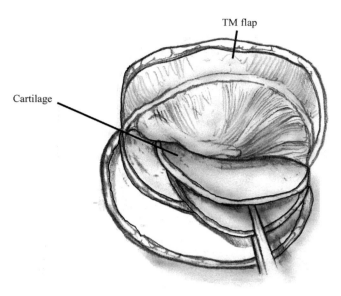

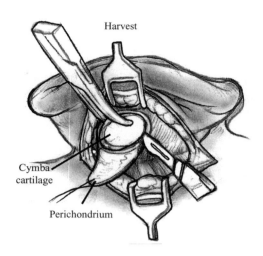

FIGURE 6–7 Harvesting of cymba cartilage with post-auricular incision (right ear).

FIGURE 6–5 Schematic of palisade technique (right ear).

al.[31] Instead of placing rectangular strips of cartilage side to side, an attempt is made to cut one major piece of cartilage in a semi-lunar fashion, which is placed directly against the malleus on top of the prosthesis (Fig. 6–8A,B). This acts to reconstruct a major portion of the posterior half of the TM and serves as a foundation for the rest of the cartilage pieces. A second semi-lunar piece is placed between this first piece and the canal wall to reconstruct the scutum precisely (Fig. 6–8C). Any spaces that result between this cartilage and the canal wall or scutum are filled in with small slivers of cartilage to prevent prosthesis extrusion and recurrent retraction (Fig. 6–8D). The reconstruction is then covered with the

previously harvested perichondrium draped over the posterior canal wall (Fig. 6–9).

Although this technique can be used for TM reconstruction without ossicular reconstruction, it is favored when ossiculoplasty is performed in a malleus-present situation and is especially suitable for cholesteatoma surgery. Because the prosthesis is placed prior to the cartilage reconstruction, this technique allows direct visualization and contact of the notched prosthesis to the manubrium handle, which has been shown to provide superior hearing results.[32] The prosthesis acts as a scaffolding on which the cartilage is placed, which serves to reconstruct the TM as well as prevent prosthesis extrusion. It likewise allows a precise and watertight fit between the reconstructed TM and the canal wall in the posterior area, where recurrent cholesteatoma most frequently occurs. Typically, in these situations, the anterior half of the TM is not altered or is grafted with conventional materials to allow cholesteatoma surveillance and possible intubation in the postoperative period if necessary.

POSTOPERATIVE CARE

Typically, the packing material of Gelfoam and antibiotic ointment is completely suctioned from the external canal 1 to 2 weeks after the surgical procedure. Antibiotic steroid-containing drops are used for an additional 2 weeks to clear the ear of residual ointment and Gelfoam, the latter of which can lead to granulation and fibrous tissue formation if inadequately removed from the TM. The adult patient is instructed to begin the Valsalva maneuver, and children are instructed to use the Otovent

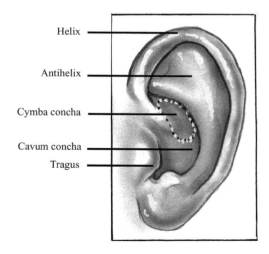

FIGURE 6–6 Schematic illustrating location of cymba cartilage (left ear).

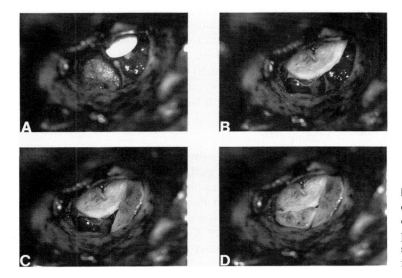

FIGURE 6–8   Series demonstrating sequence of palisade reconstruction (left ear). (A) Total ossicular replacement prosthesis (TORP) in place. (B) Initial cartilage placement. (C) Reconstruction of the scutum. (D) Reconstruction of remainder of posterior tympanic membrane.

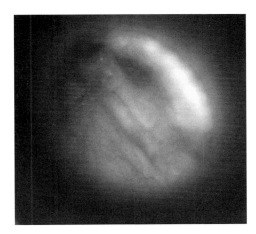

FIGURE 6–9   Postoperative appearance of tympanic membrane after palisade reconstruction (right ear).

(Invotec International, Jacksonville, FL), three times a day beginning 2 to 3 weeks after the surgery. A postoperative audiogram is obtained 6 to 8 weeks later, and the TM is examined. If the hearing result is good and the TM is clear, the ear is examined at 6 months and again at 1 year from the date of surgery. If effusion is present, nasal steroids are added, the Valsalva (or Otovent) is encouraged, and the ear is examined at 3 months. If the effusion is still present at that time, the ear is intubated. If a total cartilage reconstruction had been performed, tube insertion using traditional techniques can be difficult. In this situation, a CO_2 laser myringotomy is preferred, followed by insertion of a soft tube, such as the Goode T-tube (Medtronic Xomed Surgical Products Inc., Jacksonville, FL).

SPECIFIC INDICATIONS AND SUBSEQUENT MODIFICATIONS TO THE SURGICAL TECHNIQUE

THE HIGH-RISK PERFORATION

The high-risk perforation, defined as a revision surgery, a perforation anterior to the annulus, a perforation draining at the time of surgery, a perforation larger than 50%, or a bilateral perforation, has been shown to be associated with increased failure rates using traditional techniques. In these cases, cartilage has proven extremely valuable for reconstruction of the TM.

Revision tympanoplasty has been shown by numerous authors to be a risk factor for subsequent failure in graft take and hearing results,[33–35] and drainage at the time of surgery is considered by many to represent a negative prognostic factor.[33,34,36] Although every attempt is made to dry an ear prior to surgical intervention, it is not considered a prerequisite for tympanoplasty. Cartilage is used in this situation and has proven to yield successful results. Cartilage is likewise used for reconstruction when the size of the perforation is larger than 50%, because larger perforations in general fair less well.[34,37,38]

Age as a prognostic factor in cartilage tympanoplasty of high-risk perforations is somewhat controversial. In previous studies, a young patient age (<18 years) was not found, in and of itself, to have a negative influence on success.[28,39] There is, however, an association between young age and other significant factors, such as bilateral ear disease and drainage at the time of surgery, which are associated with immature tubal function. The general approach to pediatric patients is to avoid repairing the TM during the otitis-prone years (<3 years). If the contralateral ear is normal, routine tympanoplasty is performed at age 4.[40] If the contralateral ear is abnormal at this time, adenoidectomy is considered, and tympanoplasty is generally deferred until age 7.[41-43] If contralateral disease is still present at this time, cartilage tympanoplasty is performed on the worse ear because a perforation in the contralateral ear has been shown to be associated with a high risk for failure.[44]

Typically, the perichondrium/cartilage island flap as described above is utilized for the high-risk perforation, with the exception that the size of the cartilage is tailored to the size of the perforation. For example, if the perforation is a 50% anterior perforation, the flap is constructed with the posterior island of cartilage removed to avoid the need to modify the normal TM posteriorly, which would otherwise be necessary to facilitate this plate of cartilage. The perichondrium is typically left the same size as described above so that it still extends under the posterior TM and drapes over the canal wall under the tympanomeatal flap for enhanced stability. Gelfoam is placed anteriorly to hold the graft against the annulus, but Gelfoam is avoided posteriorly around the ossicular chain. In revision surgery, fibrosis and disrupted mucosa are frequently seen, and Gelfoam in this milieu should be avoided to alleviate further scarring and optimize hearing results.

Our results with cartilage reconstruction of the TM with a high-risk perforation have been good. In our experience with over 1000 cartilage tympanoplasties, 34% were performed for a high-risk perforation, with an average 2.9-year follow-up. Of these, 60% were performed in children (<18 years of age) and 47% were revision cases. Successful closure of the TM was seen in 96% of this group (4% incidence of recurrent perforation). The average preoperative pure tone average air–bone gap (PTA-ABG) at 500, 1000, 2000, and 3000 Hz was 21.7 ± 13.5 dB whereas the postoperative value was 11.9 ± 9.3 dB, which represented a statistically significant improvement in hearing ($p < 0.05$). Complications were few and included a 2% incidence of postoperative effusion requiring postoperative intubation of the TM and a 2% incidence of conductive hearing loss requiring revision surgery for prosthesis extrusion or dislocation.

Ears Requiring Ossiculoplasty

Reconstruction or reinforcement of the TM with cartilage is typically performed in conjunction with ossiculoplasty to prevent prosthesis extrusion, recurrent retractions, or cholesteatoma. Although the usual surgical indication is cholesteatoma in these cases, the method of cartilage reconstruction is dependent not so much on the middle ear pathology but on the presence or absence of the malleus manubrium, and will be discussed as such.

Malleus Present

When the malleus handle is present, the modification of the palisade technique, as described above, is utilized. An acoustic benefit has been shown with the incorporation of the malleus in ossicular reconstruction, possibly due to the cantenary action of the malleus in the TM.[32] Likewise, the presence of the malleus with an intact anterior malleolar ligament offers improved prosthesis stability by allowing precise length adjustments and ultimate fit, leading to optimal hearing results.[45] This has led us to abandon the use of the tragal island flap when the malleus is needed for ossicular reconstruction due to the fact that prior placement of the flap, using the underlay technique as described, obscures the malleus and makes the subsequent ossicular reconstruction less precise. Likewise, it is frequently difficult to carve the cartilage with enough precision so that the island flap fits exactly against the canal wall, which is necessary in cases involving cholesteatoma. We have seen cholesteatomas recur when even a small gap is left between the posterior cartilage and the canal wall. Thus, the palisade technique is preferred in this situation.

When the malleus handle and suspensory ligaments are present, a partial ossicular replacement prosthesis (PORP) cut to 2 mm and a total ossicular replacement prosthesis (TORP) cut to 4.0 to 4.5 mm can be consistently used for precise reconstruction when the notch of the prosthesis is placed just inferior to the insertion of the tensor tympani (Fig. 6–10). After precise ossicular reconstruction is performed, the posterior half of the TM is reconstructed with cartilage pieces, as described above for the palisade technique. The TM is pieced together like a jigsaw puzzle: the half-moon–shaped piece is placed on top of the prosthesis first, abutting the malleus handle, followed by the scutum piece. Because the usual indication for this technique is cholesteatoma, any spaces left between these two plates and the canal wall are reconstructed with slivers of cartilage cut to fit precisely in these areas. The reconstruction is then covered with perichondrium if available; however, this is not necessary in most cases if good fit is achieved. No space is left between the canal wall and reconstructed TM to prevent cholesteatoma or retraction pocket recurrence. In addition, the

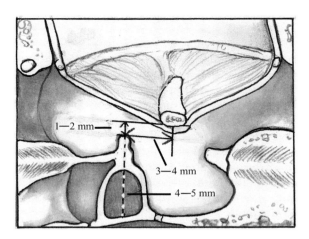

FIGURE 6–10 Schematic illustrating the relationship between the stapes and malleus for ossicular reconstruction.

anterior half of the TM is typically not reconstructed with cartilage so as to allow postoperative surveillance and tube insertion, if necessary.

If reconstruction of the anterior TM is necessary due to pathology, perichondrium is used. The technique is the same, but after precise fitting of the prosthesis to the malleus handle, the prosthesis is removed and the perichondrium is placed as an underlay graft. The prosthesis is then reinserted, with palpation of the malleus handle through the graft to facilitate precise fit. The posterior palisade technique is then performed.

Malleus Absent

The malleus-absent situation represents one of the most useful indications for cartilage tympanoplasty but one of the more challenging situations for ossicular reconstruction because there is no malleus enabling an exact fit between two essentially stable, bony platforms and allowing the surgeon to build the ossicular reconstruction to the TM. The cartilage tympanoplasty technique described below has proven useful to alleviate this problem.

The perichondrium/cartilage island flap from tragal cartilage is utilized. Even though the malleus is absent, a similar circular cartilage flap is constructed, again removing the 1- to 2-mm strip of cartilage from the center section to facilitate accurate placement of the ossicular replacement prosthesis. The cartilage is inserted in an underlay technique medial to the anterior TM remnant, with the perichondrium again toward the ear canal. Several pieces of Gelfoam are inserted to support the graft securely to the anterior annulus and the bony ledge just lateral to the supratubal recess. With the anterior portion of the cartilage graft held securely in place,

the posterior half is folded out to expose the trailing edge of the anterior piece of cartilage, which acts, in effect, as a neo-malleus (Fig. 6–11). The distance between the stapes footplate or superstructure and this trailing edge of the anterior cartilage is measured, and the prosthesis is cut to the appropriate length.

For ossicular reconstruction, a prosthesis specifically designed for use with cartilage tympanoplasty techniques is used. For example, the Dornhoffer HAPEX TORP or PORP has a head that notches the malleus, or the edge of the cartilage if the malleus is absent, and broadens posteriorly to shift the center of gravity over the shaft, acting as a scaffold for the cartilage reconstruction.[45] The notched portion of the prosthesis is hooked under the trailing edge of the anterior piece of cartilage, much in the same way that the malleus would be used in conventional ossiculoplasty, with the shaft placed on the stapes (Fig. 6–12).[46] The posterior half of the cartilage is folded back and is supported by the broader posterior head of the prosthesis. This technique allows accurate length measurement and placement of the prosthesis, with direct visualization to the stapes superstructure or footplate. Once the freestanding prosthesis is accurately positioned, supporting Gelfoam is placed to provide extra security during the postsurgical healing phase.

Our results for cartilage reconstruction of the TM after ossiculoplasty have been encouraging. We have performed this type of reconstruction with the stapes superstructure present (PORP) in 499 cases, of which 43% were revisions. The average preoperative PTA-ABG was 26.7 ± 12.5 dB, and the postoperative PTA-ABG was 14.5 ± 8.7 dB. This

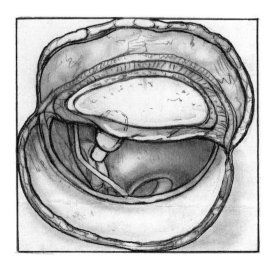

FIGURE 6–11 Line drawing illustrating reconstruction technique when malleus is absent (right ear).

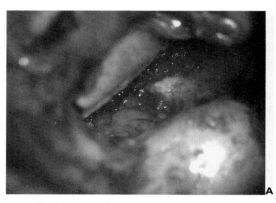

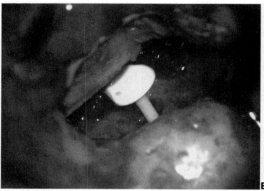

FIGURE 6–12 (A) Placement of cartilage graft (left ear), with posterior piece of cartilage folded laterally, revealing posterior edge of anterior cartilage (neo-malleus). (B) Placement of total ossicular replacement prosthesis (TORP), notching the neo-malleus (left ear).

difference was statistically significant ($p < 0.05$). Ossicular reconstruction was performed with no stapes superstructure (TORP) in 282 cases, of which 72% were revision cases. The average preoperative PTA-ABG was 34.4 ± 11.9 dB, and the postoperative PTA-ABG was 16.6 ± 10.5 dB, which was statistically significant ($p < 0.05$). The average follow-up was 2.7 years, and the overall prosthesis extrusion rate was 1%. We have found no statistical difference in results due to age (average patient age of 30 years; range, 4 to 88 years). Overall, there was a 3% incidence of recurrent conductive hearing loss due to displaced prostheses, requiring revision surgery. Most of the displaced prostheses occurred in the malleus-absent group, however, which had an 8% incidence of prosthesis displacement. At revision surgery, the most common cause of prosthesis displacement was thought to be lateralization of the cartilage graft during healing, causing the prosthesis to be slightly too short. Typically, minimal graft elevation and a prosthesis cut 1 mm longer at the time of revision surgery rectified this problem and gave good results.

THE ATELECTATIC EAR

The atelectatic ear represents the first and most well-described situation in which cartilage techniques have been utilized. Perichondrium and fascia have been shown to undergo atrophy after use in this situation[11]; however, numerous reports have established the efficacy of cartilage in TM reconstruction of the atelectatic ear.[19,22,23] Much of the confusion associated with this disorder stems from a poor understanding of the underlying pathophysiologic conditions that ultimately lead to changes in the TM, resulting in atrophy, diffuse or local retractions, and cholesteatoma formation.[47,48] The controversy over whether or not the patient should proceed with surgery is augmented by the fact that, early in the course of the disease, and even in the presence of incus necrosis, hearing loss is frequently minimal, and patients for the most part are asymptomatic. Because of this controversy, a grading system was developed, which was a modification of that described by Sadé,[49] to develop a treatment algorithm for this condition.[39] Once a decision is made to proceed with surgery (grade III with adhesions and grade IV), the perichondrium/cartilage island flap is generally used to reconstruct the TM.

There are two potential pitfalls specific for the atelectatic ear with an intact chain. The first is the medially rotated malleus, which can make insertion of the flap quite difficult. This can be overcome in one of two ways. The first is to remove 1 mm of the manubrium at the umbo with the malleus head amputator (malleus "nippers"). This does not affect hearing and allows medial placement of the graft. Attempting to lateralize the malleus with an intact chain should be discouraged due to the possibility of acoustic trauma. The second is to remove a slightly wider strip of cartilage (2 mm) to facilitate the malleus handle. This allows the more medial malleus to indent further into the perichondrium, allowing the cartilage plates to move more laterally in the reconstruction and avoiding contact with the promontory. This also allows the anterior island of cartilage more flexibility in positioning, which is necessary to make good contact with the anterior annulus.

The other pitfall specific to the atelectatic ear concerns management of the atrophic TM. After elevating the atrophic TM off the promontory, it is tempting to insert the cartilage medial to the intact TM. It is important, however, to remove at least a portion of the atrophic TM anterior and posterior to the malleus to ensure that the cartilage flap is incorporated into the reconstructed TM. We have experienced situations where the cartilage can be seen through the reconstructed TM and has fallen away from the TM when this removal of excess skin has not been performed, especially anteriorly.

The results with regard to graft take and hearing after reconstruction of the atelectatic ear with cartilage have been reported previously and have been excellent.[39] In our series of over 1000 cartilage tympanoplasties, an atelectatic eardrum was the surgical indication in 15% of cases, with 21% being revision cases. Two-thirds were performed in children (<18 years of age), with an average time since surgery of 3 years. The average preoperative PTA-ABG was 20.2 ± 10.9 dB, and the average postoperative value was 14.2 ± 10.2 dB. This difference was significant ($p < 0.05$). Complications included a 1% incidence of perforation, a 2% incidence of local retractions around the cartilage graft, conductive hearing loss requiring revision in 2% of cases due to a displaced or extruded prosthesis, and the need for postoperative tube insertion in 7% of cases. Because the entire TM is typically reconstructed with cartilage for this indication, tube insertion in the postoperative period can be difficult. It is frequently necessary to take the patient to the operating room for tube insertion after a small ellipse of cartilage is removed anteriorly. Recently, we have used the CO_2 laser in the clinic to create a myringotomy with some success.

MANAGING CHOLESTEATOMA

Cholesteatoma represents one of the most controversial but important pathologic conditions where cartilage is used. The primary purpose of cholesteatoma surgery is to eradicate disease and provide a safe, hearing ear. The magnitude of the controversy with regard to optimal surgical management is beyond the scope of this discussion, but cartilage should arguably be involved in each technique.

A technique involving partial canal wall removal for cholesteatoma extirpation, followed by cartilage reconstruction, is recommended.[50] For TM reconstruction, the cartilage palisade technique is preferred as this allows precise placement of the prosthesis against the malleus, with the prosthesis acting as a scaffold to support the cartilage posteriorly. This also allows excellent approximation between the canal wall and TM reconstruction, creating a watertight fit, which has greatly reduced recurrent disease. With this technique, it is also preferable to leave the anterior portion of the TM without cartilage to allow observation and possible tube placement should this be necessary in the postoperative period. For reasons that are not totally understood, the posterior portion of the TM tends to be much more prone to retraction than the anterior portion, so leaving this area without cartilage has not

proven to be a problem with recurrent cholesteatoma.[51,52]

One serious disadvantage of cartilage in this scenario is that it creates an opaque TM posteriorly, which could potentially hide residual disease. This is a problem that should be recognized, and surgical discretion should be used. If major disruption of the cholesteatoma sac occurs at extirpation, one must consider the advisability of performing a second-look surgery at a later date. This also applies to cholesteatoma surgery in general, however, not just to cases where cartilage is used in the reconstruction. One must also recognize the fact that most residual disease occurs in the epitympanum, an area that is hidden by the bony canal wall and scutum when canal-wall-up surgery of any type is performed.[53] Although posterior cartilage TM reconstruction can delay the diagnosis of residual cholesteatoma, the disease will become manifest either anteriorly or as a recurrence of a conductive hearing loss and there should be no major complications as a result of this delay in diagnosis.[54,55]

When reporting results with cholesteatoma surgery, it is essential to discuss both recurrence and residual rates. Residual disease is that which is left behind after initial surgery and is determined by the method of cholesteatoma exposure and removal. Seventy-five percent of all residual disease is thought to manifest by 2 years after surgery.[56] Recurrent cholesteatoma, on the other hand, is caused by recurrent retractions from the reconstructed TM and is dictated by the method of reconstruction and presence of continued eustachian tube dysfunction, a problem that is difficult to assess preoperatively. One must also keep in mind that "second-look" surgeries 1 year after primary surgery affect only the rate of residual disease, and these two-stage surgeries are still associated with a 10 to 12% recurrence rate due to retractions in the reconstructed eardrums with traditional reconstruction techniques.[57,58] Our study of 75 ears with 4-year average follow-up showed a recurrence rate of less than 10%, which is acceptable and considerably better than the previous results obtained at our institution using traditional techniques without cartilage reconstruction of the TM.[50,59]

MANAGING PERVASIVE EUSTACHIAN TUBE DYSFUNCTION

We have developed distinct criteria for primary intubation of cartilage tympanoplasties that comprise craniofacial abnormalities, including Down syndrome; previous head and neck cancer involving

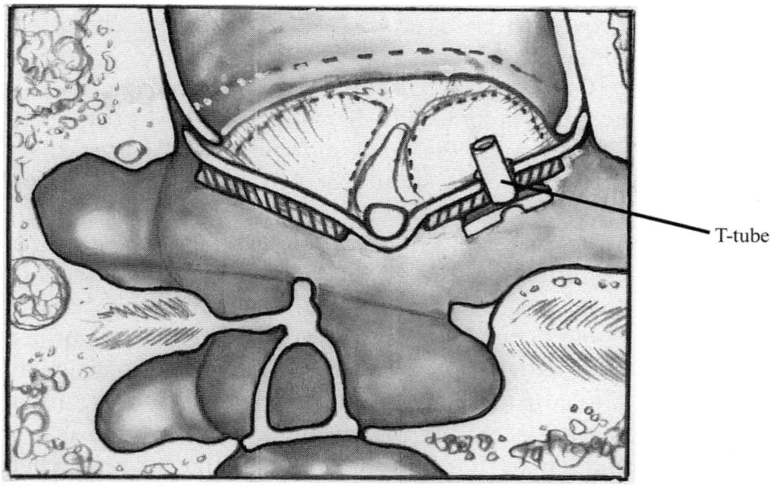

FIGURE 6–13 Schematic showing technique of cartilage tympanoplasty with intraoperative placement of T-tube.

the nasopharynx; and patients with a history of multiple ear surgeries with demonstrated eustachian tube dysfunction.

The perichondrium/cartilage island graft is harvested and prepared as previously described. Using a round knife, a window that is large enough to allow placement of a Xomed Modified Goode T-tube is cut into the anterior cartilage island. A straight pick is then placed into the cartilage window to dilate the perichondrium to allow tube placement. Using scissors, the tube is remodeled by trimming the flanges to approximately 3 to 4 mm. Prior to insetting the graft, the tube is placed into the cartilage window and brought out through the perichondrial surface. If the malleus is present, the end of the tube is first angled under the manubrium with small alligator forceps. After hooking the tube under the malleus, the graft is slid forward into place. If the malleus is absent, the graft/tube complex is slid directly into its final position (Fig. 6–13).

Should the tube be removed either accidentally or purposely, the TM heals with a monomeric membrane; however, the cartilage defect remains. If tube reinsertion is needed, a myringotomy is first performed through the monomeric membrane. The tube is then re-inserted at the original site by grasping the end of the T-tube with alligator forceps and pushing the flanges through the cartilage defect. Because the TM is relatively rigid from the cartilage reconstruction, it does not medialize when pressure is placed laterally. This increased rigidity greatly facilitates secondary tube insertion. The procedure is well tolerated by the patient because the island flap remains insensate after healing, possibly due to the cartilage preventing reinnervation from the caroticotympanic plexus.

SUMMARY

Cartilage is proving to be a very effective material for the reconstruction of the TM in cases of advanced middle ear pathology. It is it particularly useful for the management of the atelectatic ear, cholesteatoma, and high-risk perforation, and for reinforcement of the TM in conjunction with ossiculoplasty. Functional results in each pathologic group in our experience have been good, with a statistically significant improvement in hearing generally appreciated. Although the need for postoperative tube insertion is relatively rare, it can prove to be difficult when the entire TM is reconstructed with cartilage, emphasizing the need to optimize tubal function and continue research to better predict outcome based on preoperative parameters.

REFERENCES

1. Zoellner F. The principles of plastic surgery of the sound-conducting apparatus. *J Laryngol Otol* 1995;69:567–569.
2. Wullstein HL. Funktionelle Operationen im Mettelohr mit Hilfe des Freien Spaltlappentransplantates. *Arch Otorhinolaryngol* 1952;161:422–435.
3. Nissen AJ, Nessen RL, Yonkers AJ. A historical review of the use of bone and cartilage in otologic surgery. *Ear Nose Throat J* 1986;65:493–496.
4. Hermann H. Tympanoplasty with fascial tissue taken from the temporal muscle after straightening the anterior wall of the auditory meatus. *Hals Nas Ohren* 1961;9:136–137.
5. Storrs LA. Myringoplasty with the use of fascia grafts. *Arch Otolaryngol* 1961;74:45–49.
6. Shea JJ. Vein graft closure of eardrum perforations. *Arch Otolaryngol* 1960;72:445–447.

7. Tabb HG. Closure of perforations of the tympanic membrane by vein grafts: a preliminary report of twenty cases. *Trans Am Laryngol Rhinol Otol Soc* 1960;191–207.

8. Preobrazhenski TB, Rugov AA. The employment of preserved dura mater graft in tympanoplasty. *Vestn Otorinolaringol* 1965;5:38–42.

9. Albrite JP, Leigh BG. Dural homograft (alloplastic) myringoplasty. *Laryngoscope* 1966;76:1687–1693.

10. Sheehy JL, Glasscock ME. Tympanic membrane grafting with temporalis fascia. *Arch Otolaryngol* 1967;86:391–402.

11. Buckingham RA. Fascia and perichondrium atrophy in tympanoplasty and recurrent middle ear atelectasis. *Ann Otol Rhinol Laryngol* 1992;101:755–758.

12. Goodhill V. Tragal perichondrium and cartilage in tympanoplasty. *Arch Otolaryngol* 1967;85:35–47.

13. Glasscock ME, Jackson CG, Nissen AJ, Schwaber MK. Postauricular undersurface tympanic membrane grafting: a follow-up report. *Laryngoscope* 1982;92:718–727.

14. Milewski C. Composite graft tympanoplasty in the treatment of ears with advanced middle ear pathology. *Laryngoscope* 1993;103:1352–1356.

15. Loeb L. Autotransplantation and homotransplantation of cartilage in the guinea pig. *Am J Pathol* 1926;2:111–122.

16. Peer LA. The fate of living and dead cartilage transplanted in humans. *Surg Gynecol Obstet* 1939;68:603–610.

17. Kerr AG, Byrne JET, Smyth GDL. Cartilage homografts in the middle ear: a long-term histologic study. *J Laryngol Otol* 1973;87:1193–1199.

18. Don A, Linthicum FH. The fate of cartilage grafts for ossicular reconstruction in tympanoplasty. *Ann Otol Rhinol Laryngol* 1975;84:187–191.

19. Levinson RM. Cartilage-perichondrial composite graft tympanoplasty in the treatment of posterior marginal and attic retraction pockets. *Laryngoscope* 1987;97:1069–1074.

20. Yamamoto E, Iwanaga M, Fukumoto M. Histologic study of homograft cartilage implanted in the middle ear. *Otolaryngol Head Neck Surg* 1988;98:546–551.

21. Hamed M, Samir M, El Bigermy M. Fate of cartilage material used in middle ear surgery light and electron microscopy study. *Auris Nasus Larynx* 1999;26:257–262.

22. Sheehy JL. Surgery of chronic otitis media. In: English G, ed. *Otolaryngology*. Vol. 1. Revised ed. Philadelphia: Harper and Row; 1985:1–86.

23. Glasscock ME, Hart MJ. Surgical treatment of the atelectatic ear. In: Friedman M, ed. *Operative Techniques in Otolaryngology-Head and Neck Surgery*. Philadelphia: WB Saunders; 1992:15–20.

24. Eviatar A. Tragal perichondrium and cartilage in reconstructive ear surgery. *Laryngoscope* 1978;88(suppl 11):1–23.

25. Adkins WY. Composite autograft of tympanoplasty and tympanomastoid surgery. *Laryngoscope* 1990;100:244–247.

26. Amedee RG, Mann WJ, Riechelmann H. Cartilage palisade tympanoplasty. *Am J Otol* 1989;10:447–450.

27. Duckert LG, Mueller J, Makielski KH, Helms J. Composite autograft "shield" reconstruction of remnant tympanic membranes. *Am J Otol* 1995;16:21–26.

28. Dornhoffer JL. Hearing results with cartilage tympanoplasty. *Laryngoscope* 1997;107:1094–1099.

29. Gerber MJ, Mason JC, Lambert PR. Hearing results after primary cartilage tympanoplasty. *Laryngoscope* 2000;110:1994–1999.

30. Zahnert T, Huttenbrink KB, Murbe D, Bornitz M. Experimental investigations of the use of cartilage in tympanic membrane reconstruction. *Am J Otol* 2000;21:322–328.

31. Heermann J, Heermann H, Kopstein E. Fascia and cartilage palisade tympanoplasty: nine years' experience. *Arch Otolaryngol* 1970;91:228–241.

32. Dornhoffer JL, Gardner EK. Prognostic factors in ossiculoplasty: a statistical staging system. *Otol Neurotol* 2001;22:299–304.

33. Black B. Ossiculoplasty prognosis: the spite method of assessment. *Am J Otol* 1992;13:544–551.

34. Albu S, Decreaemer W, Ars-Piret N. Tympano-ossicular allografts: morphology and physiology. *Am J Otol* 1987;8:148–154.

35. Goldenberg RA. Hydroxylapatite ossicular replacement prostheses: preliminary results. *Laryngoscope* 1990;100:693–700.

36. Bellucci RJ. Dual classification of tympanoplasty. *Laryngoscope* 1973;83:1754–1758.

37. Booth JB. Myringoplasty: factors affecting results. *J Laryngol Otol* 1973;83:1079–1084.

38. Jurovitzki I, Sadé J. Myringoplasty: long term follow-up. *Am J Otol* 1988;9:52–53.

39. Dornhoffer JL. Surgical management of the atelectatic ear. *Am J Otol* 2000;21:315–321.

40. Buchwach KA, Birck HG. Serous otitis media and type I tympanoplasties in children. *Ann Otol Rhinol Laryngol* 1980;89(suppl 68):324–325.

41. Strong MS. The eustachian tube: basic considerations. *Otol Clin North Am* 1972;5:19–27.

42. Bailey HAT. Symposium: contraindications to tympanoplasty. Part I: absolute and relative contraindications. *Laryngoscope* 1976;86:67–69.

43. Berger G, Shapiro A, Marshak G. Myringoplasty in children. *J Laryngol Otol* 1974;88:1223–1236.

44. Raine CH, Singh SD. Tympanoplasty in children: a review of 114 cases. *J Laryngol Otol* 1983;97:217–221.

45. Dornhoffer JL. Hearing results with the Dornhoffer Ossicular Replacement Prostheses. *Laryngoscope* 1998;108:531–536.

46. Dornhoffer JL. Surgical modification of the difficult mastoid cavity. *Otolaryngol Head Neck Surg* 1999;120:361–367.

47. Lim D. Human tympanic membrane: an ultrastructural observation. *Acta Otolaryngol* 1970;70:176–186.

48. Pfaltz C. Retraction pocket and development of cholesteatoma in children. *Adv Otorhinolaryngol* 1988;40:118–123.

49. Sadé J. Atelectatic tympanic membrane: histological study. *Ann Otol Rhinol Laryngol* 1993;102:712–716.

50. Dornhoffer JL. Retrograde mastoidectomy with canal wall reconstructions: a single-stage technique for

cholesteatoma removal. *Ann Otol Rhinol Laryngol* 2000;109:1033–1039.

51. Sekula J. Meatotympanoplastyka. *Otolaryngol Pol* 1968;22:397–401.

52. Wehrs RE. Symposium on ear surgery. III: reconstructive mastoidectomy with homograft knee cartilage. *Laryngoscope* 1972;82:1177–1188.

53. Smyth GDL. Cholesteatoma surgery: the influence of the canal wall. *Laryngoscope* 1985;95:92–96.

54. Parisier SC, Hanson MB. Pediatric cholesteatoma: results of individualized single surgery management. In: Sanna M, ed. *Cholesteatoma and Mastoid Surgery. Proceedings of the Fifth International Conference on Cholesteatoma and Mastoid Surgery, Alghero-Sardinia, Italy.* Rome: CIC Edizioni Internazionali; 1997: 375–385.

55. Hirsch BE, Kamerer DB, Doshi S. Single-stage management of cholesteatoma. *Otolaryngol Head Neck Surg* 1992;106:351–354.

56. Roger G, Denoyelle F, Chauvin P, et al. Predictive risk factors of residual cholesteatoma in children: a study of 256 cases. *Am J Otol* 1997;18:550–558.

57. Smyth GDL. Surgical treatment of cholesteatoma: the role of staging closed operations. *Ann Otol Rhinol Laryngol* 1988;97:667–669.

58. Sanna M, Zini C, Scandellari R, et al. Residual and recurrent cholesteatoma in closed tympanoplasty. *Am J Otol* 1984;5:227–282.

59. Stern SJ, Fazekas-May M. Cholesteatoma in the pediatric population: prognostic indicators for surgical decision making. *Laryngoscope* 1992;102:1349–1352.

Chapter 7

TRANSCANAL APPROACHES TO CHOLESTEATOMA

Jay B. Farrior

Transcanal procedures for the removal of cholesteatoma are the most direct approach for the removal of disease originating in the middle ear and epitympanum, and the hypotympanum. Frequently the cholesteatoma is confined to this area of the temporal bone and does not involve the mastoid. The exposure of disease involving the epitympanum and middle ear using a transcanal approach permits the complete removal of cholesteatoma, reconstruction of the tympanic membrane, and ossicular chain, avoiding unnecessary mastoid surgery.[1,2] If more extensive disease is encountered, however, then these approaches can be expanded to allow the removal of cholesteatoma involving the mastoid.

TRANSCANAL ANTERIOR ATTICOTOMY

INDICATIONS

The anterior atticotomy is used when cholesteatoma originates from an attic retraction pocket, which is not thought to extend beyond the aditus into the mastoid antrum, or if the extent of disease is unknown. It is also useful in the management of cholesteatoma associated with tympanic membrane perforations, or involving the ossicular chain, and congenital cholesteatoma originating in the middle ear. Other indications include the management of congenital conductive hearing loss with middle ear reconstruction, ossicular chain problems, and facial nerve injuries in the middle ear and mastoid segments.[3-7]

PREOPERATIVE EVALUATION

In the evaluation of an attic retraction pocket computed tomograms of the middle ear and attic may be useful, but not mandatory, in determining the extent of the disease process and whether the mastoid is involved. Complete audiometric evaluation should be confirmed by tuning fork test.

EXPOSURE

The anterior atticotomy allows direct visualization of disease involving the epitympanum for the aditus, fossa incudis, and forward to the eustachian tube. Removal of the body of the incus and head of the malleus permits direct visualization of all disease in the epitympanum and protympanum. In the middle ear the posterior extent of the approach is the vertical facial nerve. The use of the 30-degree and 70-degree 4-mm endoscopes, following the removal of cholesteatoma, allows for direct inspection of the mastoid antrum, sinus tympani, and posterior tympanic recesses, ensuring the complete removal of the cholesteatoma.[8]

SURGICAL PROCEDURE

Intraoperative facial nerve monitoring is useful in the transcanal removal of cholesteatoma, particularly as one approaches the level of the drum. The anterior atticotomy may be performed using an endaural (preferred) or postauricular incision. It is necessary to have wide exposure of the external auditory canal. The tympanomeatal flap is extended anterior to the short process of the malleus, at the 2 o'clock position in a right ear and the 10 o'clock position in a left ear (Fig. 7–1). Depending on the extent of middle ear involvement, the tympanomeatal flap may be folded inferiorly or removed completely, ensuring adequate exposure of the pathology. The skin of the anterior and inferior canal may be elevated lateral or medial depending on the surgeon's preference.

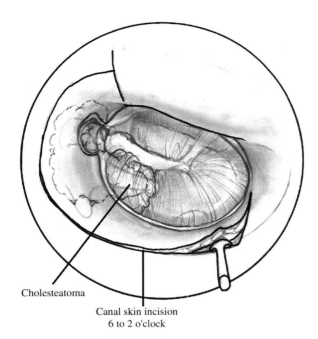

Cholesteatoma

Canal skin incision
6 to 2 o'clock

FIGURE 7–1 For the anterior atticotomy, the tympanomeatal flap is extended anterior to the short process of the malleus. In a right ear the tympanomeatal flap is made circumferentially around the posterior canal from the 6 o'clock position to the 2 o'clock position.

The ear canal is circumferentially enlarged with straightening of the anterior canal wall to expose the anterior drum and annulus. The posterior canal wall is thinned until air cells are seen through a thin layer of bone. Do not drill into the mastoid air cells, as this may lead to postoperative drainage. The roof or the canal is elevated to the level of the tegmen. The tegmen is followed medial to the scutum and lateral attic wall. The tympanic membrane and short process of the malleus are guides to the depth of bone removal. The scutum, the lateral attic wall, is thinned using a diamond or polishing bur rotating away from the malleus, clockwise in a left ear and counterclockwise in a right ear. The egg-shelled lateral attic wall is elevated away from the cholesteatoma sac and the heads of the malleus and incus, which are 0.5 to 1 mm medial to the lateral attic wall[2] (Fig. 7–2). With removal of the scutum, cholesteatoma is exposed in the attic from the fossa incudis, the aditus, and forward to the protympanum, above the eustachian tube.

Once the drum is elevated, the incudostapedial joint is separated and the incus removed. Cholesteatoma is dissected from the epitympanum. The head of the malleus is amputated to access disease in the protympanum.

Greater exposure of the oval window, posterior middle ear, and sinus tympani can be obtained by removing the posterior annulus and medial bony

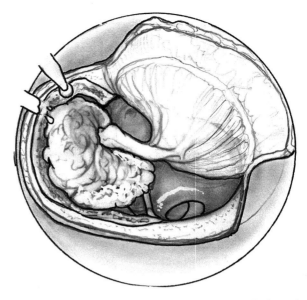

FIGURE 7–2 The tegmen is followed medial to the level of the drum and short process of the malleus with thinning of the scutum and posterior canal wall. The scutum and posterior canal wall are egg-shelled and then elevated away from the cholesteatoma and ossicles. Cholesteatoma is exposed in the middle ear and epitympanum from the aditus, the fossa incudis, forward to the protympanum, above the eustachian tube.

canal wall back to the vertical facial nerve. The pyramidal segment of the facial nerve, superior to the oval window and the chordae tympani nerve, serves as a guide to the vertical facial nerve (the lateral genu of the facial nerve is approximately 1 to 3 mm posterior to the tympanic annulus at the fossa incudis and up to 8 mm posterior to inferior tympanic annulus).[9] The technique for safely removing the posterior annulus is with the drill rotating away from the stapes, clockwise in a right ear and counterclockwise in a left ear. Strokes with the drill are from inferior to superior, toward the stapes. This reduces the risk of the drill running into the stapes and facial nerve.[5] With anterior thinning of the posterior canal wall and removal of the annular rim, wide exposure of the middle ear and attic are obtained (Fig. 7–3).

Cholesteatoma is dissected out of the aditus, epitympanum, and middle ear using blunt dissection with a small sponge. Stapes instrumentation and higher magnification may be necessary to dissect cholesteatoma from a mobile stapes. After removing all visible cholesteatoma, the middle ear and tympanic membrane are reconstructed. The aditus is obliterated with bone, cartilage, or muscle to prevent secondary retraction pocket formation.[3] The epitympanum is lined with fascia to create a smooth cavity (Fig. 7–4).

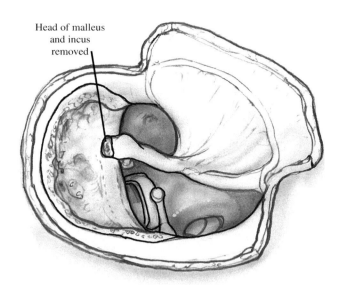

Head of malleus
and incus
removed

FIGURE 7–3 The surgical defect after removal of cholesteatoma, incus, and head of the malleus allows wide exposure of the epitympanic and middle ear spaces. The mastoid antrum and posterior tympanum recesses may be inspected for residual disease using 30-degree and 70-degree 4-mm nasal endoscopes.

If the cholesteatoma extends beyond the aditus into the mastoid antrum, the anterior atticotomy may be extended to an anterior-posterior mastoidectomy by combining the transcanal approach with an intact canal wall and complete simple mastoidectomy. Care must be taken not to thin the posterior canal wall, which has been thinned on its anterior surface.[10,11] If there is a long history of chronic ear problems or a sclerotic mastoid with extensive

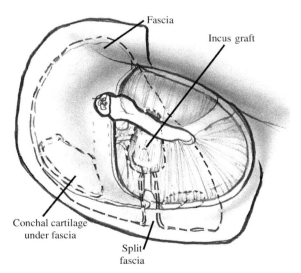

Fascia

Incus graft

Conchal cartilage
under fascia

Split
fascia

FIGURE 7–4 Reconstruction of the tympanic membrane and ossicular chain is performed. The aditus is obliterated with free conchal cartilage graft, to prevent secondary retraction pocket formation. The epitympanum is lined with fascia to promote reepithelialization.

cholesteatoma, the transcanal anterior atticotomy is converted to a modified radical mastoidectomy with tympanoplasty, by removing the posterior canal wall.[12] The attico-antrostomy where the atticotomy is extended posterior to the antrum is not recommended, because of a frequently draining cavity and problems with postoperative care due to a deep mastoid antrum with exposed mucosa.

Over time, 15% of patients develop a secondary mastoid cholesteatoma from retraction pocket formation. Should this occur and there is good postoperative hearing, a Bondy modified radical mastoidectomy may be performed without disturbing the middle ear.

WULLSTEIN'S OSTEOPLASTIC FLAP

Sabrina Wullstein has popularized the creation of an epitympanic osteoplastic flap.[13] This elegant procedure gives wide exposure of the epitympanum and mastoid antrum. Variations in the technique are more popular in the United States and Europe.[14,15]

The osteoplastic flap approach is begun like an anterior atticotomy, as previously described. The scutum is thinned but not drilled away as in the atticotomy. The scutum, the lateral epitympanic

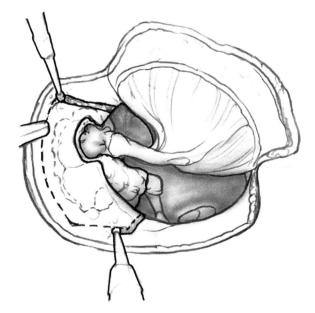

FIGURE 7–5 The external ear canal is enlarged as in the anterior atticotomy to the level of the tegmen with thinning of the lateral attic wall, the scutum. The bone cuts for the osteoplastic flap are outlined. The anterior, superior, and posterior bone cuts are made with a pointed diamond bur, using the tegmen as a guide. The posterior inferior cut at the fossa incudis is made with a small round diamond bur from lateral to medial to minimize the potential of injury to the incus or facial nerve.

wall, is cut as an osteoplastic flap using a file-pointed diamond bur. Beginning anterior to the malleus, a vertical cut is made up to the level of the tegmen. The second cut is made from the anterior bone cut back to the aditus, following the tegmen. The third bone cut is from the tegmen down to the fossa incudis. The bone in the fossa incudis is cut from lateral to medial using a small round diamond bur, reducing the potential risk to the incus and facial nerve (Fig. 7–5). Once the bone cuts are complete, the lateral attic wall is elevated to expose the epitympanum and mastoid antrum. Anterior and posterior bony shelves are created that will support the bone flap after removal of cholesteatoma (Fig. 7–6). The osteoplastic flap is replaced using Gelfoam to support the bone flap abutting the anterior and posterior bony buttresses and prevent it from contacting the ossicular chain. The bone flap may be placed lateral to its normal position to create a larger attic space if desired.

Wullstein's technique has not been popular in the United States, though a variation of her approach has been. The scutum is removed as previously described for the anterior atticotomy. Small bony buttresses are preserved above the eustachian tube and at the fossa incudis. After the cholesteatoma is removed, the lateral attic wall is reconstructed with a free cartilage or bone graft allowing re-aeration of the mastoid[14,15] (Fig. 7–7). This technique is useful if the ossicular chain is intact. Over time, however, patients with persistently poor eustachian tube function may develop a secondary attic retraction pocket cholesteatoma.

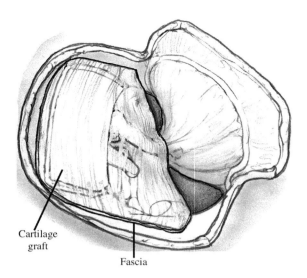

Cartilage graft

Fascia

FIGURE 7–7 The lateral attic wall, osteoplastic flap, is replaced or may be reconstructed with cartilage. Filling the epitympanum with absorbable packing and fascia graft supports it.

ANTERIOR HYPOTYMPANOTOMY

The anterior hypotympanotomy is indicated for the removal of cholesteatoma primarily involving the hypotympanum and sinus tympani, which develop as a complication of adhesive otitis media or an atelectatic drum.[1] As a result of the cholesteatoma removal and chronic eustachian tube dysfunction, the middle ear frequently heals with fibrosis, despite the best efforts to preserve a middle ear air space. Following a hypotympanotomy, the middle ear

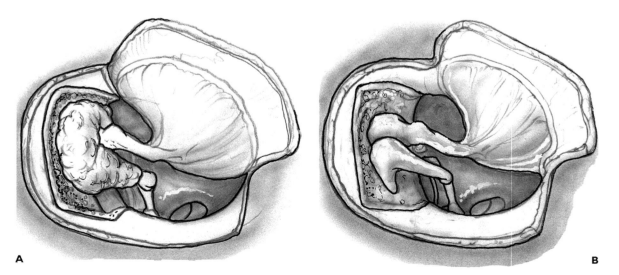

A   B

FIGURE 7–6 (A) The cholesteatoma and ossicular chain are exposed in the epitympanum with the removal of the lateral attic wall. (B) Note the anterior and posterior bony buttresses, which will support the bone flap or cartilage graft after removal of the cholesteatoma.

space frequently collapses resulting in a significant conductive hearing loss. Therefore, recurrent or chronic infection, not the need for hearing improvement, should be the primary indication for this procedure.[3]

SURGICAL PROCEDURE

The surgical approach for removal of a cholesteatoma involving the hypotympanum or sinus tympani is similar to that used for removal of a small glomus jugulare tumor of the middle ear or drainage of a petrous apex cholesterol granuloma.[16] A post-auricular incision is preferred with the inferior portion carried interiorly, allowing the pinna to be retracted anteriorly and superiorly. A short tympanomeatal flap is created extending around the posterior canal from the short process of the malleus at the 12 o'clock position to the 4 o'clock position in a right ear and the 8 o'clock position in a left ear (Fig. 7–8), allowing elevation of the posterior and inferior annulus and drum. The tympanomeatal flap and drum, if present, are pedicled on the malleus. The anterior canal wall skin is elevated medial or lateral, depending on the surgeon's preference.

The bony canal is circumferentially enlarged and the anterior canal straightened. Using the chordae tympani nerve as a guide, the posterior canal wall is removed back to the vertical facial nerve. It is recommended that the drill should be rotating away from the stapes, clockwise in a right ear and counterclockwise in a left ear, and that strokes from inferior to superior, toward the stapes, should be

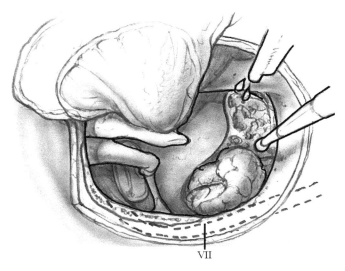

FIGURE 7–9 Removal of the posterior canal wall back to the vertical facial nerve and floor of the ear canal down to the floor of the hypotympanum exposes cholesteatoma involving the round window niche and sinus tympani. Inspection of the sinus tympani with 30-degree and 70-degree endoscopes ensures the complete removal of cholesteatoma.

used. The facial nerve is 1 to 2 mm posterior to the annulus at the fossa incudis and up to 10 mm posterior to the inferior annulus. The floor of the bony canal and annulus are lowered to the floor of the hypotympanum, reducing the potential for a postoperative reservoir for debris. By anterior removal of the posterior canal wall it may be possible to look directly into the sinus tympani, up to 10 mm posterior to the round window (Fig. 7–9). Blunt

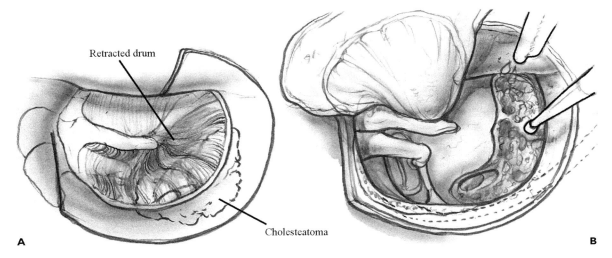

FIGURE 7–8 (A,B) Cholesteatoma developing in the hypotympanum and sinus tympani from adhesive otitis media may be removed using a transcanal hypotympanotomy. For the hypotympanotomy, the tympanomeatal flap is extended inferior and anterior. In a right ear the flap is made circumferentially from the 4 o'clock position to the 12 o'clock position. This allows bone removal from floor of the canal and posterior canal wall.

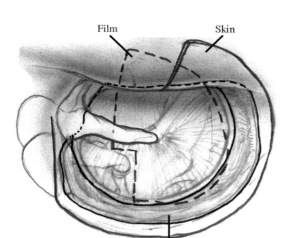

Film   Skin

Fascia

FIGURE 7–10 Reconstruction of the tympanic membrane is supported by absorbable film to reduce middle ear fibrosis. Should the eustachian tube fail to function properly following surgery, the lowered floor of the cavity will allow the drum to collapse, forming a smooth self-draining cavity, without pockets or reservoirs that may lead to chronic infections.

dissection is used to remove cholesteatoma from the middle ear, hypotympanum, and posterior tympanic sinuses. Inspection of the sinus tympani and hypotympanum using 30-degree and 70-degree 4-mm nasal endoscopes helps to ensure the complete removal of cholesteatoma.

After removal of cholesteatoma, the tympanic membrane and ossicular chain are reconstructed. Gelfilm or Silastic is placed over the promontory to reduce adhesions (Fig. 7–10). Unfortunately, many these patients have long-standing poor eustachian tube functioning, and frequently have collapse of the middle ear space. The resulting self-cleansing cavity looks like a mini-radical mastoid cavity, with a 30- to 40-dB conductive hearing loss.

MEATOPLASTY

The meatus of the external auditory canal should be enlarged to conform to the larger size of the bony ear canal following transcanal removal of cholesteatoma. A formal meatoplasty may be performed with the removal of conchal cartilage. In many transcanal procedures a relaxing vertical incision through the incisura, between the anterior helical rim and tragus, allows the external meatus to expand to the shape of the bony canal. Packing of the ear canal for 4 to 6 weeks following surgery reduces postoperative stenosis.

REFERENCES

1. Farrior B. *Tympanoplasty in 3D, Cholesteatoma in 3D.* Vol. 3. Washington, DC: American Academy Ophthalmology and Otolaryngology; 1972.
2. Farrior B, Farrior JB. *Tympanoplasty in 3D, Cholesteatoma in 3D.* Vol. 3. 2nd ed. Washington, DC: American Academy of Otolaryngology Head and Neck Surgery; 1986.
3. Farrior JB. Surgical approaches to cholesteatoma. *Otolaryngol Clin North Am* 1989;22:1015–1028.
4. Donald P, McCabe BF, Loevy SS. Atticotomy, a neglected otosurgical technique. *Ann Otol Rhinol Laryngol* 1979;83:652–662
5. Farrior JB. Management of congenital hearing loss. *Adv Plast Reconstr Surg* 1989;5:217–236.
6. Farrior JB. Anterior facial nerve decompression. *Otolaryngol Head Neck Surg* 1985;93:765–768.
7. Pou JW. Decompression of the facial nerve, a simplified technique. *Trans Am Acad Ophthalmol Otolaryngol* 1962;72:789–795.
8. Tarabichi M. Endoscopic management of acquired cholesteatoma. *Am J Otol* 1997;18:544–549.
9. Litton WB, Krause CJ, Anson BA, Cohen WN. The relationship of the facial nerve to the annular sulcus. *Laryngoscope* 1969;79:1584–1604.
10. Reddy TN, Dutt SN, Shetty A, Maini S. Transcanal atticoaditomy and transcortical mastoidectomy for cholesteatoma, the Farrior-Olaizola technique revisited. *Ann Otol Rhinol Laryngol* 2001;110:739–745.
11. Farrior B. Surgery of the pneumatic mastoid. *Trans Am Acad Ophthalmol Otolaryngol* 1970;74:1196–1207.
12. Farrior B. The radical mastoidectomy, anatomic considerations and surgical technique. *Surg Gynecol Obstet* 1949;89:328–334.
13. Wullstein SR. Osteoplastic epitympanotomy. *Ann Otol Rhinol Laryngol* 1974;83:663–669.
14. East DM. Atticotomy and reconstruction for limited cholesteatoma. *Clin Otolaryngol* 1998;23:248–252.
15. Sakai M, Shenhaua A, Mayake H, et al. Reconstruction of scutum defects (scutumplasty). *Am J Otol* 1986;7:188–192.
16. Farrior JB. Anterior hypotympanic approach for glomus tumors of the infra temporal fossa. *Laryngoscope* 1984;94:1016–1021.

Chapter 8

CANAL-WALL-UP MASTOIDECTOMY

Rex S. Haberman II and Michele St. Martin

The canal-wall-up (CWU) mastoidectomy procedure was introduced by Jansen at the House Ear Clinic in 1958.[1] His goal was to perform more conservative surgical excision of cholesteatoma or other chronic ear disease, preserving the normal anatomy of the external auditory canal. This procedure was developed as a way to address some of the disadvantages of radical and modified radical mastoidectomy, which can include a lifelong need for cleaning of the mastoid cavity and for avoidance of swimming and other water sports, and the possibility of caloric stimulation by cold air or water reaching the mastoid cavity.[1] Additionally, the CWU procedure leaves the patient with more options for hearing aids postoperatively.[2]

The main disadvantage of CWU mastoidectomies is the higher postoperative rate of cholesteatoma as compared to canal-wall-down procedures. Postoperative cholesteatoma can represent either recurrent or residual disease. Residual disease is defined as the presence of cholesteatoma due to incomplete excision at the time of initial surgery, whereas recurrent disease represents new formation of a cholesteatoma from a new retraction pocket postoperatively. Published reports suggest that residual disease is more common following CWU mastoidectomy, but rates of recurrent disease are comparable to those following canal-wall-down surgery.[3] Overall reported failure rates of the CWU procedure range from 3 to 62%; failure is more common in children.[4] Results from Sanna et al,[5] however, indicated that chances of failure can be decreased with certain preventative measures, including using Silastic sheeting, repairing bony defects of the posterior canal wall, performing a staged second look surgery, and placing pressure equalization tubes. Overall failure rates for the CWU procedure dropped to 5.2% with

the use of these measures. Many surgeons perform a planned second-look surgery at 6 to 12 months postoperatively to evaluate for residual or recurrent disease, with or without reconstruction of the ossicular chain.

Hearing results following wall-up versus wall-down mastoidectomies are difficult to interpret in the literature due to wide variation in reporting methods. Data are often not stratified to allow comparison between the two techniques, or between studies. There is evidence, however, that the status of the ossicular chain is more predictive of postoperative hearing than the type of mastoidectomy performed.[2]

Indications for a CWU mastoidectomy include complications of acute otitis media, chronic otitis media, cholesteatoma, exposure of structures within or deep to the temporal bone, cerebrospinal fluid otorrhea, facial nerve trauma, and neoplasm of the temporal bone.[6] A canal-wall-down procedure should be performed if the disease is in the only hearing ear, severe complications of otitis media or cholesteatoma are present, the surgeon is unable to remove cholesteatoma completely with the posterior canal wall intact, the eustachian tube is nonfunctional, or the patient is noncompliant or a poor anesthesia risk. A contracted or sclerotic mastoid cavity is a relative indication for wall-down surgery.[7]

Preoperative preparation for the CWU mastoidectomy involves routine audiometry as well as imaging studies. High-resolution computed tomography (CT) of the temporal bones allows for intraoperative planning and can reveal features of surgical significance, such as a dehiscent facial nerve or tegmen tympani, but it is not routinely performed by all otologists prior to the procedure.

POSITIONING AND PREPARATION

The positioning of the patient is key in all otologic surgery. For the CWU mastoidectomy, the patient should be positioned on the operating table such that the head is located at the foot of the bed. This allows the surgeon's knees to fit comfortably underneath the table when seated. Also, the bed controls should be easily within reach of the anesthetist, as rotation of the bed is necessary throughout the procedure. The patient should be securely strapped to the table to allow for rotation of the bed toward or away from the surgeon without endangering the patient. The patient's head should be located at the very end of the bed, closest to the surgeon's side, and the head should be rotated away from the surgeon.

The facial nerve monitor, if it is to be used, should be placed following the induction of anesthesia. Three pairs of electrodes are used for monitoring. One pair is placed within the fibers of the orbicularis oris muscle, less than 1 cm apart; another pair is placed in the orbicularis oculi muscle. The last pair contains a ground and a stimulating electrode. These can be placed within the frontalis muscle on the patient's forehead, or the ground electrode can be placed at the patient's shoulder with the stimulating electrode below the sternal notch. The electrodes are connected to the facial nerve monitor, which is then turned on. Electrodes are checked for proper function prior to the case.

The patient's hair should be shaved approximately 3 cm behind and above the ear to be operated upon. The surgical field should be prepped widely with the surgeon's choice of sterile solution, including inside the external auditory canal. Various methods are used to secure the patient's hair away from the field, including painting the hair with Betadine, or taping it securely away with plastic tape and benzoin. The ear should then be draped with either an iodoform plastic drape or a head drape with an ear hole. The patient is then draped in the routine fashion and placed in a slight Trendelenburg position.

The operating room should be set up with the anesthetist at the patient's feet. The bed is rotated one-quarter turn following induction of anesthesia. The surgeon should be seated at a comfortable height at the patient's head. The scrub nurse and instrument table should be located either adjacent to the surgeon toward the patient's feet or across the table from the surgeon. Finally, the operating microscope should be positioned at the patient's head. The microscope should be balanced properly before it is draped; the 200- or 250-mm lens is used for otologic surgery.

INSTRUMENTATION

Aside from the routine otologic instrumentation, a CWU mastoidectomy requires special instrumentation including a suction-irrigation system and otologic drill. The drill can be electric- or air-powered, and several different brands are available, including the Anspach MicroMax (Anspach Company, Palm Beach Gardens, FL) and the Midas Rex Legend (Medtronic corporation, Minneapolis, MN) systems for mastoid surgery. Some drill handles are convertible between a straight and an angled shaft, allowing the surgeon to optimize the angle of drilling throughout the procedure. Various sizes of cutting and diamond burs are needed to complete the mastoidectomy; they should be available for the surgeon during the procedure. Many otologic drills are cooled with sterile water delivered through plastic tubing. The tubing should be securely connected to avoid leakage and overheating during the procedure, which can cause the drill to malfunction.

A suction irrigation system is also crucial for mastoid surgery. Various-size suction-irrigation tips should be included in the instrument set. The irrigation system should be connected to a large bag of sterile saline solution, and the tubing should be primed to remove air bubbles from the line. The suction system should be set up with multiple canisters in series, to avoid having to change canisters frequently during the procedure.

Finally, other routine instruments should be available, including unipolar and bipolar cautery as well as otologic instrumentation for the middle ear.

OPERATIVE TECHNIQUE

Once the patient is prepped and draped, local injection should be performed with 1 to 2% lidocaine with 1:100,000 dilution epinephrine for vasoconstriction. A postauricular injection should be made in the postauricular crease, extending from the superiormost aspect of the auricle to the mastoid tip. Care should be taken not to extend the injection beyond the mastoid tip, because temporary paresis of the facial nerve can occur. If meatal injections are required, they should be performed in all four quadrants of the external auditory canal. Local anesthetic should be injected at the bony–cartilaginous junction while pressure is applied laterally with an ear speculum. A blanch should be apparent extending toward the tympanic membrane if the injection is performed properly.

After vasoconstriction has occurred, and canal incisions have been made if necessary, the postauricular incision should be made. The incision should begin at the superiormost aspect of the auricle in the postauricular crease; it should be carried inferiorly either in the postauricular crease or up to 1 cm posterior to it. The incision should extend to the mastoid tip, but not beyond it due to risk of injury to the facial nerve. In children, the course of the facial nerve exiting the stylomastoid foramen can be quite lateral; therefore, the postauricular incision should be shifted posteriorly.[8] The No. 15 blade should be used to make the incision. The blade should be used to carry the incision down to the level of the temporalis fascia. Blunt dissection with a finger should be easily accomplished in this plane to elevate flaps anteriorly and posteriorly. Monopolar cautery is used to control bleeding.

A cerebellar retractor is then placed to retract the ear anteriorly. If a graft is needed for tympanoplasty, now is the time to harvest one. The loose areolar tissue overlying the temporalis fascia posterosuperior to the auricle is elevated by injecting deep to it with local anesthetic. The No. 15 blade is then used to begin an incision through the tissue, and the Metzenbaum scissors and a tissue forceps are then used to harvest a generous-size graft, approximately 1 cm^2 in area. The graft is then placed on a heated block and flattened with the back end of a forceps or knife handle, and left to dry.

The monopolar cautery is then used to incise the temporalis fascia along the linea temporalis, extending from the zygomatic root posteriorly. The incision is carried down through the periosteum to the temporal bone itself. A vertical T incision is then made connecting the horizontal incision to the mastoid tip. It is important during this step to leave a sizable flap anteriorly to facilitate closure of the periosteum at the end of the procedure.

The periosteum is then elevated anteriorly, posteriorly, and superiorly with a heavy Lempert elevator until the entire mastoid cortex is exposed. Bleeding from emissaries may be controlled either with cautery or with bone wax. The cerebellar retractors are then repositioned to retract the periosteum (Fig. 8–1).

The operating microscope is then positioned such that the mastoid cortex is in view. A low-power lens should be used to visualize the entire cortex, external auditory canal, and linea temporalis for orientation during dissection. A large suction irrigator and large cutting bur are used initially to make the first cuts in the mastoid cortex. The initial cuts are made posteriorly along the linea temporalis, and inferiorly along the border of the external auditory canal extending into the mastoid tip.

Dissection should begin at the zygomatic root, at the apex of the two initial cuts. The large cutting bur should be used to extend the dissection posteriorly and inferiorly, keeping the dissection at the same depth throughout the mastoid cavity to facilitate identification of landmarks. Cuts should be made parallel to the linea temporalis and external auditory canal; the bur should also be swept posteriorly along the inferior border of the mastoid as well (Figs. 8–2 and 8–3).

During dissection, the direction of the cuts should parallel the underlying structures to be identified. When locating the tegmen tympani, the cuts should

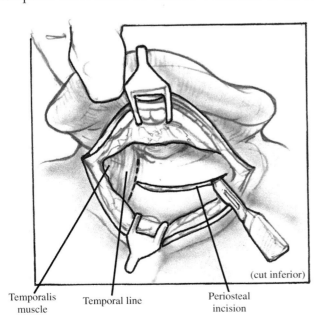

FIGURE 8–1   Exposure of the mastoid cortex.

Temporalis muscle   Temporal line   Periosteal incision   (cut inferior)

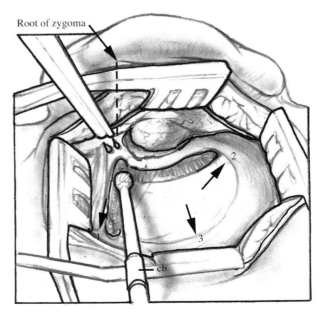

FIGURE 8–2   Exposure of the tegmen tympani.

Root of zygoma

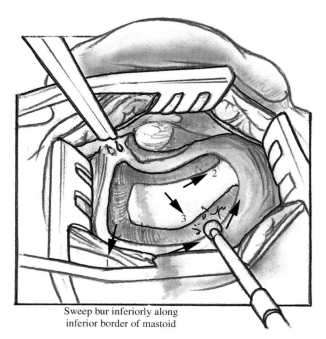

Sweep bur inferiorly along
inferior border of mastoid

FIGURE 8–3 Exposure of the mastoid tip.

be parallel and inferior to the linea temporalis to avoid injury to the underlying dura. Likewise, the sigmoid sinus is best identified sweeping posteriorly along the inferior border of the mastoid, then carrying the dissection superiorly parallel to the

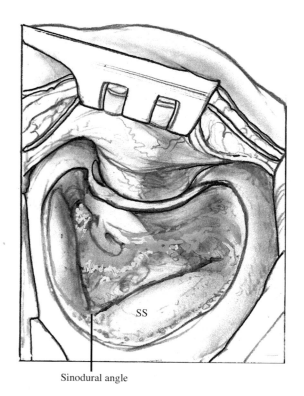

Sinodural angle

FIGURE 8–4 Tegmen tympani, sigmoid sinus, and sinodural angle.

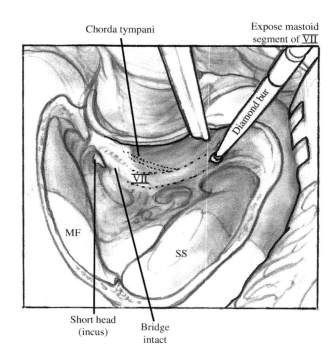

Chorda tympani

Expose mastoid
segment of VII

Diamond bur

VII

MF

SS

Short head
(incus)

Bridge
intact

FIGURE 8–5 Exposure of the mastoid portion of the facial nerve.

initial cut (Fig. 8–4). Finally, the horizontal semicircular canal should be identified by sweeping posteriorly along the border of the external auditory canal (EAC). This method avoids transection of important structures.

Once Körner's septum has been entered and the tegmen tympani, sigmoid sinus, and horizontal canal have been identified, dissection should then be focused on defining the sinodural angle and the

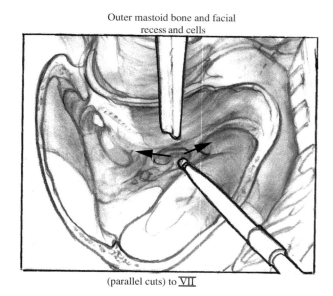

Outer mastoid bone and facial
recess and cells

(parallel cuts) to VII

FIGURE 8–6 Completed canal-wall-up mastoidectomy with facial recess.

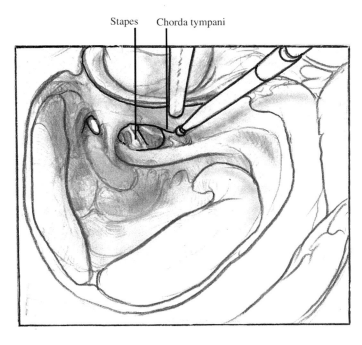

FIGURE 8–7 The facial recess is opened.

antral air cell. The surgeon should ensure that the tegmen is identified along the entire course of the linea temporalis to facilitate exposure of the antrum and fossa incudis.

The antral air cell should be identified by drilling anteriorly and superiorly at the apex of the first two bur cuts, near the root of the zygoma. At this point during the dissection, the surgeon may wish to change to a smaller cutting bur to better define the antrum. Alternatively, a curette may be used. The drill should be placed medially and pulled laterally to protect the underlying structures. The surgeon should take care not to form ledges or overhanging

bone particularly at this stage, as this may contribute to inadvertent injury. The bed may also be rotated away from the surgeon and the microscope repositioned to provide better visualization of the incus.

Once the fossa incudis and the incus have been identified, a diamond bur should be used to control any bleeding from the mastoid bone and to smooth out any rough areas remaining along the tegmen or the posterior wall of the EAC. The facial nerve should now be identified using a large diamond bur. The level of the nerve will be marked by the incus and the horizontal canal. The nerve should be identified by gently passing the drill anterior and

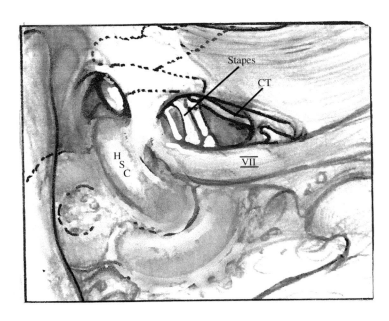

FIGURE 8–8 Extreme close-up view of facial recess.

parallel to the sigmoid sinus, then moving anteriorly. The distinct appearance of the facial nerve and the chorda tympani will appear along the posterior aspect of the EAC, coursing inferiorly (Fig. 8–5).

The facial recess is now ready to be opened if necessary. The landmarks have been identified, including the fossa incudis, chorda tympani, and mastoid portion of the facial nerve. Either a diamond bur or a cutting bur may be used to open the recess. Again, the largest bur possible should be used for this portion of the procedure. The mastoid bone and facial recess air cells are entered, taking care to avoid injury to the facial nerve by making cuts parallel to its course. Drilling is continued until the middle ear space is entered (Figs. 8–6, 8–7, and 8–8). Work in the middle ear can now be accomplished if necessary, and tympanoplasty can be carried out using standard techniques.[9]

CLOSURE

The operative wound is closed in three layers following copious irrigation of the wound to remove bone dust and fragments. The periosteum is closed using interrupted absorbable sutures such as 3-0 Vicryl. The subcutaneous tissue is also closed using interrupted absorbable suture. Finally, the skin may be closed using a number of standard techniques, including stapling, or absorbable or nylon suture. Bacitracin is then placed on the wound and a nonstick dressing such as Telfa is applied. A mastoid dressing is then placed on the patient prior to awakening, using fluffed 4 × 4's and rollergauze to create a tight pressure dressing. The patient is then awakened and taken to the recovery room.

REFERENCES

1. Naclerio R, Neely JG, Alford B. A retrospective analysis of the intact canal wall tympanoplasty with mastoidectomy. *Am J Otol* 1981;2:315–317.
2. Dodson E, Hashisaki G, Hobgood T, Lambert P. Intact canal wall mastoidectomy with tympanoplasty for cholesteatoma in children. *Laryngoscope* 1998;108:977–983.
3. Schmid H, Dort J, Fisch U. Long-term results of treatment for children's cholesteatoma. *Am J Otol* 1991;12:83–87.
4. Reddy T, Dutt S, Shetty A, Maini S. Transcanal atticoaditotomy and transcortical mastoidectomy for cholesteatoma: the Farrier-Olaizola technique revisited. *Ann Otol Rhinol Laryngol* 2001;110:739–745.
5. Sanna M, Zini C, Gamoletti R, et al. Prevention of recurrent cholesteatoma in closed tympanoplasty. *Ann Otol Rhinol Laryngol* 1987;96:273–275.
6. Schuknecht H. Simple mastoidectomy. In: Bailey, BJ, ed. *Atlas of Head and Neck Surgery: Otolaryngology.* 2nd ed. Philadelphia: Lippincott Williams & Wilkins; 2001:348–351.
7. Glasscock M, Schall D, Macias J, Widick M. Modified radical mastoidectomy. In: Bailey, BJ, ed. *Atlas of Head and Neck Surgery: Otolaryngology.* 2nd ed. Philadelphia: Lippincott Williams & Wilkins; 2001:352–355.
8. Goycoolea M. Mastoid and tympanomastoid procedures in otitis media. *Otolaryngol Clin North Am* 1999;32:513–523.
9. Sheehy J. Mastoidectomy: The intact canal wall procedure. In: Brackmann, D, ed. *Otologic Surgery.* 2nd ed. Philadelphia: WB Saunders; 2001:166–177.

Chapter 9

CANAL-WALL-DOWN MASTOIDECTOMY

Thomas J. McDonald

The goal of modern otologic surgery is to maintain or restore normal anatomy. This maxim, however, sometimes persuades surgeons performing tympanomastoid surgery to do anything to leave the canal wall intact, despite the fact that there are clear intraoperative reasons for removing it. First and foremost, in most patients having chronic otitis media with cholesteatoma, the mastoid cell system is usually significantly sclerotic, and therefore a properly done canal-wall-down (CWD) procedure results in a small, manageable mastoid bowl to maintain. Second, middle ear grafting is more than possible with a CWD procedure together with reconstruction of the middle ear and transformer mechanism when indicated and when feasible. Third, in ears with extensive cholesteatoma where disease itself and anatomic constraints indicate the need for a CWD procedure, residual disease usually results when the surgeon persists in attempting to remove disease with the wall intact. Additionally, in certain situations (for instance, low-hanging middle fossa tegmen), complications such as injury to the tegmen and dura and/or sigmoid sinus can occur when attempts are made to remove disease without removing the canal wall.

The controversy continues and was discussed in two landmark papers by Sade[1] in 1987 and Paparella et al[2] in 1989. Three distinct periods in the evolution of mastoidectomy are outlined. In the 1950s, surgery for cholesteatoma usually resulted in radical mastoidectomies. In the 1970s, canal-wall-up operations became very "fashionable," and otologic surgeons are now performing more CWD operations.

Another controversy continues regarding the management of cholesteatoma in the pediatric age group, and the options have been well debated in the literature.[3–9] The consensus, with which I agree, is to perform canal-wall-up operations in most children.

INDICATIONS FOR CANAL-WALL-DOWN MASTOIDECTOMY

The following are indications to remove the wall to accomplish a modified radical mastoidectomy. This option is defined as exteriorizing the ear canal with the mastoid while maintaining or grafting the middle ear space.

1. *Large, bony defect.* A large, bony attic defect or a posterior superior bony defect is almost always caused by cholesteatoma. In removing disease from such a defect, additional bone is usually curetted from its margin, thus further enlarging the defect. If a decision is then made to leave the wall intact (and in view of the fact that continued eustachian tube dysfunction is a given), then attic retraction, despite measures such as bone or cartilage graft placement, will usually occur. Therefore, in these situations the wall should be removed.

2. *Extensive disease.* This is another important reason for removing the canal wall. In a sclerotic mastoid, the middle fossa tegmen is always low and the surgeon's ability to remove cholesteatoma from any part of the epitympanum (particularly anteriorly in the sinodural angle) will result in two common problems: injury to the tegmen and/or dura with cerebrospinal fluid (CSF) leak and bleeding, or thinning and eventual penetration of the superior part of the bony canal wall. A second site where disease is difficult or impossible to remove is in the facial recess. Even with removal of the incus and

enlarging the facial recess, disease can be trapped on both sides of the superior part of the recess with resulting difficulty in total removal. Doing extensive facial recess enlargement can result also in a retraction pocket.

3. *Recurrent disease.* A new attic retraction pocket with disease following a previously performed canal-wall-up procedure should have a CWD operation.

4. *Lateral semicircular canal fistula in the only hearing ear.* This is an absolute indication for removing the canal wall in surgery for chronic otitis media. It is often, but not exclusively, a situation in an older patient who has no hearing in the opposite ear due to an earlier childhood event affecting that ear. These patients present with dizziness, positive fistula testing, large cholesteatomas, and strong evidence clinically and radiographically of a lateral semicircular canal fistula. There is often no measurable hearing in the other ear, and the hearing in the available ear often has compromised sensorineural components due to the fistula and because of the age of the patient. The best surgical strategy in these patients is to clean the middle ear in the usual manner and then graft it, and then upon exploring the mastoid, remove the canal wall and leave the squamous epithelium or matrix over the lateral canal fistula. In patients with good to normal hearing in the opposite ear, different strategies can be pursued, including lifting up the matrix and repairing the canal directly and then lining the area with fascia and then leaving the canal wall up. In instances where there is no hearing in the opposite ear, it is absolutely mandatory to avoid exposing the fistula and instead leave it covered with the matrix.

PROCEDURE

PREOPERATIVE EVALUATION

The preoperative evaluation of patients undergoing CWD mastoidectomy with or without tympanoplasty has some very special components. Examination should be done with the microscope, making sure that the other ear is also examined and evaluated. An audiogram confirmed by tuning fork testing is also essential. Vestibular evaluation is not done routinely unless there is a question of a semicircular canal fistula. In this instance, vestibular evaluation is extremely important because one wants to document not only the integrity of the peripheral labyrinth on the side of the disease, but also, and as importantly, the function of the labyrinth on the opposite side. It would obviously be a difficult

problem if the patient had vestibular impairment following tympanomastoidectomy with CWD to repair a lateral canal fistula, while the other ear had undetected labyrinthine hypofunction.

Imaging by computed tomography is also important and magnetic resonance imaging is usually not necessary. Culture of material in the ear canal is not done routinely, but if there is purulent material, the ear is cleaned with the use of the microscope and treatment is initiated using topical drops (Cipro HC drops), and also broad-spectrum antibiotics for 7 to 10 days. At that time, the ear is reevaluated, which allows (1) reassessment of the situation, and documentation that the ear is now ready for surgery; and (2) another opportunity for a discussion with the patient and family.

PREOPERATIVE DISCUSSION

The preoperative discussion is of paramount importance and should contain the following elements: (1) an explanation with diagram that the underlying problem in the ear with chronic otitis media with or without cholesteatoma is eustachian tube dysfunction; (2) an explanation that this dysfunction is not going to be corrected, but that the disease caused by this problem will be corrected; and (3) an explanation that the goal of the operation is not hearing improvement but hearing maintenance and prevention of complications.

Unlikely complications such as injury to the central nervous system (CNS), facial nerve, labyrinth, and cochlea are important to mention, but not to overly stress. A useful approach is to point out that the likelihood of any of these injuries occurring during surgery is much less than complications due to the disease process itself. The fact that there is perforation of the eardrum with disease and ossicular discontinuity because of disease is clearly pointed out preoperatively so that the patient is alerted that the conductive loss is established. However, a clear plan is outlined that everything (removal of disease and reconstruction) will either be done at the first setting (my preference) or at a "second-look" operation. It is important to stress more than once that the goal is a safe ear and not necessarily a better-hearing ear. The best way to put this to patients is to tell them that the opposite ear (assuming this is normal) will be their "better hearing ear."

SURGICAL PROCEDURE

The procedure is done under general anesthesia, and the key steps are as follows. After complete preparation and draping, the postauricular region and the meatus is injected with 1% Xylocaine with epinephrine, with a 1:10,000 concentration of epinephrine. It is wise to alert the attending anesthesiologist that this high concentration of epinephrine is being used. A postauricular incision is made without performing any transcanal dissection first. Before the incision is made, an imaginary line is drawn through the roof of the ear canal and brought back postauricularly; this is a landmark for the insertion of the temporalis muscle whose overlying fascia is harvested easily. The upper part of the incision is gently carried down so the fascia is visualized, and then a rake is inserted. With a small scissors, a plane is created between the subcutaneous tissue and the fascia. Finger dissection is very useful at this point. A large piece of fascia is harvested and the area lightly cauterized. The rake is removed and then the lower part of the incision is carried down to the mastoid bone, identifying the spine of Henle. At this time, a retractor is introduced and the posterior canal skin is partially elevated. Using a No. 69 blade, a transverse incision is made in the canal skin and then the anterior "jaw" of the retractor is now placed in the upper flap while the posterior part of the retractor is placed in the inferior flap. The microscope is then brought into place, the

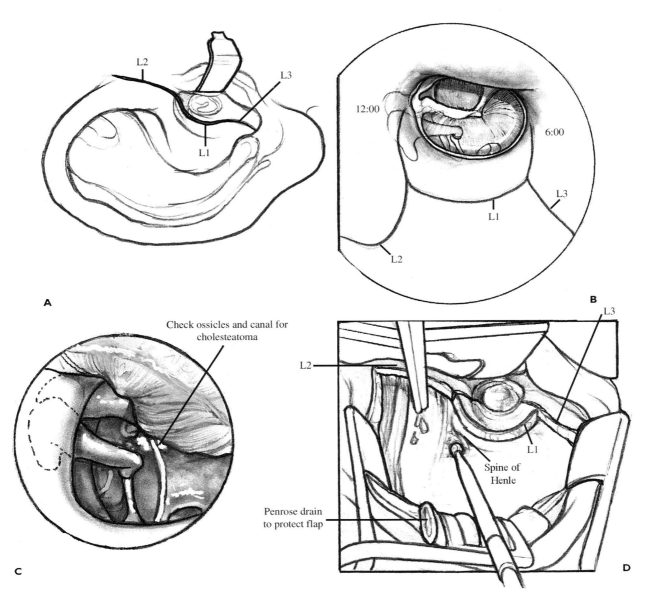

FIGURE 9–I (A) Canal incisions. (B) Tympanomeatal flap. (C) Check ossicles. (D) Exposure. L1, L2, L3, endaural incisions.

incision enlarged, and the ear canal and eardrum are now completely visualized.

THE IMPORTANCE OF PERFORMING THE MIDDLE EAR WORK FIRST (FIG. 9–1)

In patients having a large attic or posterior superior retraction pocket with cholesteatoma (reasons for considering a CWD procedure), this area is debrided and the disease removed directly. A tympanomeatal flap is then elevated, carefully preserving the canal skin, and the middle ear is entered. Examining and dealing with the middle ear disease as the initial step has many different advantages. First, it establishes the condition of the ossicles, and, in most cases where extensive cholesteatoma is present, the long process of the incus has eroded, and thus the incus can be separated and removed from the malleus. The malleus head can then be amputated, allowing further removal of disease. The status of the stapes is then established, and the precise position of the facial nerve is confirmed with its normal bony covering. The middle ear is then completely cleaned of disease, and the mastoid dissection is then commenced.

THE MASTOIDECTOMY (FIG. 9–2)

The temporalis muscle is dissected superiorly from the dural line so that the root of the zygoma is well exposed. Here, the first cut of the drill with the largest cutting bur is made, brought back posteriorly and gently carried down so that the first landmark seen is always the level of the middle fossa tegmen. This structure will have a slight bluish to purplish hue. The rest of the mastoid dissection in the classical shape is then made, preserving the canal wall at first and establishing the degree of cellularity in the mastoid. There are two possibilities at this point. Due to lifelong eustachian dysfunction, the mastoid may be completely sclerotic with a very low-hanging middle fossa tegmen, almost touching the superior wall of the canal. If this is the case, then the canal wall is brought down as the mastoid dissection progresses, entering the antrum, which will always be present (Fig. 9–3). In this case, the wall is lowered to the level of the facial ridge (Fig. 9–4). Again, this brings up the advantage of doing the middle ear work first because one is able to see the middle ear portion of the facial nerve as one approaches the antrum. The second possibility is that the mastoid is somewhat cellular, allowing the mastoid dissection to take place, preserving carefully the integrity of the middle fossa tegmen and performing a small mastoid dissection.

It is very rare to have a fully cellular mastoid with a cholesteatoma, although it can occur and poses a problem when taking the wall down because a large mastoid bowl has to be maintained and cleaned. So, most of the time a small cavity results when the wall is taken down for cholesteatoma. The cholesteatoma is then removed as much as possible, and, for the reasons stated earlier in the chapter, the wall is then taken down. A double-action biting forceps is used, and then with a smaller drill the wall is lowered

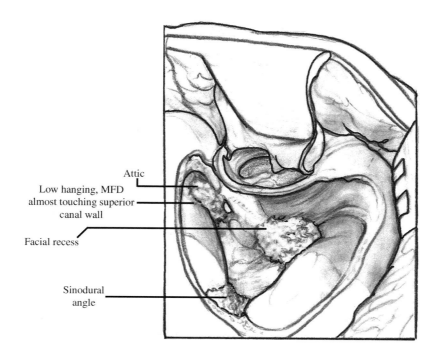

Attic

Low hanging, MFD almost touching superior canal wall

Facial recess

Sinodural angle

FIGURE 9–2 Mastoidectomy.

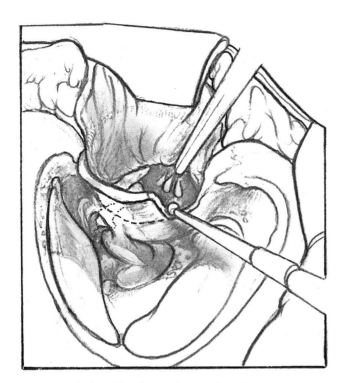

FIGURE 9–3 Take down the canal wall.

completely to the level of the facial ridge. It is important not to leave any sort of "step" between the level of the middle ear and the mastoid. It is very essential not to drill out nondeveloped parts of the mastoid, because there is no disease present, and

because it adds to the size of the mastoid and scope of the mastoid maintenance that has to be carried on for the rest of the patient's life. I prefer not to obliterate mastoids but to leave them open, lower the wall to a safe level, polish the mastoid cavity, and then, finally, cover all exposed bone with fascia, even returning to the upper part of the postauricular incision to obtain more fascia if needed.

The middle ear, in my practice, is always reconstructed (Fig. 9–5). Over the years, transposed incus grafts have been used, followed by Plasti-Pore, then by hydroxyapatite. Currently in my practice, I use exclusively the Kurz prosthesis interposed between the footplate in the absence of a stapes superstructure or on the stapes head to the new eardrum or to the malleus, depending on the anatomic relationships. Banked homograft rib graft cartilage or autograft tragal cartilage is interposed between the Kurz prosthesis and stapes. I do not use Silastic or Gelfoam in the middle ear. I graft the middle ear with a medially laid piece of fascia brought out over to completely line the exposed bone (Fig. 9–6). Then, Silastic is introduced over the eardrum and fascia. A meatoplasty is then performed and the ear is packed with gauze containing Cortisporin ointment. The incision is closed with interrupted buried catgut sutures. A pressure dressing is applied, and the patient is discharged from the hospital either that day or the next morning.

ADEQUATE MEATOPLASTY

Meatoplasty is an important part of a CWD procedure and is performed as follows: an assistant grasps the ear and pulls it laterally. Using a new No. 69

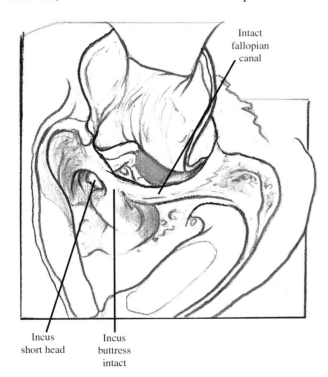

Intact
fallopian
canal

Incus
short head

Incus
buttress
intact

FIGURE 9–4 Facial ridge is lowered.

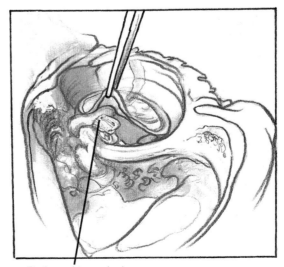

Replace with prosthesis

FIGURE 9–5 Reconstruct the middle ear.

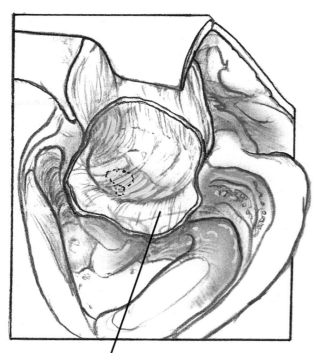

Fascia graft over ossicles,
then overlay with canal skin

FIGURE 9–6 Fascia graft.

blade, I transect the posterior skin and then remove as much subcutaneous fat from the flap and all of the conchal cartilage that is available. I then pedicle this inferiorly and, with a 4-0 chromic suture, sew it to the adjacent muscle. This now allows a pedicled flap to be everted and allows a layer of skin to start the epithelialization process of the mastoid bowl. It

should be made quite large to assure aeration, self-cleaning, and the ability to inspect and clean in the office.

REFERENCES

1. Sade J. Treatment of cholesteatoma. *Am J Otol* 1987;8:524–533.
2. Paparella MM, Morris MS, DaCosta SS. A one stage compromise of the open vs. closed method: the IBMC intact-bridge tympanomastoidectomy procedure. In: Tos M, Thomsen J, Peitersen E, eds. *Cholesteatoma and Mastoid Surgery.* Amsterdam: Kugler & Ghedini; 1989:885–892.
3. Algarra JM, Gimenez F, Mallea I, Armengot M, Fuente L. Cholesteatoma in children: results in open versus closed techniques. *J Laryngol Otol* 1991;105:820–824.
4. Dodson EE, Hashisaki GT, Hobgood TC, Lambert PR. Intact canal wall mastoidectomy with tympanoplasty for cholesteatoma in children. *Laryngoscope* 1998;108:977–983.
5. Edelstein DR, Parisier SC, Ahuja GS, et al. Cholesteatoma in the pediatric age group. *Ann Rhinol Laryngol* 1988;97:23–29.
6. Arriaga MA. Cholesteatoma in children. *Otolaryngol Clin North Am* 1994;27:573–591.
7. Sheehy JL. Cholesteatoma surgery in children. *Am J Otol* 1985;6:170–172.
8. Lau T, Tos M. Cholesteatoma in children: recurrence related to observation period. *Am J Otolaryngol* 1987;8:364–373.
9. Iino Y, Imamura Y, Kojima C, Takegoshi S, Suzuki J. Risk factors for recurrent and residual cholesteatoma in children determined by second stage operation. *Int J Pediatr Otorhinolaryngol* 1998;46:57–65.

Chapter 10

INTACT-BRIDGE MASTOIDECTOMY: A VERSATILE ONE-STAGE OPERATIVE TECHNIQUE

Hamed Sajjadi

From about 1965 to 1985, many otologists, notably Sheehy and Patterson,[1] Jansen,[2] and Smyth,[3] recommended either the closed-cavity, intact-wall tympanomastoidectomy or a combined approach, accomplishing each approach usually in two or three stages. First the pathologic conditions were eradicated, then 8 to 12 months later the hearing apparatus was reconstructed via tympanoplasty; sometimes a separate exploratory procedure later searched for residual cholesteatoma. At the First International Conference on Cholesteatoma (held in Alabama in 1977), McCabe and colleagues[4] noted rising enthusiasm for two-stage techniques using intact-canal-wall mastoidectomy. Farrior[5] and Paparella and Kim[6] recommended occasional selection of an intact-canal-wall tympanomastoidectomy, depending on existing anatomic and pathologic findings in each patient.

By 1982, when the Second International Conference on Cholesteatoma was held in Tel Aviv, discussion had reverted to the high rate of recurrent or residual cholesteatoma found with intact-wall procedures,[7] requiring revision of the surgery in 38.1%, compared with 9.4% for open procedures. Recommendations swung back to open-cavity techniques. Brown,[8] comparing 1142 consecutive cases of cholesteatoma treated surgically with open and with closed techniques, concluded that closed methods produced better hearing results but higher rates of recurrence.

In Paparella and Kim's[6] study, most patients with chronic otitis media and mastoiditis had sclerotic and hypocellular mastoids. On the basis of this observation, Paparella and Jung[9] developed a surgical technique called the intact-bridge tympanomastoidectomy (IBM) procedure. This procedure produced excellent long-term results by preserving desirable elements of both open-cavity (intact canal-wall) and closed-cavity (canal-wall-down) techniques, allowing eradication of diseased tissue, better reconstruction of the middle ear and ossicles, enhanced tympanoplastic methods, and enhanced obliteration of the mastoid (when indicated), all within a single stage. From then on, Paparella and Sajjadi have performed more than 1200 IBM procedures with excellent results. It remains the treatment of choice for chronic otitis media and mastoiditis where there is a canal wall or bridge.[10]

SURGICAL TECHNIQUE

The IBM is indicated for patients with chronic otitis media and mastoiditis, intractable cholesteatoma, cholesterol granuloma, or granulation tissue in the mastoid, middle ear, or attic, either as a first operation or, if there has been prior surgery, to revise where the earlier procedure has left an intact posterior canal wall or bridge. Because most patients with chronic otitis media and mastoiditis do have small, sclerotic, hypocellular mastoids, they are ideal candidates for the IBM.[11] In the rare patient with a well-pneumatized mastoid, excellent results can be obtained by adding some techniques from combined-approach tympanoplasty to the intact-canal-wall tympanomastoidectomy. For the most difficult cases of severely contracted, sclerotic mastoids, however, an intact-canal-wall tympanoplasty may be unnecessarily hazardous even in the hands of experts and it does not offer much alleviation of open-cavity postoperative problems. The IBM techniques result in a very small cavity.

Incision

In a well-pneumatized mastoid, a postauricular incision is used to expose mastoid and middle ear; sometimes, if the meatus is small, a limited endaural incision is added. In the more frequent sclerotic or diploic mastoid, however, Lempert endaural incisions I, II, and III are begun 5 to 7 mm from the tympanic annulus in the bony ear canal (Fig. 10–1). Then incisions are made at the 6 o'clock and 12 o'clock positions with a sickle knife, and a No. 1 knife at the tympanic annulus, to connect with the Lempert I and delineate a tympanomeatal flap (Fig. 10–2). The flap is separated from the mastoid flap at the Lempert I incision, using a duck-billed knife/elevator, and is elevated down to the annulus, but the middle ear is not yet entered. A Lempert elevator is used to further elevate the Lempert I incision with the mastoid flap, and the mastoid flap is put inside a self-retaining retractor with a Penrose drain between retractor and flap to protect the integrity of the flap (Fig. 10–3). Then from the Lempert II incision, with self-retaining retractors, we harvest temporalis muscular fascia, put it into a fascial press for 10 minutes, and then open the press and allow it to air-dry.

Canaloplasty

Most patients with chronic otitis media have small external ear canals that bulge into the anterior and often also the posterior canal. Generous canaloplasty, tailored to each patient, is usually required. Using self-retaining retractors, skin of the anterior canal is elevated in a laterally based flap, and skin of the posterior canal in a medially based flap. A high-speed cutting drill under suction/irrigation is used to enlarge the circumference of the posterior canal, removing the spine of Henle and all overhangs to achieve a straight, direct, unobstructed approach to the tympanic annulus (Fig. 10–4).

If there is prominent bulging into the anterior canal that obscures the view of the drumhead, an incision is made in the anterior canal with a No. 2 knife lateral to the tympanic annulus in a semicircle from the 6 o'clock to 12 o'clock positions. The skin of the anterior canal is very carefully elevated using a duck-billed knife/elevator; then just past the bone–cartilage junction a thin skin flap is carefully raised with a larger, round, duller periosteal elevator (Fig. 10–5), being careful not to amputate the flap. A high-speed cutting drill with suction/irrigation is then used to make two grooves in the anterior canal wall, inferiorly and superiorly, and then connect them with drilling. This allows full visualization of the anterior drumhead by removing the bulge in the canal. Apparent distance to the temporomandibular

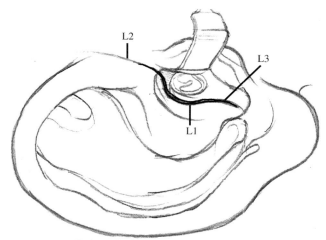

Endaural incisions (Lempert 1, 2, 3)

FIGURE 10–1 Lempert incisions.

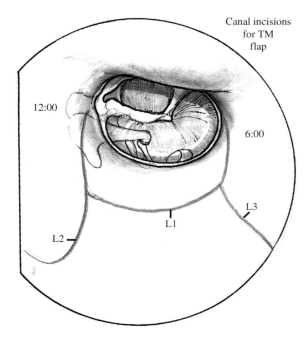

Canal incisions for TM flap

FIGURE 10–2 Canal incisions and tympanomeatal (TM) flap.

joint may be deceptive, so care must be taken not to enter the joint or, if its endosteum is entered, to cease drilling.

Optional Mastoidotomy

In most of these patients, intractable cholesteatoma or granulation tissue in a sclerotic mastoid indicates that the surgeon should proceed directly to mastoidectomy, but in a few patients the status of the mastoid is unclear. For these patients, mastoidotomy,

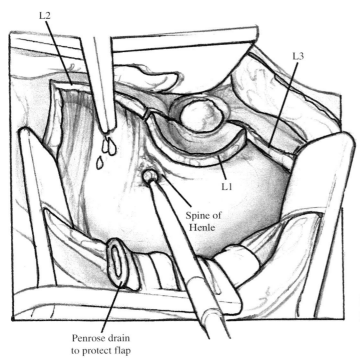

FIGURE 10–3 Retractors in place. Penrose drain protects flap.

either through the posterior wall of the ear canal through a small opening or under Macewen's triangle if preoperative radiographs show adequate pneumatization, can help safely identify the extent of the pathologic tissue. In extremely sclerotic mastoids, mastoidotomy is not indicated.

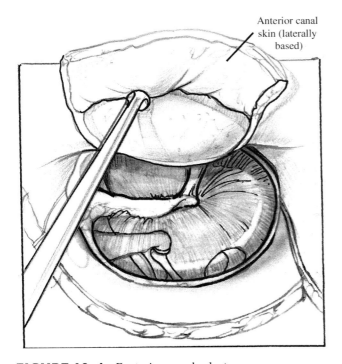

FIGURE 10–4 Posterior canaloplasty.

ATTICOTOMY AND CLEANING OF THE MIDDLE EAR

After canaloplasty, the middle ear can be entered by elevating a tympanomeatal flap inferiorly, elevating the annulus out of its groove, and extending the elevation superiorly to the notch of Rivinus. Then using a stapedial curette, a customized anterior atticotomy is achieved by removing the posterior canal wall at the level of the annulus. If the anatomy necessitates fuller visualization of diseased tissues, to eradicate them and enlarge the middle ear space, the atticotomy can be extended to include the junction of the malleus and incus, and the fallopian canal.

MASTOIDECTOMY

It should now be easier to determine the need to enter the mastoid. The intact-wall (IBM) mastoidectomy begins with drilling the wall of the posterior ear canal from canal toward mastoid. Drilling the other way, mastoid to canal, results in a smaller, not larger, middle ear space and locates the bridge more anteriorly than is desirable for good reconstruction. Putting the bridge as far posterior as possible in an enlarged middle ear with a smaller mastoid is best (Fig. 10–6A).

In the IBM, air cells of the facial or suprapyramidal recess are usually not drilled open, which helps to avoid postoperative retraction pockets. The incus buttress is left intact, overlying and posterior to the

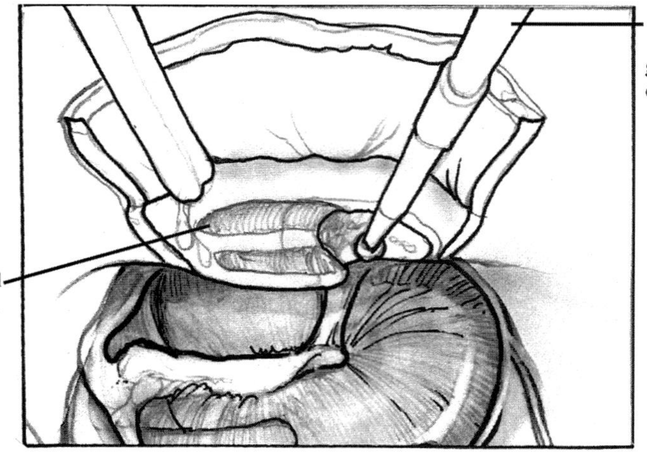

FIGURE 10–5 Elevate anterior canal skin and anterior canaloplasty.

tympanic annulus, and this bony circumferential platform then allows reconstruction of the ossicular chain and eardrum with minimal development of posterosuperior retraction (Fig. 10–6B). When all diseased tissue has apparently been eradicated, the undersurface of the bridge is carefully examined with a rigid otic endoscope (30 and 70 degrees) to evaluate for total removal of cholesteatoma or other diseased tissue.

The mastoid cavity is reduced in size by lowering its walls with a cutting drill as much as possible. To remove all angulations and achieve a smooth outer cortex, air cells of the mastoid tip and outer mastoid cortex are completely saucerized and lowered to allow for collapse of posterior skin tissue into the mastoid and to achieve a much smaller mastoid long-term. Mastoid cortical bone superior to the level of the dura of the middle fossa is drilled completely to obliterate this area. Drilling is continued posteriorly to the lateral sinus and inferiorly through the mastoid tip. This may seem to develop a larger mastoid cavity, but the opposite occurs once the postauricular wound heals and collapses inward.

The undersurface of the bridge is cleaned of all residual diseased mucosa or cholesteatoma using $\frac{1}{8}$-inch umbilical tape passed from the middle ear into the mastoid and moved very gently back and forth to remove all diseased tissue without fracturing the bridge; then full removal is checked using an endoscope. A free graft of temporalis muscle and periosteum is used to obliterate the defect from the posterior atticotomy, obliterate the mastoid, and separate the mastoid air-cell system from the middle ear space, thus "exteriorizing" the mastoid so that it is no longer dependent on the eustachian tube for drainage. This helps keep the middle ear space well pneumatized and free of discharge from the mastoid.

RECONSTRUCTION OF THE MIDDLE EAR, OSSICULOPLASTY, AND INSERTION OF TUBES

Finally, an ossiculoplasty may be performed in the newly cleaned space; the techniques for this are discussed elsewhere in the literature. The malleus is lateralized by visualizing it endoscopically or microscopically, or feeling for it with the incudostapedial joint knife; then the tensor tympani tendon is severed. When the stapes is stabilized, the handle of the malleus can be lateralized 1 or 2 mm to allow for a larger middle ear space, but lateralization must be carefully balanced with pressure on the stapedial joint to avoid subluxation of the incudostapedial or the incudomalleal joint. Then silicone sheeting (Silastic 0.005 to 0.13 mm thick) is custom cut to cover the mucosa of the promontory and the opening of the eustachian tube, taking care to keep it outside the eustachian tube and not touching the stapedial crura. The ossicles are assessed for the need for partial or total reconstruction. It is preferable to insert any prosthesis for partial ossiculoplasty under the handle of the malleus for better connection and reduced risk of extrusion. The prosthesis would then be surrounded by Gelfoam soaked in a combined solution of sulfa, steroids, and antibiotics.

Myringotomy is performed in the anteroinferior tympanic remnant or any remnant available. A small (type 1) Paparella ventilation tube with internal diameter of 1.1 mm is inserted, avoiding insertion through fascial grafts of temporalis muscle, if possible. However, it may not be possible to avoid it with a severely dysfunctional eustachian tube and ossiculoplasty, and putting the tube in the graft may then be necessary to prevent postoperative effusion, retraction, or rejection of the implant. In most patients who receive tubes in the fascial graft, it may be in position permanently.

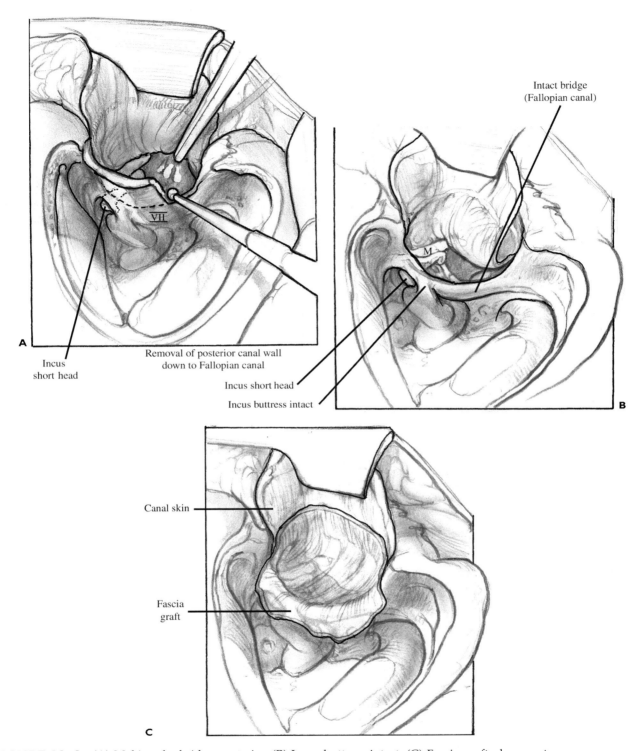

FIGURE 10–6 (A) Making the bridge posterior. (B) Incus buttress intact. (C) Fascia graft placement.

GRAFTING THE TYMPANIC MEMBRANE

The harvested temporalis muscle-fascia (see step one above) is now semiparchment-like. It is rehydrated using the same sulfa-steroid-antibiotic solution and immediately reinserted in the middle ear space as an underlay or as an overlay or in a combined grafting technique, as the needs of the patient indicate, to cover the drumhead anteriorly and even cover the middle ear. In most patients, what is required is a lateral graft reflected onto the mastoid cavity over the obliterated aditus and over the intact bridge. Anteriorly the graft is reflected up the anterior canal wall 1 to 2 mm, then secured in position by reinserting the flap of anterior canal skin over the fascial graft (Fig. 10–6C).

MASTOID OBLITERATION

If there is still a sizable mastoid at this stage, a Palva flap or other obliteration may be used, but we have found that the IBM technique lets most patients avoid any significant obliteration of the mastoid. When the aditus is closed with a free graft of temporalis muscle (see above), the resulting mastoid cavity is rather small.

MEATOPLASTY

This step is essential to prevent entire failure of any open cavity or IBM procedure. A large cotton ball is soaked in the sulfa-steroid-antibiotic solution and then inserted in the mastoid to cover the reconstructed area, collect any blood running toward deeper structures, and prevent blood from obstructing the reconstructed area. Using sharp dissection, a generous subcutaneous piece of conchal cartilage (but not much conchal skin) is removed to allow wide exposure of the meatus. It is difficult to remove too much cartilage, because meatal skin rests on the bony walls below, and the meatus always narrows postoperatively. It is necessary to preserve as much meatal skin as possible, to be used to line the mastoid cavity, but it is very important to remove as much conchal cartilage as needed to allow for wide meatoplasty.

OPTIONAL THIERSCH SKIN GRAFTING

Patients who undergo IBM procedures mostly have small mastoid cavities devoid of squamous epithelium. Lack of sufficient lining may lead to long-standing postoperative drainage and a poorly healed surface easily broken down on superficial contact with devices such as hearing aids or Q-tips. Poorly healed mastoid cavities without a tough epithelium make patients prone to postoperative otorrhea, upper respiratory infections, and more. If raw mastoid surfaces remain longer than 2 or 3 weeks, and if there is aggressive response by granulation tissue, then Thiersch grafting should be done, unless (as in rare cases) meatal skin has covered the mastoid adequately.

The author usually performs Thiersch grafting 3 or 4 weeks postoperatively, either in the office or in an outpatient setting under local anesthesia. Delaying grafting avoids disrupting postoperative packing or jeopardizing a fragile graft when packing is removed. Delayed grafting has been shown to be more effective because the graft can be laid on a bed of granulation tissue, allows for contraction of a healed wound so as to graft a much smaller mastoid cavity, and accommodates those few patients who may heal without need for a graft. A 0.009-inch-to 0.23-mm-thick skin graft is obtained from the medial surface of the ipsilateral upper arm. It is placed over silk gauze soaked in gentamicin ointment, then placed in the mastoid cavity in strips, to line all raw surfaces.

DISCUSSION

Patients who have never had otologic surgery or whose prior surgery preserved the bridge or canal wall can undergo an IBM procedure. Our results with it have been gratifying when compared with results for either open-cavity or closed-cavity tympanomastoidectomy. The IBM can achieve improved hearing (as in intact-wall techniques) and eradicate cholesteatoma (as in open-cavity techniques). In the small, sclerotic mastoid common to these patients, the IBM approach allows wide exposure of the middle ear space and mastoid.

Because the temporal bones used in dissecting laboratories to teach techniques for intact-wall mastoidectomy often come from patients who have died of nonotologic causes and may have well-pneumatized mastoids, students and practicing otolaryngologists may become comfortable performing these procedures on well-pneumatized temporal bones, which are not to be seen in patients with chronic otitis media. The tight, sclerotic, hypocellular mastoids with cholesteatoma in varying and difficult-to-reach places found in live patients make the procedure difficult in actual practice, and many young otolaryngologists then become frustrated with the approach, which seems to work less well in live bones than it did as they learned it as residents. They may abandon otologic surgery. The IBM procedure allows both otologic experts and other well-trained otolaryngologists to eradicate disease competently, with efficiency, accuracy, and safety. Exposure of a tight sclerotic mastoid is much easier, using this technique, which (due to the preserved facial buttress) allows for excellent reconstruction of the apparatus of the middle ear and the circular bony annulus. Unlike traditional canal-wall-down techniques that remove the bridge and may lead to retraction of the tympanic membrane into the attic and thus to large conductive hearing losses, the IBM allows a larger middle ear space. This is essential for ossiculoplasty that will remain successful postoperatively. The IBM also totally sequesters structures of the middle ear from the mastoid air-cell system and its diseases.

Adding to this protocol the optional delayed Thiersch grafting allows for full epithelialization of the small mastoid cavity that results from the IBM. In fact, postoperatively, patients may commonly appear to have only a very large ear canal and not much of a mastoid cavity. These patients require minimal care of the mastoid cavity, and it may be a year or more before they need removal of any wax. Most achieve completely self-cleaning mastoids.

This method provides desirable features from closed-cavity, intact-wall, and open-cavity techniques. Holmquist and Bergstrom[11] noted that the resultant reservoir of air after an IBM is smaller than that retained in intact-wall techniques, but most patients needing an IBM have reduced mastoid air cells in the first place, and the IBM extends the air-containing cavity of the mesotympanum. This is more useful to these patients, who have dysfunctional eustachian tubes that would not be significantly improved by creation of a new pseudo-mastoid cavity. The enlarged mesotympanum enhances reconstruction of the middle ear and enhances ossiculoplasty, leading to better long-term hearing results than those achieved in intact-wall or closed-cavity mastoidectomy.

It is important that the IBM be accomplished in a single stage, avoiding purposeful planning of costly, inconvenient, and painful additional stages with the attendant risk of complications. It becomes medically and financially difficult to justify two- and three-stage procedures on patients with chronic ear disease when the one-stage IBM can provide a safe, functioning middle ear and mastoid—ideal for patient, physician, and insurer. The technique has served this author well for 18 years, producing hearing results equal to or better than those from intact-wall tympanomastoidectomies, especially where an intact ossicular change can be preserved. Residual rates of postoperative return to cholesteatoma have been comparable with rates for canal-wall-down techniques, and with the advent of endoscopic techniques we can hope for total eradication of cholesteatoma using the one-stage IBM.

REFERENCES

1. Sheehy J, Patterson ME. Intact canal wall tympanoplasty with mastoidectomy: a review of eight years' experience. *Laryngoscope* 1967;77:1502–1542.

2. Jansen C. The combined approach for tympanoplasty: report on ten years' experience. *Otolaryngol Head Neck Surg* 1968;82:779–793.

3. Smyth G. Combined approach tympanoplasty. *Arch Otolaryngol* 1969;89:250–251.

4. McCabe BF, Sadé J, Abramsen M, eds. *Cholesteatoma: First International Conference.* Birmingham, AL: Aesculapius; 1977.

5. Farrior JB. The canal wall in tympanoplasty and mastoidectomy. *Arch Otolaryngol* 1969;90:706–714.

6. Paparella MM, Kim CS. Mastoidectomy update. *Laryngoscope* 1977;87:1977–1988.

7. Yanagihara N. Surgical treatment of cholesteatoma: problems in indications and technique. In: *Cholesteatoma and Mastoid Surgery.* Amsterdam: Kugler; 1982:483–480.

8. Brown JS. A ten-year statistical follow-up of 1142 consecutive cases of cholesteatoma: the closed vs. the open technique. *Laryngoscope* 1982;92:390–395.

9. Paparella MM, Jung TK. Intact bridge tympanomastoidectomy (IBM): combining essential features of open vs. closed procedures. *J Laryngol Otol* 1983;97:579–585.

10. Alleva M, Paparella MM, Morris M, daCosta SS. The flexible/intact-bridge tympanomastoidectomy. *Otol Clin North Am* 1989;22:41–49.

11. Holmquist J, Bergstrom B. The mastoid air-cell system in ear surgery. *Arch Otolaryngol Head Neck Surg* 1978;82:779–793.

Chapter 11

REVISION MASTOIDECTOMY

John F. Kveton

Persistent or recurrent drainage from the ear after canal-wall-up (CWU) surgery may be related to surgical technique or patient disease. Drainage indicates the presence of chronic otitis media, but the exact cause of the chronic otitis media must be determined. Factors that may help determine the cause of recurrent aural drainage include the timing of the appearance of the drainage in relation to the original surgery; the frequency of the drainage; the pathology in the original surgery; the status of the tympanic membrane; the development of symptoms such as hearing loss, vertigo, or facial palsy; and other associated patient disease. The development of aural drainage immediately after surgery suggests failure to exenterate all active disease at the time of the original mastoidectomy. This is usually related to poor surgical technique. Recurrent drainage weeks to months after the initial procedure may also be due to poor technique, but may also be secondary to residual cholesteatoma, or may be due to organisms resistant to standard therapies. Intermittent drainage, rather than constant drainage, suggests the presence of cholesteatoma or eustachian tube dysfunction related to allergy. Recurrent drainage after CWU surgery for cholesteatoma indicates recurrent cholesteatoma until proven otherwise.

The presence of drainage with tympanic membrane perforation and granulation tissue may indicate poor technique with residual disease, inadequate eustachian tube function, or cholesteatoma. Retraction of the tympanic membrane with drainage indicates poor eustachian tube function and possible development of cholesteatoma. The development of hearing loss, vertigo, or facial palsy in the presence of an intact tympanic membrane indicates cholesteatoma, whereas the presence of these symptoms with a perforated tympanic membrane may also be due to activation of significant bacterial disease. The appearance of aural drainage in a seasonal timeframe indicates an allergic factor causing poor eustachian tube function. Aural drainage during exacerbation of connective tissue disorders is related to the proliferation of granulomatous tissue within the middle ear and mastoid, while poor control of serum glucose in diabetes will result in the worsening of any existing chronic infection.

EVALUATION

Evaluation of the draining ear should begin with inspection of the auricle and the mastoid region. Postauricular swelling is a sign of acute mastoiditis, whereas tenderness over the mastoid region suggests a subacute process. Swelling of the external auditory canal indicates that the chronic otitis media has produced otitis externa as well. This situation is usually found in long-standing chronic disease with extensive granulation tissue formation in the middle ear or in immunocompromised patients. The status of the tympanic membrane can provide clues as to the cause of failure of the previous procedure and so guide in future surgical decision making. A total tympanic membrane perforation with granulation tissue filling the middle ear suggests widespread disease throughout the temporal bone. An anterior, dry perforation may indicate poor eustachian tube function, but more likely reflects inadequate surgical technique. A retracted tympanic membrane, with or without an attic retraction, reveals eustachian tube dysfunction. In this situation, especially after a first-stage intact-canal-wall procedure for cholesteatoma, it is impossible to determine whether residual or recurrent cholesteatoma is present prior to surgery.

Audiometric evaluation is mandatory prior to revision mastoidectomy. Conductive hearing loss should be expected in these cases. Asymmetric sensorineural hearing loss should raise concern. Sensorineural hearing loss indicates that inner ear damage may have occurred at the previous procedure, but such hearing loss is also suggestive of fistulization of the inner ear caused by aggressive disease. Sensorineural hearing loss should therefore alert the surgeon to proceed cautiously around the labyrinth and cochlea during surgery. The degree of conductive hearing loss can also be helpful in surgical planning and counseling. Mild conductive hearing loss suggests that the ossicular chain is intact and that removal of disease and repair of the perforation should restore hearing to normal. A hearing loss greater than 40 dB usually indicates ossicular chain disruption or fixation. The ultimate hearing result in such cases is always more variable.

In addition to audiometric testing, imaging of the temporal bone should be performed prior to most revision mastoid procedures. This is usually not necessary in planned second-stage procedures for cholesteatoma. Noncontrast high-resolution computed tomography (CT) scan of the temporal bone is the imaging procedure of choice. Plain films of the mastoid should be performed only when CT scans are not available. Magnetic resonance imaging (MRI) should be used as a secondary imaging modality. It is indicated when there is concern of an intracranial complication of mastoiditis such as meningoencephalocele, intracranial abscess or inflammation, or venous sinus thrombosis. CT scans aid in diagnosis and surgical planning. Although the appearance of soft tissue within the mastoid defect is not uncommon, complete opacification of the operative mastoid defect, especially with obstruction of the attic, is evidence of active disease. Soft tissue involvement of residual air cells suggests persistent disease. Especially in the attic region, these air cells may be responsible for chronic ear drainage. Erosive changes in the temporal bone are important to note, because erosion suggests cholesteatoma in the vast majority of cases, and rarely, neoplasm. In particular, the otic capsule should be examined for fistula.

Tegmen defects should be identified, both for their diagnostic significance and surgical planning. The absence of the tegmen at the cortex must be recognized prior to revision surgery to avoid dural injury during initial exposure of the mastoid defect. Tegmen defects deep within the temporal bone indicate progressive disease if such defects were not present after the initial procedure. The fallopian canal should be examined to determine possible facial nerve exposure. Although it is difficult to identify dehiscence precisely, especially of the horizontal segment, the proximity of soft tissue or bone erosion near the fallopian canal should alert the surgeon to the possibility of facial nerve exposure during the revision procedure. The status of the ossicular chain may be implied by identification of the structures on CT scan, but the presence of soft tissue surrounding the ossicles in most cases produces averaging artifact that makes positive identification of ossicular continuity impossible.

CANAL WALL UP OR DOWN

When confronted with a revision mastoid procedure, the most important decision to be made by the surgeon is whether to preserve or remove the posterior canal wall. The differences between CWU and canal-wall-down (CWD) procedures should not be minimized. Hearing loss, aftercare, and the caloric effect produced by the exposed bony labyrinth are major drawbacks to the CWD procedure. On the other hand, a well-done CWD procedure results in a safe, dry ear, whereas a well-done CWU mastoidectomy may result in recurrent cholesteatoma or mastoiditis. The challenge for the surgeon is to recognize those factors that should alert the surgeon to perform the one procedure that will result in a successful outcome, that is, that obviates the need for another revision procedure in the future.

The clues that will direct the surgeon to perform a CWU procedure or a CWD procedure can be found preoperatively on the physical exam and in the location and extension of disease intraoperatively. Any signs of cholesteatoma on physical exam that would indicate the need for a second procedure after the initial revision should prompt the surgeon to consider performing a CWD procedure. Such situations include cholesteatoma extending into the external auditory canal, filling the middle ear space with extensive granulation tissue, visualized in a perforation with extension medial to the remaining tympanic membrane, or impacted in the posterior-superior quadrant with or without scutal erosion. The appearance of a granulation polyp in the external auditory canal invariably indicates that cholesteatoma is present medial to the polyp. Retraction of the tympanic membrane, with or without an attic defect, is a sign of eustachian tube dysfunction. Eustachian tube dysfunction is an indication for CWD surgery because the ultimate result of poor middle ear aeration is retraction and development of cholesteatoma.

The challenge for the surgeon arises when the degree of retraction at the time of surgery is minimal or even moderate. In such instances it may be difficult for the surgeon to determine whether eustachian tube function is poor but stable, or whether the eustachian tube dysfunction is progressive and so will result in further retraction as time passes. If the moderate retraction is found in a recently operated ear, the likelihood is that the retraction will continue and CWD surgery should be considered. Slight or even moderate retraction in an ear operated on 10 to 15 years earlier would suggest a more stable middle ear condition that would more likely benefit from a CWU procedure. Complete retraction of the tympanic membrane with drainage is an indication for a CWD procedure. The size of the attic defect can also dictate the need for a CWD procedure. Complete attic retraction after an initial CWU procedure warrants a CWD procedure, but if the complete retraction had not been addressed in the initial mastoid procedure, a revision CWU procedure may be considered. A wide atticotomy with partial removal of the posterior canal wall often contributes to chronic drainage after the initial mastoid procedure. Only by converting the ear into a CWD mastoid defect can drainage be controlled in this situation.

In other circumstances, the decision to preserve or remove the posterior canal wall can be made only when cholesteatoma is uncovered during surgery. Cholesteatoma in the middle ear is the most common site for development of recurrence. The sinus tympani region is traditionally the area most mentioned for possible recurrence, but extension of cholesteatoma into the hypotympanum must also be considered. Both of these regions are accessible through a facial recess or extended facial recess exposure, but full exposure is not possible. A CWD procedure affords better exposure of both regions, and so with extensive disease, the CWD procedure is indicated. Residual cholesteatoma is often found anterior to the cochleariform process and anterior to the cog in the anterior epitympanum, abutting the semicanal of the tensor tympani. This region can usually be exposed by a CWU procedure with disarticulation of the incus and amputation of the head of the malleus. In poorly pneumatized temporal bones, removal of the posterior canal wall may be necessary to exenterate all disease in this area. Other situations that warrant a CWD procedure in revision mastoidectomy include cholesteatoma infiltrating the perilabyrinthine air cells, petrous apex extension of cholesteatoma, and fistulization of the bony labyrinth.

SURGICAL TECHNIQUE OF REVISION MASTOIDECTOMY

The initial surgical approach in revision mastoidectomy is not dependent on whether a CWU or CWD procedure is to be performed. The ear canal should be injected and a vascular strip should be outlined as in an initial tympanomastoidectomy. The postauricular incision should be carried down through the previous incision. If extensive scar tissue or keloid formation is present, the scar should be excised. A plane over the temporalis muscle should be identified and temporalis fascia should be harvested. This is often easiest recognized by dissection posterior and superior to the mastoid defect to identify a plane over the temporalis fascia free of scar tissue and following this plane anterosuperiorly to obtain an adequate piece of fascia for grafting. A T incision is next made in the musculoperiosteal layer over the mastoid defect. Prior to making the incision, the blunt end of a knife handle or a Freer dissector should be used to palpate for bone over the tegmen region to avoid penetrating through the dura on the incision. The vertical incision over the mastoid defect should be done in layers, with occasional blunt palpation to avoid entering an exposed sigmoid sinus. In most revision mastoid cases, the musculoperiosteum is scarred into the mastoid defect. The periosteum can be elevated from the mastoid bone with a Freer dissector. It is easiest to develop a plane between the bone and periosteum above the sinodural angle, insinuate the dissector between the undrilled mastoid cortex and periosteum, and sweep the dissector into the mastoid defect to separate the fibrous bands holding the periosteum into the previously dissected mastoid region. At times the scarring within the mastoid is quite thick, and in these cases, once the periosteal thickness has been identified posteriorly, the fibrous tissue can be sharply dissected from the musculoperiosteal flap, leaving the adherent tissue in the mastoid to be removed when drilling begins.

Once mastoid retractors are placed, attention should be directed to the middle ear and ear canal. The canal is inspected for cholesteatoma or erosion. If a large attic defect is present, surface debridement may be carried out, but complete removal of all disease should be avoided. If a perforation is present, the margins of the perforation should be freshened and all granulation tissue removed. If present, the remaining tympanic membrane should be elevated from the posterior tympanic ring so that the middle ear space can be inspected. The annular ligament should be elevated into the anteroinferior quadrant to allow complete visualization of the hypotympanum. Superiorly the tympanic membrane is elevated out of the notch of Rivinus (or any attic defect if present), away from the neck of the malleus, and often detached from the handle of the malleus to provide complete exposure of the anterosuperior portion of the tympanum. All disease should be removed from the tympanum, except the posterosuperior quadrant. Epinephrine-soaked Gelfoam is packed into the middle ear for hemostasis. The posterosuperior quadrant should now be inspected. Any disease, whether granulation tissue or cholesteatoma, should be debulked, the presence or absence of ossicles confirmed, and Gelfoam placed.

The technique for bone dissection in a revision mastoid procedure does not depend on whether a CWU or CWD procedure is the ultimate goal. The middle cranial fossa dura should be identified along the tegmen, and the tegmen plate should be skeletonized, removing all air cells in the process. The sinodural angle is opened to remove any residual air cells and the sigmoid sinus is skeletonized, removing any diseased air cells overlying the sinus. Most often in revision cases, the mastoid tip air cells are infected, and thorough drilling down to the digastric ridge must be carried out. The lateral semicircular canal should be identified by removing any granulation tissue or cholesteatoma from it. In the case of cholesteatoma, the possibility of a fistula must always be considered. Perilabyrinthine disease should be removed, and skeletonization of the labyrinth is often necessary. Once the lateral semicircular canal has been identified, soft tissue disease and involved air cells should be removed to identify any ossicles within the epitympanum. If chronic mucosal disease without cholesteatoma is present in the epitympanum, disease removal can continue in this region, carefully working over the horizontal segment of the facial nerve into the middle ear.

If cholesteatoma is present in the epitympanum, the middle ear, or the mastoid region, a facial recess approach must be started at this point. This is accomplished by first identifying the vertical segment of the fallopian canal. Especially in severely diseased ears, the safest method to identify the vertical segment begins by following the digastric ridge to the stylomastoid foramen, and then progressing proximally toward the lateral semicircular canal. If a facial recess approach has been previously performed, careful dissection with a smooth diamond drill along the vertical segment will identify the fallopian canal without injury to the nerve. Once the fallopian canal has been identified in the vertical segment, the chorda tympani nerve is located, usually about 5 mm from the stylomastoid foramen.

Using progressively smaller diamond burs, the facial recess is opened between the chorda tympani and the fallopian canal. The facial recess now provides access to the posterior middle ear space and actually allows for easier exposure of the anterior epitympanum.

Once the facial recess has been opened, the decision regarding the necessity of a CWD procedure can be made. A labyrinthine fistula greater than 2 mm, unretrievable cholesteatoma in the sinus tympani, petrous apex cholesteatoma, cholesteatoma tracking between dura and tegmen plate, extensive posterior canal wall destruction, and recurrent cholesteatoma after well-performed two-stage procedures indicate the need for removal of the canal wall. Recurrent cholesteatoma may take two forms. The most obvious form is the presence of cholesteatoma matrix in the mastoid or middle ear space regardless of the status of the tympanic membrane. The more difficult situation arises when a severe retraction pocket occurs after an initial CWU procedure. This retraction pocket generally involves the attic region and/or the sinus tympani/facial recess region and indicates poor eustachian tube function. Such a retraction will ultimately result in the development of cholesteatoma, and so the appropriate procedure to eliminate the need for future procedures is to perform a CWD mastoidectomy.

Removal of the posterior canal wall requires little time once a facial recess approach has been performed. A small rongeur may be used to remove the canal wall quickly. The most important aspect of the CWD procedure is to make the transition from the anterior tympanic ring to the mastoid as smooth as possible. This involves removal of any remnants of the canal wall inferiorly and superiorly that might serve as an area for accumulation of keratin once the ear has healed. Especially superiorly, this "transition zone" requires removal of attic air cells so that the anterior canal wall blends into the plane of the tegmen tympani region. The purpose of the CWD procedure is to make the middle ear and mastoid regions continuous so that reepithelialization of the defect is uniform, and the possibility of accumulation of keratin debris is reduced. The mastoid bowl should be saucerized to allow the auricle to lie closer to the skull, which reduces the amount of reepithelialization that must occur in the mastoid defect. The decision to graft the middle ear space depends on the extent of cholesteatoma in the middle ear, especially the sinus tympani. In the vast majority of cases, removal of the canal wall results in complete removal of cholesteatoma from the sinus tympani by improving visualization, allowing for grafting of the middle ear to occur. In cases of unresectable cholesteatoma, usually involving penetration into the petrous apex, the middle ear should remain open to aid in follow-up care and debridement.

COMPLICATIONS OF REVISION MASTOIDECTOMY

Complications associated with revision mastoid surgery are the same as in an initial mastoid procedure, but the incidence of complications is higher due to the increased anatomic distortion caused by the previous surgery or residual disease. The surgeon must therefore maintain a disciplined approach to performing the revision procedure to avoid complications. As in any mastoid procedure, the surgeon should identify systematically important structures within the temporal bone in this order: middle fossa dura, sigmoid sinus, lateral semicircular canal, ossicles within the epitympanum, and the facial nerve. Such a disciplined identification of these structures eliminates most complications in revision surgery.

Facial nerve injury is the most likely complication associated with revision mastoid procedures.[1] Facial nerve monitoring may be helpful in avoiding such complications, but a successful outcome is most dependent on the surgeon's knowledge of temporal bone anatomy. Although the most common location of injury is at the second genu in initial procedures, in revision cases injury in the horizontal segment due to preexisting dehiscence of the fallopian canal is more likely. Such injury occurs during removal of disease around the lateral semicircular canal and oval window regions. The key to avoiding facial nerve injury revolves around early identification of the fallopian canal during the revision procedure. Once the lateral semicircular canal and any remaining ossicles in the epitympanum have been identified, attention should be directed to identification of the vertical segment of the facial nerve. Especially in severely diseased mastoids and previous facial recess exposures, the safest way to identify the vertical segment of the fallopian canal is to first dissect out the digastric ridge in the mastoid region. Following the digastric ridge anteriorly will lead to the stylomastoid foramen. The fallopian canal can then be uncovered at the stylomastoid foramen and followed along the vertical segment to the lateral semicircular canal. In revision facial recess cases, there is often disease or fibrosis present in the facial recess. By identifying the whole vertical segment, the surgeon can remove this disease with direct visualization of the integrity of the fallopian canal.

Identification of the fallopian canal in the vertical segment also helps the surgeon avoid injury to the horizontal segment. In revision cases, the likelihood of disease in the oval window region is almost guaranteed, and the possibility of a dehiscent facial nerve is extremely high. Injury to the nerve occurs when the surgeon has not recognized the nerve, so careful identification of the nerve distal to the disease aids in facial nerve preservation. Working, therefore, from the second genu, the surgeon should carefully dissect disease away from the fallopian canal, paying attention to the integrity of the fallopian canal. By focusing on the relationship of the lateral semicircular canal ampulla, the cochleariform process, the horizontal segment of the fallopian canal, and the oval window and the footplate or stapes superstructure (if present), the surgeon should be able to identify any dehiscence of the fallopian canal and dissect disease away from the exposed facial nerve. It is highly unlikely that complete removal of cholesteatoma from an exposed facial nerve cannot be accomplished using this technique.

The horizontal segment of the facial nerve is then followed to the geniculate ganglion region using high-power magnification. In most cases the geniculate ganglion is not dehiscent, but in well-pneumatized temporal bones, disease may be infiltrating into this region. Important landmarks during dissection in this region include the tegmen tympani, the ampullated region of the superior semicircular canal, and the cochleariform process.

Cerebrospinal fluid (CSF) leak is an unusual event. This is usually iatrogenic, being caused by overaggressive use of a cutting bur on the tegmen plate, but it may occur due to dural erosion secondary chronic inflammation or cholesteatoma. Iatrogenic injury may occur during the incision of the temporalis muscle as the T incision is made at initial mastoid exposure. This type of injury is easily avoided by palpation of the temporalis muscle with the blunt end of the knife handle prior to making the incision. Damage to the dura with resultant CSF leak is more common with the otologic drill. This complication usually occurs because the surgeon has failed to identify the middle cranial fossa dura plate at the onset of the revision mastoidectomy.

Tearing the dura in this manner may result in parenchymal hemorrhage, so care must be taken to examine the area for any bleeding prior to repair. CSF leak caused by removal of disease occurs when the disease has eroded through the dura completely and is contacting pia arachnoid. Removal of the disease invariably tears the delicate pia arachnoid, producing the CSF leak. This type of leak rarely is associated with bleeding, and can be overlooked if it is not a brisk leak.

Repairing the tegmen plate defect with hydroxy-apatite cement can effectively control CSF leaks.[2] A neurosurgical pledget should be placed over the defect until the procedure has been completed. The reconstruction of the tegmen defect should be done prior to the tympanoplasty. The tegmen plate should be removed around the site of the leak, and the dura around the defect cauterized with a bipolar. This will shrink the dura and allow better exposure of the defect. Hydroxyapatite cement is applied over the defect with a Freer dissector, and the cement is applied widely over the tegmen plate as well to stabilize the hardening of the cement in the defect. Gentle compression with neurosurgical pledgets aids in hardening of the cement prior to performing the tympanoplasty and wound closure. If paren-chymal bleeding was present at the time of the dural injury, CT of the brain should be performed on the first postoperative day to rule out significant hemor-rhage.

A tear of the sigmoid sinus is another complica-tion that may occur on reexposure of the mastoid defect. Blunt palpation of the scarred musculoperi-osteal layer should be performed before any incision is made. Whether using a cautery or knife, the vertical arm of the T incision should be made in layers rather than plunging directly through the soft tissue. Often bleeding is encountered during this incision; it should be controlled with a bipolar cautery as the posterior portion of this flap is elevated out of the mastoid. If the sinus is entered, direct compression should be applied, avoiding suctioning directly into the defect. Oftentimes appli-cation of bone wax controls the bleeding. If bleeding persists, a large piece of Gelfoam should be com-pressed over the site of injury with a neurosurgical pledget. Any bone or fibrosis surrounding the defect can then be removed to assess the extent of injury to the sigmoid sinus. Serial compression and gentle bipolar cautery of the sinus control small tears. Larger tears may require a small vascular suture followed by application of Gelfoam. If the defect is large, extraluminal obliteration may be necessary to control the hemorrhage. If injury to the sigmoid sinus has occurred, it is inadvisable to perform a CWD procedure.

Sensorineural hearing loss and vertigo are com-plications that can occur if there is violation of the perilymphatic space. Inadvertent opening of a labyr-inthine fistula is the most common cause of this type of complication. Once the mastoid defect is opened, any granulation tissue should be removed carefully over the labyrinth with a blunt dissector. If choles-teatoma is present, the matrix should be first palpated with a gimmick or sickle knife to identify a small bone defect. Using high-power magnification and a 20-gauge suction, the cholesteatoma matrix should be slowly rolled away from the labyrinth, being watchful for a blue line, which denotes a prefistulous condition. If a fistula smaller than 2 mm is identified, the matrix overlying the fistula may be removed and a piece of soft tissue immediately placed over the fistula. Care must be taken not to suction over the fistula once the matrix has been removed. Fistulas larger than 2 mm must be mana-ged by leaving the matrix over the fistula and converting the mastoid procedure to a CWD proce-dure.[3] Cochlear fistulas should be managed simi-larly, although the removal of matrix should be performed in a more conservative fashion.

Inadvertent damage to the footplate or round window membrane is another cause for violation of the perilymphatic space. Round window mem-brane injury is rare, because in most cases the round window membrane is thickened due to inflamma-tion associated with the chronic middle ear disease, and so it is less prone to injury. The footplate region, on the other hand, is more prone to injury. Often granulation tissue is impacted into the oval window region, with the tissue adherent to the footplate itself. Dissection of this granulation tissue or choles-teatoma from the oval window region may disrupt the annular ligament of the footplate, removing the footplate with the granulation tissue. This may lead to a dead ear unless quick action is taken. A 20-gauge suction should be used on the margin of the oval window only to keep blood from entering the vestibule, and a piece of fascia should be placed immediately over the oval window. A piece of Gelfoam may be placed over the fascia and removal of remaining disease from the middle ear can be completed. Ossicular reconstruction can be per-formed just as if a footplate were still present.

POSTOPERATIVE CARE

Postoperative care varies depending on whether the canal wall has been preserved. In a CWU procedure, the patient returns in 3 weeks for debridement of the external auditory canal. Under the operating micro-scope any crusting is removed from the ear canal, and evidence of infection is noted. The tympanic membrane is inspected with removal of any debris. Antibiotic otic drops are used if infection is present. Only in the case of extensive canal swelling should oral antibiotics be considered. Water precautions are continued for 6 weeks, when the second visit occurs. An audiogram is performed at this time to assess hearing. If the ear canal and tympanic membrane are healed, water precautions are lifted and the patient is allowed to fly and resume all activities. Patients are evaluated at 3-month intervals for the first year, and then annually for the next 2 years.

Postoperative management of a CWD procedure is more intensive. If packing was used in the mastoid defect, the patient returns in 1 week for packing removal and instillation of a broad-spectrum antibiotic ointment into the mastoid defect. In this case and in cases in which ointment was used at the time of surgery, the patient returns in 2 to 3 weeks for mastoid debridement. At this time crusting and granulation tissue in the mastoid bowl is removed under the operating microscope. The neomembrane over the middle ear is manipulated minimally. The mastoid defect is painted with gentian violet for its bacteriostatic effect. Antibiotic otic drops are used two to three times per day for the next 2 weeks, and this routine is continued until the mastoid bowl reepithelializes. Acetic acid washes may be substituted for antibiotic drops, especially when granulation tissue is minimally purulent. The reepithelialization process usually takes 8 weeks. Once the cavity has healed, an audiogram should be performed to assess residual hearing. Long-term follow-up after a CWD mastoidectomy usually requires annual visits.

SUMMARY

Revision mastoid surgery requires careful planning to achieve a successful outcome. Computed tomography is a necessary tool to identify factors that contribute to recurrence of disease, to avoid complications, and to decide to preserve the posterior canal wall. Knowledge of the surgical anatomy of the temporal bone is the key to a safe and successful surgical procedure.

REFERENCES

1. Kveton JF. The facial nerve in revision mastoid surgery: avoiding complications. *Oper Tech Otolaryngol Head Neck Surg* 1992;3:69–72.
2. Kveton JF, Goravalingappa R. Control of CSF otorrhea using hydroxyapatite cement. *Laryngoscope* 2000;110: 1116–1119.
3. Gacek RR. The surgical management of labyrinthine fistula in chronic otitis media with cholesteatoma. *Ann Otol Rhinol Laryngol* 1974;83:1–19.

Chapter 12

RECONSTRUCTION OF THE POSTERIOR EAR CANAL

Peter S. Roland and Joseph L. Leach

The canal-wall-down (CWD) mastoidectomy finds favor with otologists primarily for one reason: the technique reduces the risk of persistent or recurrent cholesteatoma. Whether one takes the posterior canal wall down or not, there is a significant incidence of epithelial pearls that remain behind and can form the nidus of new disease.[1] These pearls may or may not cause clinically detectable findings. Smythe[1] reported that recurrent cholesteatoma from a retraction pocket occurred in 14% of intact canal-wall ears as compared with 1% of ears treated with mastoid obliteration and tympanic reconstruction. He concluded that the best way to reduce the incidence of cholesteatoma complications to the greatest possible degree long-term was to remove the posterior canal wall.

Nevertheless, after a CWD mastoidectomy, a patient is left with several problems inherent in the open cavity. The exposed bone of the mastoid leaks tissue fluid, which is a rich medium for bacterial growth. Unlike other areas of the head and neck, the mastoid, and in particular the sclerotic mastoid, is not particularly well vascularized.[2] The combination of mediocre blood supply and weeping tissue fluid means that control of bacterial ingrowth can be challenging. Not only may healing be marginal or delayed, but also the patient may need to avoid moisture for life. Recurrent aural discharge afflicts 10 to 60% of patients with an open mastoid cavity.[3,4] Other complications, such as perichondritis of the pinna, have been reported.[4] It is widely taught that the incidence of discharge or other infectious complications can be minimized by lowering the facial ridge, making the cavity large, and providing a generous meatal opening,[3] but these maneuvers also have their drawbacks. For one, hearing aids are often required in these patients. Although it is undesirable to fit a hearing aid in a discharging

mastoid cavity, it is also a problem to construct a mold for an enlarged meatus.[3,5] In addition, lowering of the facial ridge may decrease the depth of the middle ear space, which makes ossicular reconstruction difficult and hearing less than optimal.[6] Although a large meatus may reduce the incidence of postoperative drainage, it is often cosmetically unappealing (Fig. 12–1). A large mastoid cavity can draw the pinna inward, causing a noticeable deformity of the auricle. It may also draw the medial concha inward and displace the pinna laterally.

The dizziness associated with caloric stimulation is another drawback of a large open mastoid, and patients sometimes have to limit their exposure to water and wind. The ear loses its natural ability to clean itself, and wax and squamous debris build up over time. A foul smell can develop, which can be an irritation and source of embarrassment. In most cases, the mastoid bowl needs to be cleaned on a routine basis every 6 to 12 months. Water exposure can lead to infection. This is especially disappointing to patients who wish to swim regularly. In fact, it is not the size of the cavity that is crucial. In a comparative study, ears with a small open mastoid bowl have fared no worse than those with an obliterative flap.[1] It is believed that the critical issue is the adequacy of the meatal opening as determined by the ratio of the meatal circumference to the volume to the mastoid cavity. One must have an opening sufficient to allow free circulation of air.

Therefore, many reasons exist not only for CWD mastoidectomy, but also for reconstruction of the posterior ear canal and obliteration of the mastoid. Hearing aids are easier to fit into an obliterated cavity than into an open cavity. The obliterated cavity is also more likely to retain its epithelial migratory potential and be self-cleaning because it is smaller.[3] Obliteration of the mastoid cavity leaves a smaller

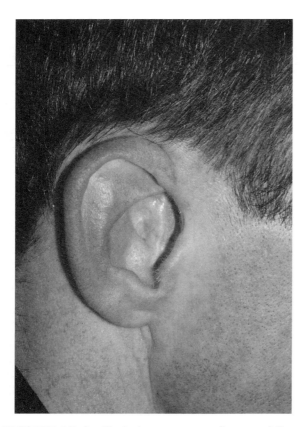

FIGURE 12–1 Typical appearance of an ear following canal-wall-down mastoidectomy with large meatoplasty.

surface area. Healing is therefore theoretically faster, and there is a reduced likelihood of developing granulations. Obliteration has been shown to significantly reduce the symptoms associated with the open mastoid. In a survey of patients with recurring mastoid disease, groups were treated either with revision mastoidectomy or obliteration.[3] The preoperative symptom scores were not significantly different, but the patients treated by obliteration had a significantly lower postoperative symptom score.[3] Some recommend mastoid obliteration as a routine procedure in all mastoid surgery.[7]

Nevertheless, mastoid obliteration should not be undertaken lightly, because it carries a risk of enclosing cholesteatoma within the cavity. Computed tomography (CT) may or may not be effective in detecting these residua. A study was conducted in cadaver temporal bones in which cholesteatoma pearls were covered either with hydroxyapatite or muscle.[8] Scanning was effective in detecting small pearls within the cavity obliterated with hydroxyapatite, but not so effective when muscle was used. In practice, however, obliteration has been safe. When CT was performed on 31 ears after mastoid obliteration with hydroxyapatite, there was no residual

cholesteatoma in the obliterated area.[8] A muscle flap may have an advantage over hard tissue replacement because an epithelial cyst may present as a swelling beneath the flap.

Mastoid obliteration may be contraindicated if there has been removal of a malignant tumor, if there are otogenic intracranial complications, if cholesteatoma has not been totally removed, or when air cell removal has been incomplete.[9] Although there are many options for mastoid obliteration, all depend on a rich blood supply for success. Well-vascularized flaps are the best options when there has been extirpative surgery for cancer or osteoradionecrosis.

The goal of reconstruction of the posterior external auditory canal is to provide a safe, dry mastoid and restore hearing to near-normal levels. No single procedure has yet been devised that entirely accomplishes these purposes consistently. Various materials have been used to fill the mastoid, including fascia, fat, muscle, cartilage, bone paste, cancellous bone strips, bioactive glass ceramics, Proplast (a combination of polytetrafluoroethylene and glassy carbon fibers) methylmethacrylate, and ionomer-based bone substitutes.[5] Most biologic tissues have a tendency to atrophy over time, and some otologists recommend overfilling the cavity to compensate for the expected loss of the volume of the obliterating tissues over time.[10] Because the final shape and size of the obliterated mastoid cavity cannot be predicted, using biologic tissues for obliteration can be a drawback.

The earliest obliteration techniques involved flaps of local tissue. One of the early methods was that of Mosher[11] in 1911. He used soft tissues from the back of the auricle and pedicled toward the temporalis muscle. Mosher always performed a simple mastoidectomy first, and then lowered a greater part of the posterior canal wall, leaving a bridge of bone external to the aditus in place. Popper[12] described another early method in which he used periosteum to line the mastoid. He made a postauricular incision through the skin and subcutaneous tissues, retracting the posterior skin flap as far back as possible. He then made a horseshoe-shaped incision through the periosteum, creating an anteriorly based flap. Popper's aim was not to entirely obliterate the cavity but to provide a viable lining with good blood supply to facilitate healing. Meurman and Ojala[13] described filling the lower part of the cavity by using an inferiorly and caudally based postauricular musculoperiosteal flap. Guilford[14] attempted a more complete obliteration by combining the Meurman and Ojala flap with a superiorly pedicled postauricular flap.

These early flaps all demonstrated variable viability and some atrophy of tissue over time. In an effort to provide more consistent and longer-lasting results, Palva[15] in the early 1950s began using a meatally based musculoperiosteal flap for obliteration and simultaneous reconstruction of the posterior canal wall. This flap retained the essential form of Popper's flap but included all the tissues between the skin and bone. For the Palva flap, the skin incision is made 1.0 to 1.5 cm behind the postauricular fold to facilitate liberation of the tissues posteriorly (Fig. 12–2). The horseshoe-shaped incision includes all the subcutaneous tissues from the retroauricular area down to the bone, theoretically preserving the facial nerve branches to the postauricular muscles and forestalling atrophy of the tissues.[7,15] The flap could be made broad and long to allow obliteration of even large mastoid cavities.

Despite its good viability, the Palva flap demonstrated gradual atrophy in patients over years of follow-up. New methods of obliteration were sought. The soft tissue flaps mentioned above are all based on a random-pattern blood supply. If they are raised with a length-to-width ratio of greater than 1:1, ischemia of the distal portion is a risk, and subsequent necrosis and contraction of the flap would result in inadequate coverage and fill of the cavity.[4] Another drawback to these local flaps is that they rarely have sufficient bulk or plasticity to completely line and fill a large mastoid.[4] Another flap used to obliterate the mastoid has been the temporalis muscle flap, which is pedicled anteriorly.

Experience has shown that these flaps have a tendency to undergo atrophy, and the majority shrink down to the point that the resulting cavity is as large as it was originally.[9] This is probably because the muscle becomes denervated and the blood supply becomes compromised, making the flap in effect a free muscle graft.[4]

In an effort to overcome such problems, practitioners have advocated the use of vascularized temporalis fascia. Both the deep and superficial temporalis fascia have been used. The deep temporalis fascial flap, "the Hong Kong flap," is based on the middle temporal artery. It is thin, strong, and pliable, with more than adequate surface area to line the entire mastoid cavity.[16] Its proponents claim that because it is translucent in nature, detection of recurrent disease is not compromised.[16] Although the flap is adequate for achieving a healthy dry ear, it does not completely obliterate the mastoid or reconstruct the posterior canal wall.

The superficial temporalis or temporoparietal fascial flap is a good option for mastoid obliteration. The flap is thin, pliable, and can accept skin grafts.[17] It also provides enough bulk for the obliteration of large mastoid defects.[17] To avoid compression on the pedicle of the flap when it is rotated into the cavity, the middle fossa dura can be skeletonized above the ear canal at the ridge formed by the root of the zygomatic arch.[4] A vertical incision is made through the scalp in the temporal area. Dissection is carried out just deep to the hair follicles, and bipolar cautery is used to avoid damage to the vessels. Care must be

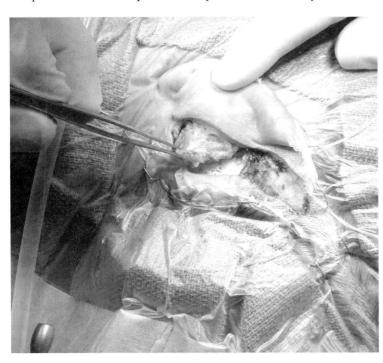

FIGURE 12–2 The Palva flap.

taken not to damage the frontal branch of the facial nerve. The flap incorporates an area of temporoparietal fascia 8 × 7 cm.[4] A small absorbable tacking suture is used to anchor the flap to the temporalis muscle so that it will not pull away from the mastoid cavity. The temporoparietal fascia flap has shown its utility in patients who have undergone partial temporal bone resection for the treatment of a variety of neoplasms and revision surgery for chronic otitis media.[17] In these cases, the standard pedicled muscle and periosteal flap reconstruction was not possible due to scarring, radiation damage, and disruption of vascularity resulting from previous surgery.[17] Because the flap does not contain muscle, it should not shrink, but experience shows that some shrinkage can occur.[4,18]

Because vascularized tissue may not provide adequate long-term obliteration of the mastoid cavity and secure reconstruction of the posterior ear canal, biologic and nonbiologic implants have been used to afford bulk and stability. Fat grafts to the mastoid were first described in the late 1940s, but consistent success was not reported in subsequent articles.[19] Guilford[20] found that diced cartilage was effective in reducing the size of fenestration cavities, but not helpful following mastoidectomy for chronic otitis media. Dornhoffer[6] has had success using cartilage for partial mastoid obliteration. Mastoid disease is removed, and the cavity is contoured. Cartilage is harvested from the concha and the meatus, and perichondrium is included. The cartilage is pressed and morcellized with a scalpel. Obliteration is carried out only to the level of the facial ridge. Although reconstruction of the posterior auditory canal and complete mastoid obliteration were not attempted, problems with an open mastoid such as drainage or debris collection were ameliorated. After 2 years, it appeared that the cartilage became well incorporated into the mastoid, and ingrowth of fibrous tissue took place between the cartilage chips, which increased the volume of obliteration.[6] Dornhoffer thought that the contour of the cavity was more critical than the amount of obliteration achieved. One disadvantage with this technique is that the amount of cartilage that can be obtained from the concha and tragus is limited. The use of autogenous iliac bone strips for cavity obliteration has been reported to be successful, but problems in resorption of the bone grafts were reported.[18,21] There is associated incapacitating pain at the donor site, and prolonged bed rest of 12 to 14 days was recommended.[18,21]

A simpler method of adding bulk to the reconstruction is to collect bone chips and bone paste during the mastoidectomy. To avoid collecting any cholesteatoma matrix or infected tissue, it is important to collect the bone before entering the diseased portion of the mastoid. Along with a large cutting bur and continuous irrigation and suction, the paste is collected in a specialized bone paste collector or in an ordinary trap bottle connected to the suction tubing within the sterile field.[18,22] Covering the walls of the mastoid with bone paste may inhibit the process of transudation of tissue fluid and reduce the risk of subsequent infection.[3] In addition to bone paste, bone chips from the mastoid have been used. Guilford[20] reported using bone chips taken from the mastoid for obliteration prior to 1957. He felt that they acted as foreign bodies, however, and discontinued their use. Despite Guilford's experience, others have continued to use native bone fragments with better results.[23] Bone fragments are mixed with either fibrin glue[24] or bone paste[15] to add stability. Some advocate keeping periosteum to the bone chips to enhance survival.[15,25] With this technique, a new bony posterior canal has been observed after 6 to 8 weeks.[25] To harvest the bone, undermining is carried out posteriorly, allowing removal of cortex over a broad area with a chisel.[25] Bone from the mastoid tip can be removed by a rongeur. Removing bone in this area has the added benefit of allowing the mastoid cavity to partially collapse.

Reconstructing the posterior ear canal with an autogenous, bilaminar membrane (soft wall reconstruction) has also been described.[26] This method, unlike others, allows inspection of the underlying cavity for residual or recurrent disease due to the fact that the soft canal wall is semitransparent. The canal is reconstructed in such a way as to allow aeration of the mastoid from the middle ear. A large fascia graft is draped from the tympanic membrane underneath the posterior canal skin, which is preserved (Fig. 12–3). The mastoid cavity is packed with gelatin foam, which supports the fascia graft. Laterally, a Palva flap underlies and supports the fascia. Over 2 years, retraction of the posterior canal wall was observed in about half the cases, but functional results were good.[26] In some of these cases, significant eustachian tube dysfunction persisted and the soft wall retracted into the mastoid defect, but the ear usually remained dry. The resulting cavity tended to be smaller than the classic modified radical mastoidectomy cavity.[26] The technique is not recommended for patients with extremely small, sclerotic mastoids or for those with aggressive cholesteatomas involving multiple small cell tracts, or if there was hypertrophy of the mucosa of the protympanum.[26]

The mastoid contains not only bone but also air. Intuitively, it would seem difficult, at best, to restore

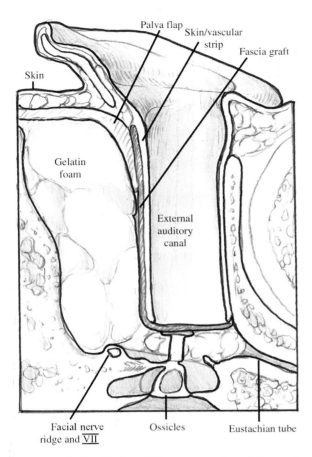

FIGURE 12–3 "Soft wall" reconstruction of the posterior canal.

the entire volume of the mastoid by replacing only the native bone, whether that would be in the form of paste or chips, and given that it could be collected efficiently and free of disease. Adding local cartilage grafts might help, but their volume is limited as well. Fascia, fat, and muscle are often not sufficiently bulky or long lasting to sufficiently reconstruct the posterior canal in the long term. In the past this problem was dealt with by use of homograft cartilage and bone, but the fear of transmitting infectious diseases, especially AIDS, has curtailed their use.[6] Citing the fact that obliteration of the mastoid with bone makes sense because it utilizes the material natural to the area, Shea et al[27] used bone chips from the femoral heads in bone banks. They broke the bone up into chips about 3 mm in diameter, and applied a layer of autogenous bone paste to the surface of the bone chips to develop a hard smooth surface on the new posterior canal wall. It resulted in a canal wall with a natural texture and appearance. Guilford[20] used heterogeneous bone paste for mastoid obliteration, but found it to be unsatisfactory. These experiences with homograft

tissues laid the groundwork for the later use of allografts.

Most alloplastic implant materials, such as plastic mesh, Proplast, and porous polypropylene, have not been successful long-term due to difficulties in the face of infection.[5,28] Although there was initial enthusiasm for Proplast, it was subsequently discovered that the material caused a lasting giant cell reaction.[28] Antibiotics could not clear the infection when the organisms became harbored in the pores.[29] A two-stage tympanoplasty was necessary so that the area could be relatively sterile. Postauricular fistulas, persistent drainage, and purulent granulation tissue led to gradual disuse of plastics.[2] The mastoid bone is a problematic site for alloplasts because it is devoid of cancellous bone and its stem cells and has marginal vascularity.[2] An implant that elicits a marginal foreign body reaction cannot stimulate neovascularity by intimation in such an environment.[2]

Hydroxyapatite is the main constituent of living bone and is a natural choice as a bone substitute for mastoid obliteration and canal-wall reconstruction. The use of hydroxyapatite avoids donor-site morbidity and is well tolerated in an infected field. Ideally, it osseointegrates into surrounding bone, leaving a stable canal wall that does not retract with time. Because hydroxyapatite is bioactive, graft failure and extrusion in the long term should not be observed. Unlike bone paste, there is no risk of implanting cholesteatoma. Hydroxyapatite has been used in four different forms, including granules, cement, preformed canal-wall prostheses, and in a block form, which is sculpted to fit the individual defect. The most common complication that accompanies the use of hydroxyapatite is incomplete covering of the material with viable tissue in the healing phase.[23]

Hydroxyapatite cement, unlike granules, can be confined relatively easily to the operative site. The cement comes as a powder that is mixed with sterile water and hardens within 20 minutes.[30] Risk to the surrounding tissue is minimal, because the reaction is essentially isothermic and occurs at a physiologic pH.[30] Hydroxyapatite cement is microporous, with a pore size of approximately 8 to 12 μm.[30] When implanted in a subperiosteal location, new bone formation occurs.[30] When exposed to cerebrospinal fluid or blood, conventional hydroxyapatite cement takes a long time to set, but this can be reduced to 5 to 8 minutes when the calcium phosphate powder is mixed with a phosphate solution instead of water.[31] The material was used in a series of 21 patients, including two involving the mastoid, with no complications.[31] With a mean follow up of 15 months, there were no infections or extrusions.

Blocks of ceramic hydroxyapatite share the excellent tissue compatibility and osseointegrative potential found with hydroxyapatite granules and cement. The blocks, however, are brittle, and the material is difficult to contour. Sculpting the blocks takes additional operating room time. Nevertheless, sculpted hydroxyapatite blocks were used in a series of nine patients with 78% success.[5] There was one failure due to granulation and one due to stenosis. Canal-wall reconstruction with the preformed hydroxyapatite prostheses should overcome the problem of sculpting encountered with hydroxyapatite blocks. Nevertheless, the prostheses generally do require some amount of shaping. Instability has also been a problem.[5] This is especially true when attempting to reconstruct a previously drilled radical cavity when the tegmen and the inferior tympanic bone were smoothed appropriately. In these cases, a notch can be drilled in the zygomatic area to stabilize the prosthesis. Although some prefer hydroxyapatite reconstruction at a second stage if the ear is free of cholesteatoma,[32] others implant the material at the time of mastoidectomy.[5,33] Reconstruction of the posterior canal with the hydroxyapatite prosthesis without obliteration is possible, but there is the risk that retraction will occur and that the hydroxyapatite will cut through the skin of the auditory canal.[33]

When reconstructing the posterior ear canal at the time of CWD mastoidectomy, it is helpful to leave the facial ridge high, if this is possible without compromising disease eradication. The high facial ridge acts as a posterior margin for the obliteration and helps to retain the obliteration material. As a general rule, one should ensure that the middle ear is sealed off with a temporalis fascia graft.[18] If a CWD mastoidectomy is already present, the flap of skin that used to line the mastoid cavity is used to line the reconstructed posterior ear canal wall. The edge of the mastoid cavity is then identified, and the skin lining is carefully elevated forward to a point just short of the facial ridge. Any excess or poor-quality skin is excised. Filler (bone chips, bone paste, hydroxyapatite granules, or hydroxyapatite cement) is then placed into the mastoid cavity, behind the skin flap and fascial lining, so as to fill the cavity and leave an ear canal of near-normal size (Fig. 12–4).

When using hydroxyapatite granules, Yung[10] advocates covering them with an inferiorly based periosteal flap that can incorporate temporalis fascia at its superior margin. He also recommends soaking the granules in an antibiotic solution for 10 minutes. When a hydroxyapatite canal-wall prosthesis is used, it should be burred to the exact size using a diamond bur. One should then fashion a groove in

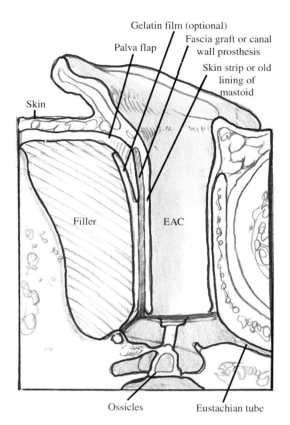

FIGURE 12–4 A typical method of reconstructing a posterior ear canal. EAC, external auditory canal.

the residual bony buttresses, which allows for dovetailing of the prosthesis and stabilizing it. Estrem and Highfill[5] recommend covering the prosthesis with fascia and skin or fascia or homograft dura. Grote[32] recommends covering the canal-wall prosthesis at the canal side with a cranial-based periosteal flap, which is then covered by the vascular strip and the tympanomeatal flap. In the case of previous CWD mastoidectomy, the mastoid lining and a vein graft are used anterior to the periosteal flap.[28] Gelatin film is placed on the other side of the prosthesis. Grote and Van Blitterswijk[28] warn that if the periosteal flap is not used, and if poor attention is paid to the epithelial remnants, there can be erosion between the implant and the bony canal.

Postoperatively, the principles of wound care that are followed with other otologic procedures make good sense for the patient who has undergone posterior ear canal reconstruction. A good postauricular closure and a mastoid dressing are used. Although there is some argument that keeping packing in place for 3 weeks may allow better epithelialization than removing the packing at the usual 7 to 10 days,[23] one has to keep in mind the possibility of overgrowth of organisms in the dressing. Eardrops are generally used to maintain an acidic pH in the ear, prevent infection, and promote rapid healing. When granulation tissue forms in the ear canal postoperatively, it is sometimes necessary to treat these patients with application of dilute silver nitrate solution.

When implants are used in the mastoid along with a flap, there is always the possibility that partial or total loss of the flap could occur or that the implant could become exposed. These complications seem to be more common if obliteration is attempted in an old open mastoid.[4,23] Local wound debridement, cleaning, and otic drops may alleviate the problem, but occasionally reoperation is necessary. Retraction pockets and recurrent cholesteatomas are occasional reported complications of the various obliteration techniques described.[5,33]

Experience has shown that with long-term follow-up, random, muscle, and fascia flaps undergo atrophy, retraction, and fibrosis.[18,22] Temporal muscle flaps in particular tend to retract away from the cavity and do not form good support of the canal wall.[15] Despite the claim to contain innervated muscle, the Palva flap atrophies over time. Over a 13-year period, mastoid volumes were noted to increase significantly in cavities obliterated by this method.[1,9,33] Nevertheless, retraction pockets and other hidden cavities were uncommon.[33] Significantly, no recurrence of cholesteatoma was seen in more than 2000 ears that used the flap.[15]

With obliteration with bone chips alone, a significant increase in the cavity size has been observed long-term.[33] Some of these lost their self-cleaning ability and had to be taken care of as radical cavities.[33] Obliteration with bone paste, on the other hand, has demonstrated decrease of the cavity size due to osteoneogenesis.[34] Obliteration of the mastoid with hydroxyapatite granules has shown greater than 85% long-term success.[5,10] Water has been tolerated in the cavities in most patients, and the majority report no aural discharge or need to use eardrops.[10] Long-term success with hydroxyapatite canal-wall prostheses is a bit lower, at about 75%.[5,32] Although extrusion and recurrent cholesteatoma may compromise the implant, the main cause of failure in one series was recurrent middle ear infection.[32] When the implants are retrieved, they tend to show good remodeling with living bone tissue.[32] Retroauricular fistulas have occurred with hydroxyapatite prostheses, one appearing 3 years postoperatively.[33] Nevertheless, the general rule is that the cavities remain dry long-term.[33]

Because CWD mastoidectomy continues to be a commonly performed procedure, the open cavity will continue to pose problems. Mastoid obliteration and reconstruction of the posterior canal eliminate many of these problems in a majority of patients. Techniques that incorporate well-vascularized tissues into the area will continue to supplant those that do not. Exciting new materials, particularly the several forms of hydroxyapatite, hold great promise in restoring these patients to better function and appearance.

REFERENCES

1. Smythe DL. Cholesteatoma surgery: the influence of the canal wall. *Laryngoscope* 1985;95:92–96.

2. Hambley WM, Horn KL. Failure of Proplast in mastoid obliteration. *Am J Otol* 1981;2:286–288.

3. Irving RM, Gray RF, Moffat DA. Bone pâté obliteration or revision mastoidectomy: a five-symptom comparative study. *Clin Otolaryngol* 1994;19:158–160.

4. East CA, Brough, MD, Grant HR. Mastoid obliteration with the temporoparietal fascia flap. *J Laryngol Otol* 1991;105:417–420.

5. Estrem SA, Highfill G. Hydroxyapatite canal wall reconstruction/mastoid obliteration. *Otolaryngol Head Neck Surg* 1999;120:345–349.

6. Dornhoffer JL. Surgical modification of the difficult mastoid cavity. *Otolaryngol Head Neck Surg* 1999;120:361–367.

7. Palva T. Mastoid obliteration. *Acta Otolaryngol Suppl* 1979;360:152–154.

8. Yung MMW, Karia KR. Mastoid obliteration with hydroxyapatite: the value of high resolution CT scanning in detecting recurrent cholesteatoma. *Clin Otolaryngol* 1997;22:553–557.

9. Shea MC, Gardner G. Mastoid obliteration using homograft bone. *Arch Otolaryngol* 1970;92:358–365.

10. Yung MW. The use of hydroxyapatite granules in mastoid obliteration. *Clin Otolaryngol* 1996;21:480–484.

11. Mosher HP. A method of filling the excavated mastoid with a flap from the back of the auricle. *Laryngoscope* 1911;21:1158–1163.

12. Popper O. Periosteal flap grafts in mastoid operations. *S Afr Med J* 1935;9:77–78.

13. Meurman Y, Ojala L. Primary reduction of large operation cavity in radical mastoidectomy with muscle-periosteal flap. *Acta Otolaryngol* 1949;37:245–252.

14. Guilford FR. Obliteration of the cavity and reconstruction of the auditory canal in temporal bone surgery. *Trans Am Acad Ophthalmol Otolaryngol* 1961;65:114–122.

15. Palva T, Makinen J. The meatally based musculoperiosteal flap in cavity obliteration. *Arch Otolaryngol* 1979;105:377–380.

16. Soo G, Tong MCF, van Hasselt CA. How I do it: mastoid obliteration and lining using the temporoparietal fascial flap. *Laryngoscope* 1997;107:1674.

17. Cheney ML, Megerian CA, Brown MT, et al. Mastoid obliteration and lining using the temporoparietal fascial flap. *Laryngoscope* 1995;105:1010–1013.

18. Moffat DA, Gray RF, Irving RM. Mastoid obliteration using bone. *Clin Otolaryngol* 1994;19:149–157.

19. Del Canizo SR. Radical surgical treatment of the ear with implantation of free fat grafts. *Rev Clin Esp* 1949;34:403–408.

20. Guilford FR. Controlled cavity healing after mastoid and fenestration operations. *Arch Otolaryngol* 1960; 71:165–171.

21. Schiller A. Mastoid osteoplasty, obliteration of mastoid cavity using autogenous cancellous bone: final progress report. *Arch Otolaryngol* 1963;77:475–483.

22. Shea MC, Gardner G, Simpson ME. Mastoid obliteration using homogenous bone chips and autogenous bone paste. *Trans Am Acad Ophthalmol Otolaryngol* 1972;76:160–172.

23. Minatogawa T, Machizuka H, Kumoi T. Evaluation of mastoid obliteration surgery. *Am J Otol* 1995;16: 99–103.

24. Tokoro K, Chiba Y, Murai M, et al. Cosmetic reconstruction after mastoidectomy for the transpetrosal-presigmoid approach: technical note. *Neurosurgery* 1996;39:186–188.

25. Palva T. Operative technique in mastoid obliteration. *Acta Otolaryngol* 1973;75:289–290.

26. Smith PG, Stroud MH, Goebel JA. Soft-wall reconstruction of the posterior external ear canal wall. *Otolaryngol Head Neck Surg* 1986;94:355–359.

27. Shea MC, Gardner G, Simpson ME. Mastoid obliteration with bone. *Otolaryngol Clin North Am* 1972;5:161–172.

28. Grote JJ, Van Blitterswijk CA. Reconstruction of the posterior auditory canal wall with a hydroxyapatite prosthesis. *Ann Otol Rhinol Laryngol Suppl* 1986; 123:6–9.

29. Janeke JB, Shea JJ. Proplast implants used in otology and in facial reconstructive surgery. *S Afr Med J* 1976;50:781–783.

30. Friedman CD, Constantino PD, Takagi S, et al. Bone-Source™ hydroxyapatite cement: a novel biomaterial for craniofacial skeletal tissue engineering and reconstruction. *J Biomed Mater Res* 1998;43:428–432.

31. Costantino PD, Chaplin JM, Wolpoe ME, et al. Applications of fast-setting hydroxyapatite cement: cranioplasty. *Otolaryngol Head Neck Surg* 2000;123: 409–412.

32. Grote JJ. Results of cavity reconstruction with hydroxyapatite implants after 15 years. *Am J Otol* 1998;19:565–568.

33. Gyllencreutz T. Reconstruction of the ear canal wall using hydroxylapatite with and without mastoid obliteration and by obliteration with bone chips. *Acta Otolaryngol Suppl (Stockh)* 1992;492:144–146.

34. Ojala K, Sorri M Sipila P, et al. Late changes in ear canal volumes after mastoid obliteration. *Arch Otolaryngol* 1982;108:208–209.

Chapter 13

PEDIATRIC TYMPANOMASTOIDECTOMY

Weiru Shao and Frank Rimell

Treating chronic otitis media in the pediatric population remains a major challenge. Recent advances in microbiologic evaluation and antimicrobial development provide accurate identification and effective eradication of most of the offending organisms. Nevertheless, recurrent ear infection and failure of medical management continue to require surgical intervention. In addition, cholesteatoma, congenital malformations, and cochlear implantation are some of the other indications for pediatric tympanomastoidectomy.

The operative details of pediatric tympanomastoidectomy do not vary significantly from those of adult. Yet, special factors in pediatric ear surgery need to be considered preoperatively. Although tympanomastoidectomy implies a canal-wall-up (CWU) technique, canal-wall-down (CWD) mastoidectomy (also termed modified radical mastoidectomy) is briefly discussed.

GOALS AND TYPES OF SURGERY

Most ear surgeons are conservative in operating pediatric chronic ears for these reasons:

1. The disease processes in the pediatric patients are different from those in adults. Spontaneous improvement of chronic otitis media in an adult is uncommon, whereas it is the norm for young children to improve with age. It is frequently feasible to "buy time" with medical management and CWU procedures to wait for a child to become immunologically competent and their eustachian tubes to function better.[1]
2. In children less than 2 years old, the facial nerve is anatomically more vulnerable and risky in radical ear surgeries.[1]

3. A child's young age and future lifestyle dictate that the surgeon choose procedures that will last 70 years or longer and will endure the punishment of adolescent sports and sometimes swimming.
4. Minimal postoperative care is a major consideration in selecting types of ear procedures, as frightened children may not cooperate.
5. Young children themselves cannot consent to surgery. It may be prudent to delay an elective operation with significant risk and complication until adulthood.

FACIAL NERVE ABNORMALITY

A discussion of the facial nerve embryology is beyond the scope of this chapter. Nevertheless, certain points are worth stressing. The facial nerve and many ossicular parts, notably the stapedial crura, the manubrium of the malleus, and the long arm of the incus, are derived from the second branchial arch. Malformation in one may suggest defect in another.[2]

The occasional ear surgeon is more likely to operate on ears with minor malformations or with no apparent abnormality at all. Such operations actually pose a greater risk of facial nerve injury than do operations on major malformations because the surgeon may not suspect congenital abnormality. During a routine middle ear or mastoid exploration, extra caution must be paid to dissect "fibrous tissue bands" or "adhesions," because they may actually represent a dehiscent and aberrant facial nerve. During the preoperative period, subtle or "soft" signs, such as abnormal-looking auricles, preauricular pits, a short and blunt malleus, and small tympanic membrane, should alert the surgeon to a congenitally abnormal ear. In children with identifiable congenital middle ear malformations, expect facial nerve abnormalities. Intraoperatively, to avoid facial nerve injury, be suspicious of any soft tissue tubular structure regardless of its location.[3]

Keen observation skills, quality imaging modalities, and a thorough knowledge of temporal bone embryology and anatomy are critical in preventing facial nerve injury. The surgeon must understand malformation-related variants of nerves and vessels to avoid catastrophic events. Jahrsdoerfer and Hall[4] reported that 24% of ears with congenital anomalies of the middle ear had an aberrant course of the facial nerve.

Types of Congenital Malformations of the Facial Nerve

In the middle ear, two most common facial nerve anomalies are nerve displacement (Fig. 13–1) and fallopian canal dehiscence. The nerve may be found at the level of the promontory and covered only by respiratory mucosa. It may be found inferior to or at the level of the stapes or oval window. Sometimes the stapes superstructure ends blindly in the soft tissue substance of the facial nerve. The facial nerve may also bifurcate around an intact stapes, and the split nerve may or may not remain separate (Fig. 13–2). Discovering a malformed stapes during the operation should immediately alert the surgeon that the facial nerve could be out of position. If the oval window is absent, in almost 80% of the cases there is facial nerve displacement.[5] Lastly, an uncovered and displaced facial nerve may be found in association with a congenital cholesteatoma.

An inferiorly displaced facial nerve may conceal the round window. It is recommended not to transpose the facial nerve simply to locate the round window. If an oval window is present, hearing preservation procedures should be attempted. It is uncommon to encounter an absent round window as an isolated anomaly. If an oval window is absent, a round window may or may not be present. If an oval window is present, a round window is almost always present.[3]

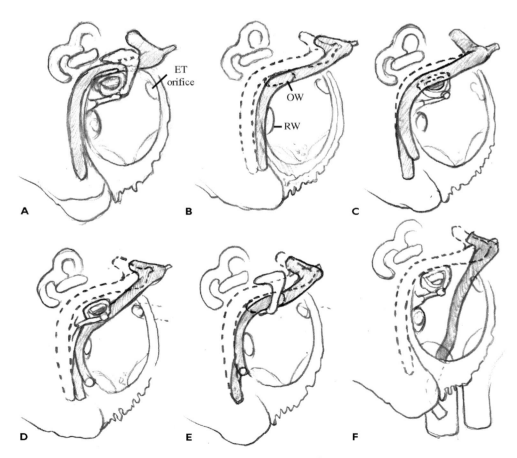

FIGURE 13–1 (A–F) Patterns of facial nerve displacement in congenital middle ear malformations. ET, eustachian tube; OW, oval window; RW, round window.

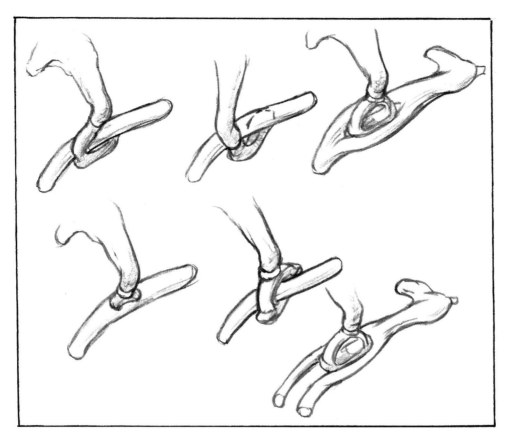

FIGURE 13–2 Patterns of stapes malformations in relation to facial nerve associated with congenital middle ear malformation.

Finding a large chorda tympani nerve warrants a pause and reappraisal of the operative condition. It is best not to sacrifice any large chorda tympani nerve because it may be the real facial nerve with a sharp anterior and lateral curving feature. At least it may herald an abnormal facial nerve. Electrical stimulation is of no diagnostic value as the chorda tympani nerve propagates the electrical stimulation to the facial nerve. The mastoid portion of the facial nerve almost always migrates anteriorly with external and middle ear anomalies.[3]

OSSICULAR ABNORMALITY

Ossicular anomalies without malformation of the external ear have been classified into three groups: malleus and/or incus fixation, incudostapedial disconnection, and stapes fixation. Combinations of these anomalies may occur and may be associated with facial nerve and otic capsule anomalies. Isolated ossicular chain malformations are often bilateral, especially in familial cases of congenital ossicular malformations. The most commonly in-

volved ossicle is the stapes; least commonly, the malleus.[6]

VASCULAR ABNORMALITY

The most significant vascular malformation is the aberrant internal carotid artery (ICA). The ICA is separated from the tympanic cavity by a thin (less than 0.5 mm) bony carotid plate. Rarely, this plate is dehiscent. A second abnormality is the persistent stapedial artery. There may or may not be an associated aberrant ICA. A third abnormality is a dehiscent jugular bulb that may protrude into the middle ear cavity.

OPERATIVE CONSIDERATIONS

PREOPERATIVE TESTS

1. Audiometry is always needed. In general, postoperative air–bone gaps are larger than preoperative ones when the stapes superstructure is involved by diseases. Though rare, operation

on the wrong ear has happened. Therefore, verify the correct ear to operate upon with the audiogram immediately before the surgery.

2. Although not a prerequisite for tympanomastoidectomy, a thin-cut computed tomography (CT) scan of the temporal bone is routinely ordered as part of the preoperative evaluation at our institution. It helps to detect defects such as scutal erosion, labyrinthine fistula, tegmen defects, disease involvement of the ossicles, and invasion or anomalies of the fallopian canal. However, CT scans do not distinguish granulation tissue, cholesteatoma, and effusion, and do not reliably determine the full extent of the disease. Therefore, the surgeon and the patient or parents all have to be prepared for intraoperative surprises.

3. Some inner ear anomalies can also be detected on CT. Inner ear defects like a wide internal auditory canal (IAC) (>10 mm in diameter), enlarged vestibular, or cochlear aqueduct predispose patients to a perilymphatic gusher during cochlear implantation. Absence of the IAC is a contraindication for cochlear implantation.

4. Magnetic resonance imaging (MRI) scanning is indicated if there is suspicion of disease involvement or invasion of the dura, sub- or epidural abscess, brain tissue herniating into the mastoid, invasion of the membranous labyrinth or facial nerve, or sigmoid sinus thrombosis.

INTRAOPERATIVE MONITORING

Facial nerve injury is the most feared complication of pediatric ear surgery. Although many ear surgeons do not think that intraoperative facial nerve monitoring is necessary, we consider it of potential benefit and routinely use it. It is almost impossible to predict an impending complication in either simple or complicated cases, such as revision operations, previous facial nerve palsy, and congenital anomalies. Using the nerve monitor on a regular basis not only provides a safety net but also offers psychological comfort to surgeons in training. On the other hand, relying solely on the nerve monitor for facial nerve identification is dangerous, as it often does not function or is not connected properly. Therefore, positive visual identification of the facial nerve and using the nerve stimulator for confirmation is the best way to avoid facial nerve injury.

After placing the surface electrodes for the nerve monitor, adjust the alarm volume. Test the function of the monitor by gently tapping the electrode and checking the alarm (no muscle paralytic agent should be used beyond this point).

TYMPANOMASTOIDECTOMY

The surgical technique of tympanomastoidectomy is summarized in this section. It would be helpful to review other chapters and illustrations in this book to compare different surgical approaches.

PREPARING THE EAR

Currently most surgeons use a postauricular incision for chronic ear disease. Exposure of the anterior middle ear, mastoid cavity, and facial recess is excellent with this approach. It can also be converted to a CWD procedure with minimal difficulty. After general anesthesia is instituted, the operated ear is positioned facing up. To improve the postauricular exposure, the hair above and behind the ear may be shaved or taped down. Under the operating microscope, wax is cleaned from the ear canal. Using a 3-cc syringe with Luer-Lok and a 25- or 27-gauge needle, 1% lidocaine with 1:100,000 epinephrine is injected into the bony–cartilaginous junction. With the largest speculum that fits the ear canal pressing firmly on the bony canal, the injected solution is directed medially toward the tympanic membrane (TM). During this process of hydrodissection, steady pressure from the syringe is more important than the volume of the injectant. When the injection is properly carried out, the needle sweats with condensation and the total volume injected at all four quadrants is less than 1 cc.

Then postauricular incision is also injected. Remember that the maximum amount of lidocaine with epinephrine to be injected in a child is 7 mg/kg. In children younger than 3 years of age, the mastoid tip may not be fully developed. As the facial nerve exits the stylomastoid foramen, it is immediately deep to the subcutaneous tissue underlying the skin. To avoid injury to the nerve, the postauricular incision should be placed more posterior and away from the mastoid tip (Fig. 13–3). As the mastoid tip and tympanic ring develop, the nerve takes a deeper position. In a young adult the nerve is protected by the mastoid tip, tympanic bone, and the fascia between the parotid and cartilaginous external canal. The postauricular incision may be placed at the auriculomastoid crease (Fig. 13–4). It is a good practice to place the surgeon's finger over the mastoid tip in a child, and between the mastoid and the angle of the mandible in a young adult, to provide added protection for the facial nerve. Excessive local anesthetic injection near the mastoid tip may render the facial nerve monitor nonfunctional during the operation.

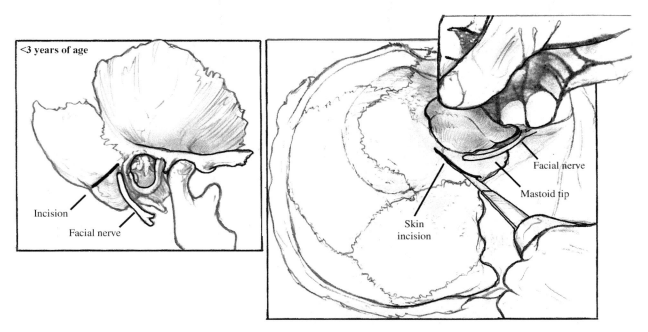

FIGURE 13–3   Postauricular incision in children younger than 3 years of age. (A) The facial nerve is immediately deep to the subcutaneous tissue underlying the skin. (B) To avoid injury to the nerve, the incision should be placed away from the mastoid tip.

The skin and the ear are prepped with sterilizing agent while the surgeon washes his or her hands.

SOFT TISSUE INCISION

After the ear is properly draped, the ear canal is irrigated with saline and suctioned. Using a No. 72 Beaver blade the canal incision is made from the 12 o'clock position to the 6 o'clock position down to the bone 5 to 10 mm from the annulus. When severe TM retraction is present, there is a tendency to overestimate the annulus medially. With an annulus elevator the precise location of the bony annulus can be palpated before the incision is made. Although a long tympanomeatal flap is usually appreciated, a flap that is too long may interfere with middle ear exposure. Using a sickle canal knife or No. 66 Beaver blade, the incision is extended laterally at the 12 o'clock and 6 o'clock positions. Gelfoam soaked with 1:1000 epinephrine is placed in the canal for hemostasis while attention is turned to the postauricular incision.

Again, to provide protection for the facial nerve the postauricular incision needs to be modified in a child (Fig. 13–3); the surgeon's finger is placed over the mastoid tip or, in a young adult, between the mastoid and the angle of the mandible. After the incision is carried through the postauricular muscle, the pinna is lifted laterally to improve visualization of the superficial layer of the deep temporalis fascia. Blunt dissection with a finger can be used to expose the mastoid, the temporalis line, and the zygomatic root. If a tympanoplasty is planned later, either an areolar or a true fascia graft can be harvested over the temporalis muscle.

Using a Bovie, a curved T incision is made at the inferior border of the temporalis line, which is the insertion site of the temporalis muscle. Cutting into the temporalis muscle causes excessive bleeding and is to be avoided. Inferiorly as the T incision approaches the mastoid tip, place a finger over the mastoid tip to protect the facial nerve. The soft tissue including periosteum is elevated off the mastoid cortex with a Lempert elevator. Such a multilayered approach prevents postauricular depression postoperatively.

After the posterior canal is exposed, the canal skin flap is gently elevated off the posterior canal wall. A Penrose drain is placed around the posterior canal skin flap and reflected anteriorly to protect and retract the flap. The Penrose drain is clamped to the drape.

REMOVAL OF MASTOID CORTEX

Using a 4- or 5-mm cutting bur, the mastoid cortex is removed in a systemic fashion, moving from one landmark to another. The suction and irrigation setup is the same as in adult surgery. The first cut is made immediately posterior to the *spine of Henle* along the *posterior canal wall* between *Macewen's triangle* and the *mastoid tip*. The second cut

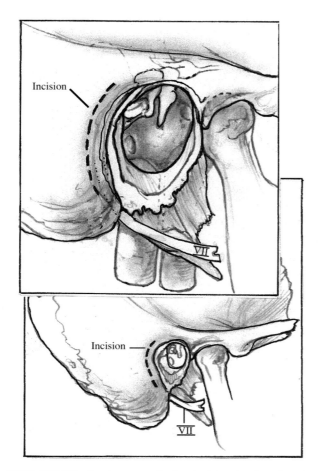

FIGURE 13–4 A postauricular incision is placed at the auriculomastoid crease in a young adult. The facial nerve is protected by the mastoid tip, tympanic bone, and the fascia between the parotid and cartilaginous external canal.

draws along the *temporalis line* toward the sinodural angle perpendicular to the first. The third cut connects the first two along the posteroinferior border of the mastoid. The mastoid cortex within the triangle is then removed superficially over the tegmen and sigmoid sinus but deeper at the Macewen's triangle where the mastoid antrum lies underneath.

Starting from the Macewen's triangle and drilling along the temporalis line, the tegmen is identified and delineated. Dissection parallel to a given landmark with a large bur is a safe technique. An eggshell-thin layer of bone needs to be preserved along the tegmen and sigmoid sinus.

CAVITY SAUCERIZATION

Wide cortical exposure is the key to adequate angular visualization of critical underlying struc-

tures. Failure to do so causes a bothersome constriction of the cavity at the medial level. Constricted dissection obscures critical landmarks and invariably leads to surgical failure and complication.[7] The mastoid cortex should be removed slightly beyond the sigmoid sinus posteriorly and the tegmen superiorly. The lateral portion of the posterior canal wall should be thinned. The sinodural angle is a common place for disease recurrence if residue air cells are inadequately removed. It has earned the name of "the angle of sorrow."

The mastoid tip in a child is often poorly developed and the facial nerve may be more superficial than the surgeon thinks. A few superficial passes by the drill to remove the cortex is usually adequate dissection for the mastoid.

ENTERING THE MASTOID ANTRUM

Dissection is concentrated at the junction of the posterior canal and the zygomatic root. After *Körner's septum* is breached, the *lateral semicircular canal (SCC)* should be identified before further dissection proceeds. When there is significant mucosal edema and concurrent mastoiditis, it may be difficult to visualize the lateral SCC. Using a curette, a small amount of trabecular bone, mucosa, and debris can be removed to identify the lateral SCC.

With a smaller bur, the tegmen is followed anteriorly and medially next to the zygomatic root. The antrum needs to be enlarged to allow adequate attic flow. The limit of anterior dissection is the *long crus of incus*. The *fossa incudis* is a useful landmark for facial recess.

MIDDLE EAR EXPLORATION

Using a weapon or No. 2 canal knife, the tympanomeatal flap is elevated up to the annulus. With a No. 2 canal knife firmly against the bony canal, the annulus and a few millimeters of mucoperiosteum of the middle ear are lifted off the bony annulus. A Rosen needle or a sickle knife is used to tear the mucoperiosteum and enter the middle ear space near the hypotympanum. With the retraction of suction tip held by the other hand, the tear in the mucoperiosteum is widened and the middle ear space is further exposed. Special care must be taken to prevent injury to the chorda tympani nerve posteriorly, the ossicles at the posterior superior quadrant, and the round window at the posterior inferior quadrant. The tympanomeatal flap is then laid anteriorly, leaving the attic widely exposed.

The integrity and the mobility of the ossicles are examined. Cholesteatoma is best removed en bloc to prevent recurrence. If ossicular erosion occurs, the decision of either a primary or staged ossicular reconstruction can be made based on the extent of the disease. Cholesteatoma at the attic and the sinus tympani can be removed using a Worlibur. To improve attic exposure, an atticotomy can be performed using a small bur or a curette. Irrigation water is placed in the middle ear and the mastoid. Free flow of water between the middle ear and the mastoid needs to be established to ensure adequate postoperative ventilation of the mastoid.

If a tympanoplasty is planned, the tympanic perforation is first postage-stamped and a rim of squamous tissue surrounding the perforation is removed with a cup forceps (this procedure is easier to perform before the tympanomeatal flap is elevated). The middle ear is packed with Gelfoam soaked with ofloxacin, or ciprofloxacin and hydrocortisone, to maintain the middle ear space. With the underlay technique, the previously harvested temporalis fascia graft can be placed under the tympanomeatal flap as far anterior to the perforation as possible. After the tympanomeatal flap is laid back onto the graft, a small amount of adjustment can be made through the perforation to ensure complete coverage of the perforation by the graft. Other options include lateral graft or a combination of the medial and the lateral technique.

If ossicular chain reconstruction is indicated, a primary or secondary operation can be carried out. The decision to delay ossicular reconstruction is often made on the basis of the severity of the disease encountered at the time of primary cholesteatoma removal. If the mucosa is edematous or is removed in a large amount, postoperative scarring and retraction are more likely to occur. Staging a reconstruction is more prudent. If a second exploration is planned, delaying the reconstruction is also appealing. If there is concern about eustachian tube dysfunction and postoperative aeration, it is often better to wait and see if an adequate middle ear space has developed and that the tympanic membrane has healed before the reconstruction. Our preference is to wait 18 months prior to reconstruction.

FACIAL RECESS

The facial recess is bordered superiorly by the fossa incudis, medially by the facial nerve, and laterally by the chorda tympani (Fig. 13–5). It occasionally allows the extension of middle ear disease into the mastoid other than from the antrum. Opening the facial recess provides additional mastoid aeration. In cochlear implantation the electrode is inserted into the cochlea through the facial recess.

The surgeon may begin drilling along an imaginary line between the digastric ridge and the horizontal SCC. The fossa incudis is a consistent and reliable landmark for identifying the level of the facial recess. Understanding that the facial nerve is most vulnerable at its second genu and at its proximal descending portion, light strokes of the bur are used at this area. The microscope is turned up in power, and copious irrigating fluid (preferably warmed to body temperature to maximize conduction to the nerve monitor) is used to flood the facial recess. It allows clear and constant visualization of the operating field and minimizes thermal injury to the facial nerve from the high-speed drill. Generally

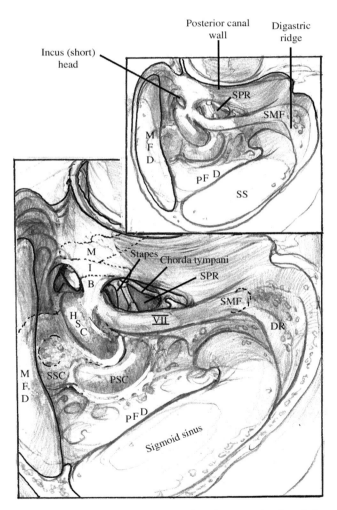

FIGURE 13–5 Approach to facial recess in the right mastoid. SPR, suprapyramidal recess; CTN, chorda tympani nerve; VII, facial nerve; SMF, stylomastoid foramen; SSC, superior semicircular canal; HSC, horizontal semicircular canal; PSC, posterior semicircular canal; B, buttress (bridge); MFD, middle fossa dura; PFD, posterior fossa dura.

a diamond bur is used to work around the nerve to allow slow but more precise thinning of the fallopian canal. A thin layer should be preserved over the facial nerve if no nerve work is intended.

Inferiorly, the nerve is skeletonized distally toward the mastoid tip to locate the take-off of the chorda tympani nerve. After it is detected, the chorda is followed into the middle ear, taking care not to disrupt the annular ridge laterally. The widest portion of the facial recess rarely exceeds 3 mm. It is necessary to use a smaller bur at this point.

With the facial recess widely opened, middle ear structures can be clearly identified. The incudostapedial joint, the capitulum of the stapes, the stapedial tendon, the round window, and the cochleariform process can be observed and checked for disease involvement.

CANAL-WALL-DOWN MASTOIDECTOMY

When compared to CWU mastoidectomy, a CWD procedure offers a lower rate of recurrent cholesteatoma at the expense of an enlarged meatus, frequent canal cleaning, difficult fitting of hearing aids, and occasional problems with water exposure. An additional disadvantage in a growing mastoid of a child is that future mastoid air cells are surgically sequestrated and may lead to suppuration due to a lack of ventilation and an inability to clean.[1]

When CWD mastoidectomy is indicated, the posterior border of the ear canal is to be removed. The medial border of the dissection is the floor of the facial recess, which is the lateral wall of the fallopian canal at the external genu. After the sigmoid sinus and middle fossa tegmen are skeletonized, the fossa incudis and horizontal SCC are identified. The anterior buttress, where the posterior auditory canal meets the tegmen, is removed to open up the epitympanum to the mastoid antrum. Next, the facial nerve is delineated by lowering the facial ridge laterally. The posterior buttress is where the posterior canal wall meets the floor of the auditory canal lateral to the facial nerve. It has to be removed well to open up the mastoid tip. The final step is an adequate meatoplasty. Considering future scar contraction, it needs to be at least twice its future size.

The removed posterior canal wall can be reconstructed in the future with a variety of material, including bone graft or synthetic bone substitutes. It has been successfully accomplished in children by the second author.

COMPLICATION MANAGEMENT

The most common facial nerve trauma is the injury to the epineurium with consequent neural edema and nerve herniation. As soon as the injury is recognized, bone overlying the nerve should be removed 5 to 6 mm both proximally and distally to the site of the injury. The epineurium may also be incised to reduce pressure on the nerve. Postoperative steroid is indicated.

Fenestrating the semicircular canal is more likely to happen in an inflamed or sclerotic mastoid. As soon as it is recognized, the mastoid should be filled with body temperature normal saline, and suctioning over the open semicircular canal is avoided. Plugging the fenestration with either bone wax or muscle fascia needs to be accomplished as soon as possible. Temporalis fascia is then used to cover the damaged semicircular canal.

Tearing the sigmoid sinus causes significant bleeding and possibly air embolism. The patient is placed in the reverse Trendelenburg position immediately. The tear should be covered with Surgicel and neurosurgery cottonoid. If bleeding continues, continuous pressure can be applied over the cottonoid. For a large tear, surgical repair with vascular sutures (5-0 Prolene) or in combination with fascial plug may be necessary.

Laceration of the tegmen can be closed with fascial plug if small. A rent larger than 1 cm is best closed with surgical sutures with or without fascia.

SUMMARY

Pediatric tympanomastoidectomy is a common procedure performed by general and pediatric otolaryngologists. Although the operative details of pediatric ear surgery are much alike those of adults, disease pathophysiology and suspicion for congenital malformation are the main reasons to pay special attention to the goal of the surgery and intraoperative observation.

REFERENCES

1. Kenna MA. Treatment of chronic suppurative otitis media. *Otolaryngol Clin North Am* 1994;27:457–470.
2. Gasser RF, May M. Embryonic development. In: May M, Schaitkin BM, ed. *The Facial Nerve.* 2nd ed. New York: Thieme; 2000:1–17.
3. Hashisaki GT, Jahrsdoerfer RA. The facial nerve and the congenitally malformed middle ear. In: May M, Schaitkin BM, ed. *The Facial Nerve.* 2nd ed. New York: Thieme; 2000:505–513.

4. Jahrsdoerfer RA, Hall JW. Congenital malformations of the ear. *Am J Otol* 1986;7:267–269.

5. Jahrsdoerfer RA. Congenital absence of the oval window. *Trans Am Acad Ophthalmol Otol* 1977; 84:904–914.

6. Briggs R, Luxford WM. Correction of conductive hearing loss in children. *Otolaryngol Clin North Am* 1994;27:607–620.

7. Nelson RA. *Temporal Bone Surgical Dissection Manual.* Los Angeles: House Ear Institute; 1991.

Chapter 14

SURGERY FOR CONGENITAL CHOLESTEATOMA

Norman N. Ge and Karen J. Doyle

Congenital cholesteatoma of the ear is cholesteatoma developed behind an intact tympanic membrane when there is no history of aural infections. House[1] first reported congenital cholesteatoma in 1953. In 1963 Cawthorne[2] postulated the congenital origin of some cholesteatomas, citing from a single case. Derlacki and Clemis[3] proposed the clinical criteria for the diagnosis in 1965. House and Sheehy[4] advocated a surgical approach for management of congenital cholesteatomas in 1980.

ORIGIN

Congenital cholesteatoma is thought to be of embryologic origin and many theories were proposed to explain the different clinical presentations. Cushing[5] suggested that many of the cholesteatomas reported by otologists were likely true dermoids originating from epidermal rests laid down in the temporal bone during embryologic development of the ear. Depending on the location of the epidermal rests, cholesteatomas may appear in the middle ear, the mastoid region, the petrous pyramid, and the cerebellopontine angle (CPA). Congenital cholesteatoma of the middle ear is the most common type. The squamous epithelial mass is found in the anterosuperior quadrant of the tympanum at the junction of the mucosa of the eustachian tube and the mucosa of the middle ear, which is the reported site of the embryologic epithelial rest. Sanna and Zini[6] suggested that congenital middle ear cholesteatoma arose from epidermal cells trapped in the posterior mesotympanum during embryologic development. This explains why the posterior mesotympanum is where congenital cholesteatoma is the most commonly presented.

Paparella and Rybak[7] proposed that ectodermal implants occurred in the fusion planes of the first and second branchial arches, which resulted in the development of epidermoid in the middle ear and other areas of the temporal bone. Michaels[8] theorized that the epidermoid formation appears early in embryonic life arising from the ingrowth of ectodermal cells from the first branchial groove, where it joins the first pharyngeal pouch. At this early primal stage of development, ectoderm and endoderm of the groove and pouch lie in close proximity to each other without intervening mesenchymal cells. Then the epidermoid formation precursor buds off from the first groove ectoderm and takes a position attached to the pharyngeal pouch.

Aimi[9] proposed that congenital cholesteatoma occurs in the middle ear because of migration of external canal ectoderm during middle ear development. Under normal circumstances the tympanic ring inhibits or restricts ingrowth of ectoderm from the external canal into the middle ear. Should this mechanism fail, migration of keratinizing epithelium into the middle ear might result in the formation of a congenital cholesteatoma.

Weber and Adkins[10] reported three cases of congenital cholesteatoma in the tympanic membrane. The authors postulated the squamous epithelial basal layer proliferation as a cause for intramembranous cholesteatoma of the tympanic membrane. If treatment is delayed, the cholesteatoma may extend into the middle ear.

PATIENT PRESENTATION

Congenital cholesteatoma is usually noted in young children. It is more common in males, with a near 3:1 preponderance in several reports.[11–13] The mean age of presentation is 4.5 years.[11–13] Doyle and Luxford[14] reported 60 cases of congenital cholesteatomas. In 24 patients, cholesteatoma was limited to the mesotympanum, 18 ears had cholesteatoma located in both the mesotympanum and epitympanum, and two patients had disease limited to the epitympanum. In 16 ears, there was extensive cholesteatoma in the mesotympanum, epitympanum, and mastoid. Classically there is no prior history of otorrhea, perforation, or otologic surgical procedures. Preoperative symptoms and signs are predominantly conductive hearing loss. Frequently, when the cholesteatoma is small, it is asymptomatic and is often discovered incidentally. Because of the silent nature of this lesion, the patient may not notice until symptoms of complication occur, such as facial nerve paralysis and intracranial extension. Landers and May[15] reported a case with facial palsy caused by a preauricular cyst associated with congenital cholesteatoma. Rapoport et al[16] reported a huge congenital cholesteatoma simulating an intracranial abscess.

Congenital cholesteatoma may occur in five sites within the temporal bone: (1) the tympanic membrane, (2) the middle ear, (3) the mastoid, (4) the petrous apex, and (5) the CPA. The mode of presentation of congenital cholesteatoma differs according to the site.

Congenital cholesteatoma within the tympanic membrane demonstrates a whitish appearance or an opaque patch on the eardrum. Hearing may not be affected or may show mild conductive hearing loss. An intratympanic cholesteatoma or patch of tympanosclerosis, when viewed binocularly, can be within or lateral to the tympanic membrane.

Congenital middle ear cholesteatoma most commonly presents as a white pearl-like structure behind the anterosuperior portion of a normal intact eardrum. Conductive hearing loss is often the first sign due to ossicular chain damage. Facial nerve palsy is also reported. Rare presentations, however, are also possible. Reilly[17] reported a case that presented as a postauricular mass. Differential diagnosis needs to be performed when a white lesion presents behind the eardrum.

Two histologic types of congenital cholesteatoma, open and closed, have been described.[18,19] The closed type is more frequent and essentially is a closed epithelial cyst. The open type involves the middle ear more diffusely and carpets the middle ear cleft with matrix and keratin debris. Both types are found in the anterosuperior quadrant of the tympanum.[20]

The majority of white lesions developing behind an intact tympanic membrane are either congenital or acquired cholesteatoma. A congenital cholesteatoma that arises from epithelial cell rests in the lateral part of the middle ear and will appear to be immediately adjacent to and in contact with the tympanic membrane. Well-developed air cells in the mastoid are often seen in congenital cholesteatoma. Most acquired cholesteatoma presents as a retraction pocket or perforation at the pars flaccida with sclerotic mastoid. A bony structure, such as an osteoma arising from the promontory or annulus may present as white lesion behind an intact tympanic membrane. But these lesions will be deep to the tympanic membrane.

Congenital cholesteatoma originating in and restricted to the mastoid process is the least common type.[21] The initial presentations are a fistula in the external auditory cannel, conductive hearing loss, and neck pain.[22] Due to its space-occupying effect, it may compress the cerebellum and the dural sinuses adjacent to it or erode the bony labyrinth. Cureoglu et al[23] reported a case of congenital cholesteatoma originating in the mastoid process and presenting as a mass that extended to the posterior fossa.

Petrous apex cholesteatoma appears in the petrous pyramid near the internal auditory canal. Early symptoms of a mass primarily arising within the petrous apex are usually nonspecific and poorly localized. Petrous apex cholesteatoma results in slow destruction of structures in and around the temporal bone. Most patients are not diagnosed until more localized symptoms appear. Gradual expansion at the petrous bone results in erosion of the adjacent carotid canal. Cholesteatoma may break into the internal auditory canal and damage the auditory and facial nerves. The semicircular canal and cochlea may be eroded, resulting in sensorineural deafness and loss of vestibular function. Nager[24] considered that the origin is aberrant neuroectodermal tissue.

The predominant symptoms of congenital cholesteatoma of the CPA were related to cranial nerves VII and VIII and headaches.[25] Signs and symptoms were divided into those caused by local involvement of the cholesteatoma, increased intracranial pressure, or both. Facial weakness/paralysis, hearing loss, tinnitus, dizziness, imbalance and headache were the most frequent symptoms. Pulec[26] reported that facial nerve twitch, hemifacial spasm, and progressive facial paralysis occurred in 15 of 19 patients. Hearing loss, tinnitus, and vertigo at some time in the course of the disease were present in all 19 cases. Pain and otorrhea occurred in six patients and were invariably associated with infection of the cholesteatoma.

Bilateral lesions are rare, affecting approximately 3% of congenital cholesteatoma patients.[27] These lesions may not present at the same time, and long-term follow-up should always include careful scrutiny of the normal ear. The finding of nearly identical lesions in each ear gives further support to a congenital etiology from similar epithelial rests.[28] Suetake et al[29] reported a case with cholesteatoma on both sides accompanied by ossicular anomalies with hypoplasia of the long process of incus and the superstructure of the stapes. Litman et al[30] reported a case of bilateral congenital cholesteatoma with middle ear effusion. Worley et al[31] reported bilateral congenital cholesteatoma in patients with branchio-oto-renal syndrome.

PREOPERATIVE EVALUATION

After careful otoscopic and otomicroscopic examinations are performed, the appearance of the lesion in its quadrant of presentation with respect to the tympanic membrane is noted and sketched. The criteria for diagnosing the congenital cholesteatoma are reviewed, which include (1) the cholesteatoma must be present behind an intact tympanic membrane, (2) the patient must have no history of aural infections, and (3) the patient must have no history of tympanic membrane perforation or surgery.[5] Audiology evaluation, including complete audiometric and impedance tympanometric studies, is performed. Radiologic studies, including noncontrast high-resolution computed tomography (CT) scanning, and magnetic resonance imaging (MRI) with special attention to the middle ear and mastoid are of value in diagnosing and managing congenital cholesteatoma.

AUDIOLOGY EVALUATION

Pure tone audiogram and speech discrimination are performed to determine the hearing level and the type of hearing loss. Hearing level is related to ossicular chain integrity, and that in turn is a function of patient age and the degree to which the cholesteatoma has extended beyond the anterosuperior middle ear quadrant. Hearing is normal in those patients whose lesion is restricted to the anterosuperior quadrant, unless the lesion has extended posteriorly with involvement of the stapes superstructure or the lenticular process of the incus. Even with ossicular erosion, however, the hearing may be normal, because the cholesteatoma may serve to complete the ossicular chain. In some cases the cholesteatoma has reached sufficient size to block the eustachian tube, in which case a middle ear effusion and a mild conductive hearing loss may be present. Posterior-superior quadrant lesions are much more likely to present with hearing loss initially and are almost always found to have ossicular damage. Impedance tympanometry shows low compliance due to the cholesteatoma mass behind the anterosuperior portion of a normal intact eardrum. Negative pressure increases when cholesteatoma block the eustachian tube. Stapedial reflex usually is absent in ears with middle ear pathology.

RADIOLOGY EVALUATION

The diagnosis of congenital cholesteatoma is usually made on otologic examination including otoscopic and microscopic study of the tympanic membrane.

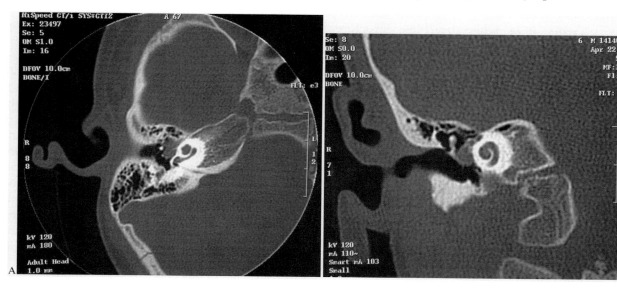

FIGURE 14–1 (A) Coronal computed tomography (CT) demonstrating a typical middle ear congenital cholesteatoma limited to the anterosuperior quadrant of the middle ear. (B) Axial CT demonstrating an anterosuperior middle ear cholesteatoma blocking the eustachian tube.

Radiologic studies, including CT scanning, and MRI, however, not only are indicated for diagnostic purposes but also are valuable in assessing the extent of the disease and the degree of bony involvement. CT can delineate the size of the cholesteatoma (Fig. 14–1), demonstrating bone erosion and smooth bone expansion associated with or without soft tissue mass. In some cases, the inferior margin of the lateral attic wall remains intact in congenital middle ear cholesteatoma in the early stage. Erosion of the tegmen, labyrinth, sigmoid sinus plate, facial nerve canal, and ossicles can be best evaluated on CT scans. Both congenital cholesteatoma and cholesterol granuloma of the petrous bone demonstrate erosion and expansion of bone, which cannot be differentiated from each other on CT scans. However, cholesteatoma appears on MRI as hypointense lesions on T1-weighted (T1W) images and hyperintense lesions on T2-weighted (T2W) images. Cholesterol granulomas are seen as homogeneously hyperintense lesions on both on T1W and T2W scans. Mafee[32] suggested that CT remains the study of choice for cholesteatomas of the middle ear cleft. MRI is superior to CT for the evaluation of infected cholesteatomas, petrous apex, and CPA cholesteatomas, as well as for evaluation of cholesteatomatous involvement of the facial nerve, membranous labyrinth, and intracranial structures.

SURGICAL TECHNIQUE

The purpose of surgical removal of congenital cholesteatoma is the elimination of disease and restoration of function. Congenital cholesteatoma within the tympanic membrane without middle ear involvement can be removed by myringotomy alone. Congenital cholesteatoma isolated in the anterosuperior quadrant of the middle ear can be completely removed with preservation of hearing using an extended transcanal tympanomeatal approach supplemented at times with an atticotomy (Fig. 14–2). Lesions involving the posterior or superior quadrants are usually much more extensive with significant ossicular involvement. Tympanomastoid surgery is required for adequate excision. Petrous apex cholesteatoma can be removed through a transmastoid approach (Fig. 14–3). The translabyrinthine-transcochlear or middle fossa approach may be required in more extensive cases.

MYRINGOTOMY

Cholesteatoma within the tympanic membrane is a rare entity. The cholesteatoma presents as a white pearl-like structure in the anterosuperior portion of

an intact eardrum. It can be removed via myringotomy incision. An incision is made on the anterosuperior portion of the tympanic membrane corresponding to the midportion of the mass. Care must be taken that the incision cuts through only the epithelium of the tympanic membrane. The cholesteatoma is visible as a spherical, yellowish-white mass seen beneath the epithelium. The mass is removed intact as a sphere without opening the matrix or spilling keratinous debris. After excision of the cholesteatoma, the epithelium is pushed back to attach the inner layer of the tympanic membrane. Packing the ear canal may avoid a pocket between the two layers of the eardrum. Early diagnosis, before the lesion affects the fibrous layer, allows a complete excision by a myringotomy approach. The cholesteatomatous pearl can be peeled off the tympanic membrane. Myringoplasty is not necessary if the fibrous layer is not violated.[33]

TRANSCANAL TYMPANOMEATAL APPROACH

This approach is to remove the isolated cholesteatoma limited to the middle ear often seen at the anterosuperior portion of mesotympanum. An incision is made on the posterior canal wall as in the stapes operation. A dissector is used to raise the posterior tympanomeatal flap to enter the middle ear (Fig. 14–2A). Exposure of the stapes, the oval and round windows, and the promontory is obtained by elevating the annulus. To expose the anterosuperior portion of mesotympanum, an incision is made on the manubrium of the malleus (Fig. 14–2B). The eardrum is then dissected and elevated off the malleus. The tympanic membrane can be completely separated from the ossicles and the middle ear widely exposed. The cholesteatoma mass can now be adequately visualized and removed (Fig. 14–2C). The congenital cholesteatoma often arises at the medial aspect of the neck of the malleus. A right-angle pick is used to dislodge the mass from its connection to the malleus. The mass is then moved inferiorly and posteriorly into the space between the manubrium of the malleus and the promontory. Once the cholesteatoma is moved through the narrow space, it can be easily removed from the middle ear. During the removal process, care must be taken not to disrupt the matrix of the cholesteatoma.

Grundfast et al[34] reported a new approach to the removal of the anterosuperior middle ear for removal of congenital cholesteatoma. They used a superiorly based tympanomeatal flap to get better exposure of the anterosuperior portion of the middle ear. They reported eight cases in which the cholesteatoma was removed without disrupting the matrix.

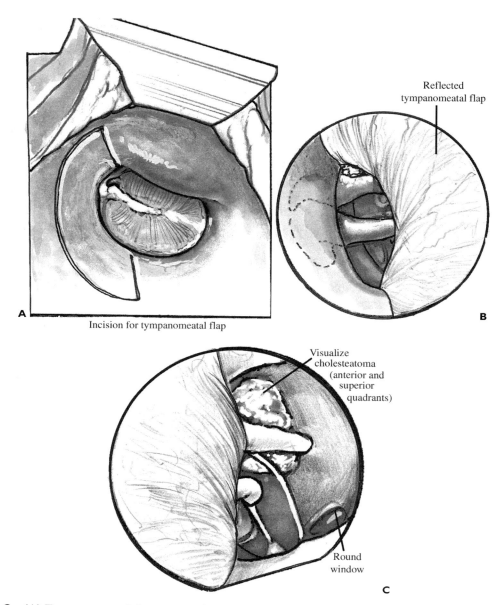

FIGURE 14–2 (A) Tympanomeatal flap approach to a middle ear congenital cholesteatoma located anteriorly in the middle ear. (B) Elevation of the flat off the malleus to approach an anteriorly based congenital cholesteatoma. (C) Complete exposure of a middle ear cholesteatoma following flap elevation.

This approach can also be extended into an atticotomy or mastoidectomy in cases in which a tympanotomy alone does not allow adequate access. Stabilization and healing of the tympanic membrane is rapid when the middle ear has been exposed via this approach.

TYMPANOMASTOID OPERATION

This procedure is for cholesteatoma involving the middle ear and mastoid; usually these cholesteatomas are more diffuse and extensive and may require a two-stage operation. The initial steps are making

canal incisions (Fig. 14–3), elevating the vascular strip, turning the ear forward, removing and dehydrating the temporalis fascia, removing canal skin, enlarging the ear canal by removing the overhanging bone anteriorly and inferiorly, and ensuring that the remnant is de-epithelialized.

Cholesteatoma should be dissected in continuity to ensure total removal of middle ear disease. All diseased tissue is dissected from the bone or mucosa, beginning in the anterosuperior quadrant, proceeding inferiorly, then posteriorly, and superiorly until the superior edge of the promontory, the lower edge of the oval window, is reached. Normal mucosa

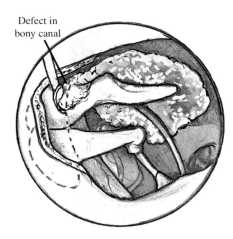

FIGURE 14–3 Vascular strip incisions to approach extensive middle ear cholesteatoma using tympanomastoidectomy approach.

should be preserved as much as possible. No attempt should be made at this time to remove cholesteatoma that surrounds the stapes or is in the oval window. Manipulations in this area should be postponed until the mastoidectomy has been completed and the facial recess is open. Removal of oval window disease should always be deferred until the end of the procedure, so that if a fistula develops inadvertently, the operation may be terminated expeditiously. Before proceeding with the mastoidectomy, if the ossicular chain is involved by cholesteatoma, the incudostapedial joint should be separated at this time. This facilitates removal of the incus after the facial recess is opened and prevents possible trauma to the inner ear, which could occur should the drill inadvertently touch the incus when the epitympanum or facial recess is being opened.

The mastoid is exenterated, under the microscope, using a drill with various-sized round cutting burs. Continuous suction-irrigation during drilling is used to cool the bone, to keep the field clean at all times, and to prevent clogging of the bur by bone dust. The initial bur cut is made along the linea temporalis. This marks the lowest point of the middle fossa dura in most cases. The second bur cut is along a line perpendicular to the one just described and tangential to the posterior margin of the ear canal. These two bur cuts outline a triangular area, the apex of which is at the spine of Henle. Projected into the mastoid, parallel to the direction of the ear canal, the apex of this triangle is directly over the lateral semicircular canal. The only structure of importance lying within this triangle as one proceeds with the exenteration is the sigmoid sinus. The deepest mastoid penetration is always at the apex of this triangle. This ensures that the antrum is

entered and the lateral canal identified before deeper penetration in other areas.

The dural plate is skeletonized superiorly and the sigmoid sinus skeletonized posteroinferiorly as the dissection proceeds. Uncovering the middle fossa or sigmoid sinus dura is not necessary but should not result in any problem. It is not considered a complication. After the lateral semicircular canal has been identified and the cortical mastoidectomy has been completed, the zygomatic root is removed to allow access to epitympanum. The posterior bony canal wall is thinned at this time. Sheehy[35] offered his experience in regard to the initial approach to the mastoid:

1. Always keep the deepest area of penetration into the mastoid at the apex of the two initial bur cuts. The direction in which one proceeds is not necessarily perpendicular to the bone; it should be parallel to the ear canal. Following parallel to the ear canal will lead to the mastoid antrum.
2. Do not dig a deep hole. One must remember to saucerize the margins, to open the exposure as one proceeds deeper. In this way, it is possible to see what one is doing and also to use the suction irrigation with the drill.
3. Always use the largest bur possible. If one should inadvertently uncover the middle fossa dura or the facial nerve or the sigmoid sinus, one is less likely to do serious damage with a large bur as opposed to a very small bur. Furthermore, if there is a problem, one will be able to see what was done.
4. If lost on the way to the antrum, go high and forward. By going high, one identifies the middle fossa dural plate. By going forward, one then squeezes into the angle between the dural plate and the ear canal. Going medial in that direction leads to the epitympanum and avoids the matter of fenestrating the lateral semicircular canal or getting into other troubles should the mastoid antrum be filled with bone.

The facial recess is one of the posterior recesses of the middle ear. It is bordered laterally by the chorda tympani, medially by the upper mastoid segment of the facial nerve, and superiorly by bone of the fossa incudis. This recess is frequently the seat of cholesteatoma, particularly when cholesteatoma is associated with a perforation below the posterior malleal fold. Bone in this area may be cellular even in a poorly developed mastoid. The landmark for opening into the facial recess is the fossa incudis. One visualizes the triangular area that is inferior to the fossa and is bordered by bone of the fossa incudis superiorly, the upper mastoid segment of the facial nerve medially, and the chorda tympani laterally. The bone is saucerized in this area with a large cutting bur. When the bony canal wall lateral to the recess has been thinned satisfactorily, bone removal is continued with a smaller cutting bur. One should always stroke with a bur parallel to the direction of the nerve, never allowing the bur to pass the bone of the fossa incudis superiorly.

The facial recess is opened from the mastoid to remove disease in the area, to gain additional access to the posterior middle ear, to obtain a better view of tympanic segment of the facial nerve, and to facilitate postoperative aeration of the mastoid. Opening into the middle ear through the facial recess is a key step in performing an intact-canal-wall tympanoplasty with mastoidectomy; with rare exceptions, it should not be omitted. Identification of the facial nerve provides an additional landmark for opening into the facial recess. A small diamond bur is used to enter into the middle ear, just lateral to the nerve, and then the opening is enlarged. It is usually possible to obtain at least a 2-mm opening. After the recess has been opened, the incus, if present, is removed along with bone of the fossa incudis. It is possible to see the pyramidal eminence, the oval and round windows, and that part of the tympanic

portion of the facial nerve lying posterior to the cochleariform process.

As disease is encountered in the mastoid, it is removed by dissecting it from behind forward. It is important to remove all the cholesteatoma matrix in continuity so that no remnant of epithelium remains. The mastoid is exenterated to the extent indicated by the disease process and to the extent necessary to obtain adequate exposure (Fig. 14–4). All mastoid and facial recess disease may be removed by elevating it and dissecting it toward the epitympanum and middle ear. Unless there is an unusually narrow angle between the tegmen and the superior wall of the ear canal, it should be possible to remove all epitympanic disease. When the cholesteatoma has contacted the malleus head, as it frequently has, the entire malleus should be removed. This exposes the opening into the supratubal recess and facilitates dissection of disease from behind and through the ear canal simultaneously.[36]

Collins et al[37] emphasized that the sinus epitympani, an anterior extension of the epitympanum, is frequently the site of hidden cholesteatoma. Surgical exploration of this area is important for complete removal of diseased tissue and improved ventilation of the attic. The areas that are most difficult to see are

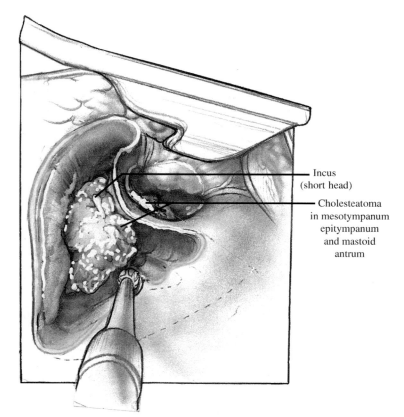

Incus
(short head)

Cholesteatoma
in mesotympanum
epitympanum
and mastoid
antrum

FIGURE 14–4 Exposure of a congenital cholesteatoma filling the posterior middle ear and mastoid using the tympanomastoidectomy approach.

the posterior middle ear recesses: infrapyramidal recess and sinus tympani. They are often the seats of cholesteatoma. The area must be cleaned with a right-angle dissector. Removal of the pyramidal process and adjacent bone with a diamond bur may be necessary at times to facilitate the cleaning. Ear or pediatric endoscopes permit visualization of the sinus tympani for cholesteatoma removal. The tympanic sinus can be approached in a well-developed mastoid from the mastoid side, medial to the facial nerve and lateral to the posterior semicircular canal. Pickett et al[38] reported the use of a retrofacial approach for removal of disease in sinus tympani.

The tympanic membrane usually is intact in congenital cholesteatoma. In case the tympanic membrane was ruptured during the cholesteatoma removal, the remnant should be grafted with dehydrated fascia. Packing is inserted and closure postauricularly is done with subcutaneous suture.

The use of the two-stage procedure is based on the removal of cholesteatoma, the mucous membrane lesion, and the status of the ossicular chain. The closed type of cholesteatoma is essentially a closed epithelial cyst. It can be completely removed without leaving a residual, and usually a two-stage procedure is not necessary. The open type involves the middle ear more diffusely and carpets the middle ear cleft with matrix and keratin debris. Total removal of cholesteatoma in the middle ear is questionable in the open type of cholesteatoma. In particular, if the epithelial matrix of cholesteatoma grows into the tympanic recess, one may not be certain of complete removal. Cholesteatoma epithelium may fill the oval and round windows or cover the stapes footplate. Excessive manipulation in these areas could result in an inner ear complication. In such cases, a two-stage procedure is necessary. The second-stage operation is planned to be performed in 9 to 12 months to inspect for possible residual cholesteatoma. By that time the residual disease may have grown to a 1- or 2-mm cyst so that it may be identified with greater ease. In the case of large areas of diseased or absent mucosa in the infected middle ear, removal of all squamous epithelium, granulations, and irreversibly diseased mucosa at the time of surgery is required. Silastic sheeting is used over the denuded areas to prevent adhesions and to allow mucosa to migrate into middle ear. A two-stage procedure is indicated to obtain the best hearing results and to prevent recurrence of cholesteatoma. If ossicular chain interruption due to cholesteatoma or stapes fixation due to tympanosclerosis or otosclerosis is present, a two-stage procedure is almost always indicated. Ossicular chain reconstruction performed in an aerated middle ear leads to a better

hearing result. A fixed stapes should not be removed during actual or potential infection. An increase in the incidence of sensorineural hearing impairment is noted in patients in whom the inner ear has been opened during cholesteatoma surgery.

Postoperatively, patients are instructed to remove their mastoid dressing on the second day and to maintain water avoidance for the ear. The initial visit is to remove the Steri-Strips from the postauricular incision in 1 week. Otoscopic examination is performed to rule out infection. Residual packing is removed at a second follow-up appointment 3 weeks postoperatively. Drops are started 1 week prior to this appointment to loosen the remaining packing. To avoid fibrosis, care is taken to completely remove all external auditory canal packing.

Patients are scheduled for follow-up on a regular bases. Reexploration is recommended if an unexplained deterioration in hearing has occurred, and the adequacy of the initial surgery is a serious concern. Recurrent disease can be managed by repeat tympanomastoidectomy. Multiple revisions may be required in those patients with extensive disease.

Complications associated with tympanomastoid surgery are related to the extent of destruction caused by cholesteatoma and surgical accidents. These complications include either dead ears or vertigo caused by inadvertently uncapping a fistula of the horizontal canal or oval window. This complication is the result both of a fistula caused by cholesteatoma and of a surgical accident in which the matrix was inadvertently removed before the surgeon recognized the presence of a fistula. Facial paralysis is one of the direst complications in cholesteatoma surgery. Facial nerve injuries usually occur when the nerve has been exposed by cholesteatoma or granulation tissue and no longer has its bony fallopian canal to protect it from the drill, suction tube, and surgical instruments. In addition, the landmarks may have been distorted by cholesteatoma or previous operation. Postoperative infections are considered a complication and can be due to poor aseptic technique or to the presence of bacteria in the ear at the time of surgery. Graft failure is a complication that is often associated with postoperative infection. Faulty undersurface grafting often results in graft failure. Lateralization and anterior blunting of the graft may occur with the overlay technique.

Most complications can be prevented by paying careful attention to aseptic technique and anatomic landmarks and by exercising good clinical judgment throughout the operative procedure. Even in the most capable hands, however, a certain percentage of complications occur. It is important to recognize complications when present and to be prepared to deal with them in an expeditious and judicious manner.

TRANSMASTOID APPROACH

Petrous apex cholesteatoma can be removed by the transmastoid approach. The translabyrinthine-transcochlear or middle fossa approach is required for surgical excision of extensive petrous apex cholesteatoma. Glasscock et al[39] reported 15 cases of petrous apex cholesteatoma. Among them, congenital cholesteatoma was described in six cases; one case was a primary attic cholesteatoma and five cases arose directly within the petrous apex. The transmastoid approach was used to surgically treat five cases, middle fossa was used in four cases, and translabyrinthine-transcochlear in six cases.

LONG-TERM PROGNOSIS

Long-term results of congenital cholesteatoma surgery including elimination of disease and restoration of function have been reported. Doyle and Luxford[14] reported 60 ears in 59 patients followed during a 15-year period. In regard to elimination of disease, cholesteatoma was considered cured in 90%. No recurrent cholesteatoma was found at the second-stage operation in all patients with initial limited cholesteatoma, and in all patients after a second-stage operation removal of residual cholesteatoma with a greater than 10-year follow-up. In regard to preservation of function, postoperative air–bone gap of 10 dB or less was found in 63% and 20 dB or less in 91% of ears, with an average postoperative speech reception threshold of 20 dB HL. Friedberg[11] reported that congenital cholesteatoma has a high rate of recurrence after removal. Substantial submucosal extension may explain the cause of recurrence. Appropriate surgical treatment, however, may reduce the residual and recurrence rates.

REFERENCES

1. House HP. An apparent primary cholesteatoma: case report. *Laryngoscope* 1953;63:712–713.
2. Cawthorne T. Congenital cholesteatoma. *Arch Otolaryngol* 1963;78:248–252.
3. Derlacki EL, Clemis JD. Congenital cholesteatoma of the middle ear and mastoid. *Ann Otol Rhinol Laryngol* 1965;74:706–727.
4. House JW, Sheehy JL. Cholesteatoma with intact tympanic membrane: a report of 41 cases. *Laryngoscope* 1980;90:70–76.
5. Cushing H. A large epidermal cholesteatoma of the parieto-temporal region deforming the left hemisphere without cerebral symptoms. *Surg Gynecol Obstet* 1922;34:557–567.
6. Sanna M, Zini C. "Congenital cholesteatoma" of the middle ear: a report of 11 cases. *Am J Otol* 1984;5:368–373.
7. Paparella MM, Rybak L. Congenital cholesteatoma. *Otolaryngol Clin North Am* 1978;11:113–120.
8. Michaels L. Evolution of the epidermoid formation and its role in the development of the middle ear and tympanic membrane during the first trimester. *J Otolaryngol* 1988;17:22–28.
9. Aimi K. Role of the tympanic ring in the pathogenesis of congenital cholesteatoma. *Laryngoscope* 1983;93:1140–1146.
10. Weber PC, Adkins WY. Congenital cholesteatoma in the tympanic membrane. *Laryngoscope* 1997;107:1181–1184.
11. Friedberg J. Congenital cholesteatoma. *Laryngoscope* 1994;104:1–24.
12. Chen JM, Schloss MD, Manoukian JJ, Shapiro RS. Congenital cholesteatoma of the middle ear in children. *J Otolaryngol* 1989;18:44–48.
13. Levenson MJ, Michaels L, Parisier SC, Juarbe C. Congenital cholesteatomas in children: an embryologic correlation. *Laryngoscope* 1988;98:949–955.
14. Doyle KJ, Luxford WM. Congenital aural cholesteatoma: results of surgery in 60 cases. *Laryngoscope* 1995;105:263–267.
15. Landers SA, May M. Preauricular cyst associated with congenital cholesteatoma: an unusual cause of facial palsy. *Am J Otol* 1994;15:273–275.
16. Rapoport PB, Di Francesco RC, Mion O, Bento RF. Huge congenital cholesteatoma simulating an intracranial abscess. *Otolaryngol Head Neck Surg* 2000;123:148–149.
17. Reilly PG. Congenital cholesteatoma presenting as a post-auricular mass. *J Laryngol Otol* 1989;103:1069–1070.
18. Michaels L. An epidermoid formation in the developing middle ear possible source of cholesteatoma. *J Otolaryngol* 1986;15:169–174.
19. McGill T, Merchant S, Healy G, Friedman E. Congenital cholesteatoma of the middle ear in children: a clinical and histopathological report. *Laryngoscope* 1991;101:606–613.
20. Michaels L. Origin of congenital cholesteatoma from a normally occurring epidermoid rest in the developing middle ear. *Int J Pediatr Otorhinolaryngol* 1988;15:51–65.
21. Luntz M, Telischi F, Bowen B, Ress B, Balkany T. Congenital cholesteatoma isolated to the mastoid. *Ann Otol Rhinol Laryngol* 1997;106:608–610.
22. Rashad U, Hawthorne M, Kumar U, Welsh A. Unusual cases of congenital cholesteatoma of the ear. *J Laryngol Otol* 1999;113:52–54.
23. Cureoglu S, Osma U, Oktay MF, Nazaroglu H, Meric F, Topcu I. Congenital cholesteatoma of the mastoid region. *J Laryngol Otol* 2000;114:779–780.
24. Nager GT. Epidermoids (Congenital cholesteatoma) involving the temporal bone. Cholesteatoma and

mastoid surgery. In: *Proceedings of the 2nd International Conference.* Amsterdam: Kugler; 1982:41–59.

25. Souza CE, Sperling NM, Costa SS, Yoon TH, Hamid MA, Souza RA. Congenital cholesteatoma of the cerebellopontine angle. *Am J Otol* 1989;10:358–363.

26. Pulec JL. Cholesteatoma of the cerebellopontine angle. *Ear Nose Throat J* 1998;77:952–959.

27. Fedok FG, Bellissimo JB, Wiegand DA. Bilateral congenital aural cholesteatoma. *Otolaryngol Head Neck Surg* 1990;103:1028–1030.

28. Bragandra RA, Kearns DB. Bilateral congenital cholesteatoma. *Am J Otol* 1993;14:191–193.

29. Suetake M, Kobayashi T, Takasaka T. Bilateral congenital cholesteatoma associated with ossicular anomalies: a case report. *Am J Otol* 1991;12:132–134.

30. Litman RS, Parisier SC, Hausman SA, Sher WH. Bilateral congenital cholesteatoma: a cause or result of chronic otitis media with effusion? *Am J Otol* 1987;8:426–431.

31. Worley GA, Vats A, Harcourt J, Albert DM. Bilateral congenital cholesteatoma in branchio-oto-renal syndrome. *J Laryngol Otol* 1999;113:841–843.

32. Mafee MF. MRI and CT in the evaluation of acquired and congenital cholesteatomas of the temporal bone. *J Otolaryngol* 1993;22:239–248.

33. Pasanisi E, Bacciu A, Vincenti V, Bacciu S. Congenital cholesteatoma of the tympanic membrane. *Int J Pediatr Otorhinolaryngol* 2001;61:167–171.

34. Grundfast KM, Thomsen JR, Barber CS. The inferiorly based superior tympanomeatal flap for removal of congenital cholesteatoma. *Laryngoscope* 1990;100:1341–1343.

35. Sheehy JL. Mastoidectomy: the intact canal wall procedure. In: Brackmann DE, Shelton C, Arriaga MA, eds. *Otologic Surgery.* Philadelphia: WB Saunders; 1994:212–224.

36. Horn KL, Luxford WM, Brackmann DE, Shea JJ III. The supratubal recess in cholesteatoma surgery. *Ann Otol Rhinol Laryngol* 1986;95:12–15.

37. Collins ME, Coker NJ, Igarashi M. Inflammatory disease of the anterior epitympanum. *Am J Otol* 1991;12:11–15.

38. Pickett BP, Cail WS, Lambert PR. Sinus tympani: anatomic considerations, computed tomography, and a discussion of the retrofacial approach for removal of disease. *Am J Otol* 1995;16:741–750.

39. Glasscock ME, Woods CI, Poe DS, Patterson AK, Welling DB. Petrous apex cholesteatoma. *Otolaryngol Clin North Am* 1989;22:981–1002.

Chapter 15

STAPEDECTOMY

Franklin M. Rizer

IN MEMORIAM

This chapter is Frank Rizer's last contribution in otology. On March 20, 2003 Frank died tragically while landing his airplane in Washington, D.C., on his way to attending the Cherry Blossom Conference. For the last 18 years, he has practiced otology and neurotology with Bill Lippy and Arne Schuring in Warren, Ohio. He was an outstanding physician and surgeon with wide interests and will be missed by his family and patients, as well as his partners and colleagues.

Stapedectomy is a remarkable operation that can be completed in an hour or less. Great hearing losses can be restored, and the steps of the operation are not terribly complicated. All of these attributes combine to describe an operation that is nearly miraculous to the observer.

The problem of stapedial fixation was identified in the 1860s.[1] Many authors considered the implications of the fixation, including those who bypassed (fenestration)[2] and those who mobilized[3] the stapes. The basic principles of stapedectomy were defined in 1958 with John Shea's[4] description of removal of the stapes and replacement of the stapes with a prosthesis. Controversy continues to exist over the best type of prosthesis, the ideal place and way to anchor the prosthesis, the importance of the stapedius tendon, the amount of the footplate to remove, the material to use to seal the oval window, and other details. The important observation is that the vast majority of stapedectomy operations are successful.[5]

Because the anatomy of the oval window tends to be consistent from case to case, and the steps of stapedectomy are well defined, each portion of the operation lends itself well to study. Thus, in stapedectomy, each portion of the operation has been studied and optimized in different ways. Surgeons have been able to define success using an optimal technique that works well in their hands.

PATIENT PRESENTATION AND INITIAL EXAMINATION

Patients present with the primary complaint of hearing loss. The hearing loss usually develops insidiously between puberty and the age of 30. Often, patients delay seeking assistance for 2 or 3 years.[6]

The family history may or may not be positive for hearing loss treated by surgery. Numerous authors in reviewing their experience have found that about 50% of patients have a positive family history.[7,8] A sibling of a patient with otosclerosis has only about a 1 in 10 chance of developing otosclerosis.[9] In spite of the changing population of the United States, these statistics have changed little over many years.

The physical examination of the ear is normal. In most patients with stapedial fixation today, there are no physical findings of note. The external ear, the canal, and the drum are all completely normal. In years past, Schwartze's sign could be seen; that is, through the tympanic membrane, a red hue of engorged blood vessels leading to an active metabolic focus of otosclerosis could be seen. Such a finding today is rare, because most disease is seen at an earlier stage.

Otosclerosis, the disease of bone that seems to cause the stapes to be fixed in the narrow oval window niche, continues to be a disease of many faces. Histologically, the disease affects 10 times more people than have clinical evidence of disease. The histologic picture is that of a basophilic focus of remodeling bone occasionally involving the cochlea and the balance canals. The occurrence of this remodeling process in endochondral bone makes otosclerosis unique. The etiology of the disease remains obscure with several theories being predominant. The first, that otosclerosis is an inherited disease, has been held for many years.[10] Genetic analysis has shed some light on the possible etiology of this situation. By comparing the components of the abnormal type I collagen gene found in osteogenesis imperfecta, with the genes found in the collagen of otosclerosis, common sequences were found, suggesting a common genetic link.[11] The second, that otosclerosis may be an immunologic reaction to a measles virus insult, is of more recent origin.[12] Modern genetic and immunohistochemical data support both etiologies.

AUDIOLOGY

There are three audiometric profiles in otosclerosis. The first is that of a progressive sensorineural hearing loss. It may be possible for these individuals to have had a small air–bone gap at some point in the past, and that gap to have resolved over time. The loss is typically progressive over a period of several decades. Such a loss can eventually result in a profound and complete hearing loss.

The second pattern of presentation is with a conductive hearing loss. In a conductive hearing loss, there has been gradual encroachment of the otosclerotic focus of bone onto the stapes. The encroachment can occur at the anterior arch or the footplate at the annulus. As there is more encroachment, the conductive hearing loss becomes greater, until a maximum conductive hearing loss is reached. Thus, a 50-dB hearing loss suggests a great deal of fixation of the footplate.

Finally, the two types of hearing loss can present together as a mixed hearing loss. That is, an individual can present with both a sensorineural hearing loss and a conductive component to their hearing loss, the combination of the two yielding the total mixed hearing loss. Carhart[13] noted an overcorrection of the hearing in many patients operated for otosclerosis. The exact mechanism of this improvement is unknown; therefore, predicting which patients will benefit in this way is difficult. Relying on such a response may prove disappointing to physician and patient.

IMPEDANCE AUDIOMETRY

Tympanometric findings are characteristic. The ear is most compliant at normal pressures, but the degree of compliance is reduced because of the ossicular fixation. Thus, the tympanogram appears relatively flat, with maximal compliance at zero pressure. The acoustic reflex patterns can be diagnostic in otosclerosis. If the stapes is firmly fixed, the reflexes will be absent. Early in the disease, the stapes will be only slightly fixed, and a biphasic "on-off" response will be elicited at the onset and the offset of the stimulus. If symptoms are present less than 5 years, 94% of patients will show the effect. Between 5 and 10 years, only 50% show the effect, and after 10 years, virtually no patients will show the effect.[14]

PATIENT SELECTION

The patient considered for stapedectomy should have two appropriately masked audiograms to confirm adequate bone thresholds and an air–bone gap in excess of 15 dB. The conductive loss must be confirmed with a reversed (bone conduction greater than air conduction) 512-Hz tuning fork, and a Weber test that lateralizes to the affected ear. The acoustic reflexes will be absent or demonstrate the on-off effect. Concomitant pathology is excluded by examination.

The poorer-hearing ear is appropriately selected for intervention. When hearing levels are similar and one ear had been previously operated, the unoperated ear should be treated rather than revising an ear. The surgery will be easier, the benefits greater, and the patient will generally be happier.

Rarely, a patient presents with otosclerosis in an only hearing ear. Much thought and consideration should be given to the decision to operate. Although one should rarely, if ever, operate on an only hearing ear, maintenance of communication and stabilization of hearing are important considerations in otosclerosis, which tends to be a progressive disease. Thus, there may be a rare patient for whom surgery might be considered in an only hearing ear. These cases should be attempted only by very experienced surgeons, and even then with trepidation.

Speech discrimination should be adequate. With a pure conductive loss, discrimination will improve to 100% if the stimulus can be made loud enough. Patients should be in reasonable health, although advanced age is not a contraindication to surgery. Stapedectomy in very young children (younger than 5 years of age) may be contraindicated until it is demonstrated that they are not prone to otitis media.

The benefits of surgery for both children and the elderly have been demonstrated.[15,16]

Stapedectomy can be beneficial in patients with far-advanced otosclerosis. These patients have a severe or profound mixed loss. Surgery may raise their thresholds into the aidable range, when previously a hearing aid could not be worn. Typically they have excellent speech production and air conduction no better than 95 dB with bony thresholds in excess of 60 to 75 dB (the limit of the audiometer). The conductive element may be detectable with the 512-Hz tuning fork applied to the teeth when it is not heard on the mastoid. The upper central incisors and the alveolar ridge give an 11-dB gain over applying the fork to the mastoid. The examiner must be sure that the fork is heard and not felt by the patient.[17]

ALTERNATE THERAPIES

SODIUM FLUORIDE THERAPY

Sodium fluoride supplements with calcium and vitamin D have been prescribed as a measure to prevent further hearing loss when it is diagnosed. Unfortunately, documentary proof of the treatment effectiveness has been scanty.[18] Because of anecdotal evidence, however, it may be appropriate to continue to prescribe the over-the-counter medication. A course of sodium fluoride (as Fluorical, two tablets twice daily for 2 years) is used.

HEARING AIDS

Any patient who will benefit from a stapedectomy will also benefit from a hearing aid. This alternative must be offered to the patient.[19] Many patients elect to try a hearing aid, but after considering the convenience of surgery versus the convenience of hearing aids, they elect to return for further consultation for surgery.

OBSERVATION

Occasionally, patients elect merely to observe their hearing loss. This can occur for many reasons, including lack of insurance coverage, other commitments, and fear. Gentle reassurance and supportive observation generally guide the patient back to the office at a later date.

CONTRAINDICATIONS

Infectious ear disease is a contraindication to surgery. This includes diseases of the middle and external ear. The presence of external otitis or a respiratory tract infection is cause to delay surgery

pending resolution of the problem. Either problem can result in entry of bacteria or viruses into the inner ear with a potentially disastrous result. Meniere's syndrome poses a potential contraindication. The dilated saccule may sit immediately beneath the footplate and be damaged upon opening the vestibule.[20]

The patient's occupation is not a contraindication to surgery. Six active-duty fighter pilots have been operated, as well as a ballerina, and they continued to perform their duties.[21] As with any surgery, however, patients should be fully informed about the potential complications as well as the benefits of surgery.

OPERATING ROOM SETUP AND PATIENT POSITIONING

It is important to perform all stapes surgery under local anesthesia with sedation. This permits less postoperative nausea and a shorter stay. Additionally, patients can inform the surgical team of any intraoperative nausea or vertigo. In revision surgery, vertigo can inform the team of adhesions between the prosthesis and the saccule, preventing complications. As a final benefit, intraoperative audiometry can be completed, allowing perfect adjustment of the prosthesis during surgery.[22]

The patient is premedicated with midazolam 1 mg IV (Versed) 1 hour prior to surgery. Upon arrival in the operating room, an air threshold audiogram is completed by the operating room nurse and compared with the results from the office. Intravenous sedation with propofol (Diprivan or Brevital) is accomplished to provide amnesia and sedation during the ear canal injections. A four-quadrant injection with lidocaine 2% with 1:10,000 epinephrine is completed. The ear is prepared with povidone iodine and any remaining prep solution is irrigated from the ear by the surgeon.

An appropriately sized speculum is introduced into the ear and rotated to dilate the ear canal. The short process of the malleus should just be visible in the speculum. Patient position should be adjusted at this point to provide an easy view of the malleus and the posterior half of the eardrum. Often, a small amount of head-down positioning with the chin moved to the contralateral shoulder suffices. A final injection of the lidocaine solution is made into the vascular strip, permitting a small amount of hydrodissection of the flap. A speculum holder facilitates the remainder of the procedure.

The surgeon sits behind the patient with the ear to be operated positioned up. The anesthetist sits across from the surgeon, allowing him or her to provide consolation for the patient and to assess the ongoing level of sedation. The scrub nurse can stand on either side of the surgeon, using his or her Mayo stand to hold the necessary instruments, and be at the surgeon's dominant hand.

SPECIFIC TECHNIQUE

THE OVAL WINDOW COVERING

What material to use for grafting the open oval window has been widely discussed. Blood, fascia, vein, and other tissues have been described. A study in the 1960s addressed the idea of the characteristics of the ideal grafting material.[23] Fascia and vein are comparable in metabolic rate. Vein creates a very thin membrane. Thick fascia may be difficult to mold to the shape of the oval window. Loose areolar connective tissue "moon glue" is one of the more ideal tissues, being composed of fascia, but more malleable.[24]

THE INCISION

A slightly dull, short sickle knife is used to make external canal incisions in the 11 and 6 o'clock positions; these incisions are joined approximately 6 mm lateral to the drum with a round knife (Fig. 15–1). Several interrupted passes with the knife are made so as to take the incision through the periosteum and cut tissue tags tethering the flap. The sickle knife crushes the edges of the flap to minimize

bleeding. It is usually possible to gradually increase the size of the speculum during this step. The final connection may be easier to make using the microscissors.

The speculum is fixed using a speculum holder. The holder is always used, as it assists with hemostasis, helps to secure the patient's head, provides a firm base against which to curette, and keeps both hands free to work. The canal elevator is passed firmly along the bone to elevate a tympanomeatal flap down to the annulus; every effort is made to avoid tearing the flap. The use of increased magnification helps to improve precision in this dissection and to avoid errors. The annulus is exposed along the entire width of the flap. The middle ear is entered in the posterosuperior quadrant, and a Rosen needle is used to dissect the annulus from its groove and identify the chorda tympani if it is not encased in the bone. An annulus elevator is inserted and the annulus freed from its sulcus inferiorly. Most tears occur here as the annulus is not clearly identified or as it is deeply embedded in bone. The chorda is dissected free from its fold of mucosa and then followed anterior and superiorly, medial to the malleus. The chorda is regularly moistened with gelatin foam pledgets soaked in saline during the procedure. This prevents many of the patient complaints of taste disturbance later.

THE MALLEUS

A gelatin foam pledget saturated with anesthetic is placed in the middle ear, serving to anesthetize the mucosa. Malleus and incus mobility are checked by vision and palpation always with the same instrument to retain the same feel (Fig. 15–2). The malleus

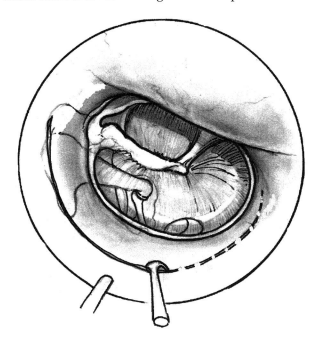

FIGURE 15–1 External ear canal incisions.

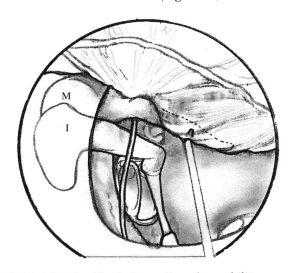

FIGURE 15–2 Check the malleus for mobility.

must be visualized from the underside of the drum, pushing the drum aside with a No. 20 suction in one hand and palpating with the other. This is done to exclude other forms of ossicular pathology, such as malleus or incus fixation. A fixed malleus can be a cause of residual conductive hearing loss.

CURETTING

Enough bone is curetted from the scutum to see the horizontal facial and the origin of the stapes tendon. A rotary motion is used to allow the curette to bite the bone and remove a small portion with each sweep. The curette is stabilized by leaning against the speculum and its holder during this process. Gross movements and biting too much bone may cause damage to other structures. The motion should be away from the incus to avoid creating a dislocation. Curetting is commenced slightly lateral to the scutum to create a furrow (Fig. 15–3). This area of bone is thinned and it subsequently allows easier removal of the annular margin where the bone is more dense. Once the curetting is finished, only a 26-gauge suction is used in the middle ear. This avoids excessive drying of the mucosa and thermal vertigo. It also prevents the inadvertent aspiration of perilymph.

THE STAPES

An assessment is made of the oval window region; any dehiscence over the seventh nerve is noted and stapes fixation is checked. Subtle fixation may be detected by palpating the footplate while observing the annular ligament for change in color or width. The footplate is also examined for the most appro-

priate site for perforation. The ideal site is a thin, blue area in the center. A thick white or an obliterated footplate may require drilling or other efforts.

Occasionally, a case with no apparent fixation will be encountered. When this happens, it is incumbent upon the surgeon to determine if there are any other causes of a conductive hearing loss. Malleus and incus fixation, or the presence of a serous otitis, are three obvious conditions to exclude.

THE INCUDOSTAPEDIAL JOINT AND THE STAPEDIAL TENDON

It can be difficult to appreciate the incudostapedial joint at first. By gently pushing on the lenticular process with the back of the joint knife, the capsule will blanch over the joint. The joint can then be easily cut with the joint knife (Fig. 15–4A). The incudostapedial joint is divided in a direction that pushes against the pull of the stapedius tendon. This motion should be gentle; care must be taken not to dislocate the incus. The tendon is divided in a convenient position with microscissors (Fig. 15–4B). Those with an inclination to preserve the tendon may tease it from the capitulum or cut it near the insertion.

Mucosa is removed from the footplate and the promontory to control any bleeding prior to proceeding with footplate removal. Bleeding may take several minutes to subside. It is important not to rush into the next step. Hemostasis is important and often takes several minutes to occur.

THE FOOTPLATE

All of the previous steps were preparatory to addressing the stapes footplate. These previous steps should have been completed without difficulty prior to proceeding. The reason for this caution is clear: No harm has been done to this point. If something

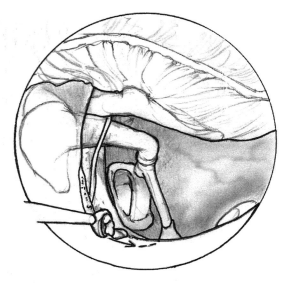

FIGURE 15–3 Curetting the bone from the scutum.

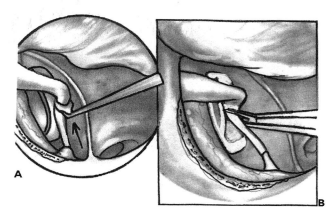

FIGURE 15–4 (A) Cutting the incudostapedial joint. (B) Dividing the stapedial tendon.

has gone awry, the procedure can be terminated, and the patient is no worse for the adventure.

In general, in addressing the footplate, there are two techniques that are used: those using the laser, and those using manual techniques. Because of the necessity to be able to directly expose certain portions of the stapes or the footplate, or because of heat transfer to surrounding structures, there are occasions where the laser cannot be used. To meet this need, two methods of dealing with the stapes footplate are described: one using the laser, and the other using manual technique.

For the first method, the posterior crus is cut using an argon laser (Fig. 15–5). The anterior crus is similarly cut using the hand-held oto-endo probe to touch the anterior crus and vaporize it directly. The superstructure is easily removed, once the crura are cut (Fig. 15–6). The footplate itself is now exposed completely. Again using the oto-endo probe, a rosette is created at the junction of the middle and the posterior one third of the footplate. This will adequately vaporize all of the bone of the footplate using 1 to 2 W and 0.1- to 0.2-second bursts (Fig. 15–7). It is easier to create the rosette by overlapping each laser burst slightly. The rosette should be two thirds of the width of the footplate, or approximately 0.8 mm. When the rosette has been completed, using a gentle motion and a small hook, the surgeon can appreciate that the bone has been vaporized, but the endosteum has not been violated. The area should be soft to touch.

If the laser cannot be used, a control hole can be created in the blue footplate at the junction of the posterior one third and the anterior two thirds of the footplate, using a Barbara needle. The control hole is enlarged across the footplate (Fig. 15–8). This frees the portion to be removed. The posterior third to one half of the footplate is removed using small hooks (Fig. 15–9). A special strong hook has been developed for this maneuver. The smaller the footplate area, the greater the proportion of the footplate that should be removed (a very small footplate should be removed entirely). This ensures the proper placement of the prosthesis and vein. Care is taken not to suction perilymph from the vestibule. Small fragments of bone falling into perilymph are left untouched, as is any bleeding or clot. More damage may be done by removing these pieces, and they cause no harm. After the footplate is removed, further mucosa is removed from the facial nerve and the area anterior to the footplate (Fig. 15–10). This further secures bleeding and provides for purchase of the graft.

Thus, the footplate can easily be handled in one of two ways. The footplate can be partially or completely removed, or a small opening can be created using a laser with a molded graft. Either technique yields satisfactory and comparable results.[25]

THE LOOSE AREOLAR FASCIA GRAFT

The graft is cut to a square about 4 × 4 mm, about the size of a cigarette in diameter. It is purposely

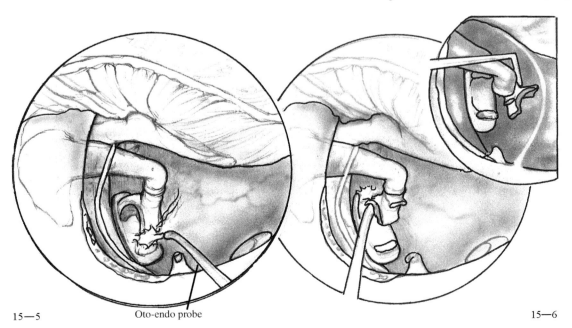

15—5   Oto-endo probe   15—6

FIGURE 15–5 Laser technique for cutting the posterior crus.
FIGURE 15–6 Laser technique for cutting the anterior crus. Remove the stapes superstructure.

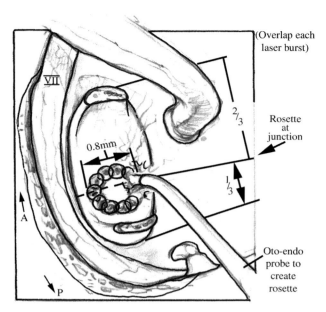

FIGURE 15–7 Laser technique for creating the rosette on the stapes footplate.

kept very thin, so that it will drape over the promontory and the facial nerve well. The graft is then placed on a glass block with a central hole measuring 1 mm deep and just fitting the size of the shaft of the prosthesis. In this case, it is about 0.8 mm to accommodate a 0.4-mm prosthesis. It is crucial that the graft generously overlaps the vestibule, as this creates a trampoline-like self-centering action for the prosthesis, and any gap may predispose to a

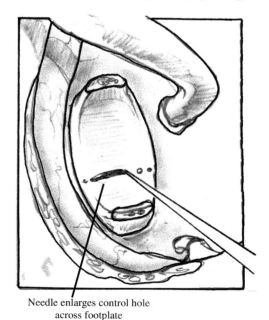

Needle enlarges control hole
across footplate

FIGURE 15–8 Manual technique for creating the control hole and dividing the anterior two thirds of the footplate from the posterior one third.

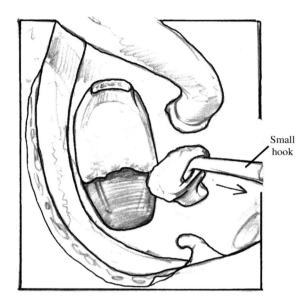

FIGURE 15–9 Remove the posterior one third of the footplate.

later perilymph fistula. By drying the graft with a prosthesis in place for a few minutes, the two can easily slip into place. The graft is placed without wetting it, centered over the opening in the footplate, and then the prosthesis is placed in the opening on top of the graft (Fig. 15–11).

THE PROSTHESIS

The microscope is positioned to allow a good view of both the incus and footplate. This is best accomplished by pulling the head of the microscope toward the surgeon and then refocusing. A 4.0-mm Robinson prosthesis is placed in the depression of the graft and rested against the incus (Fig. 15–12). It is not necessary to measure the distance between the

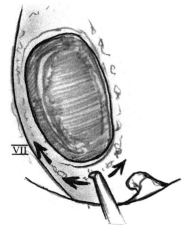

FIGURE 15–10 Scarification of the mucosa around the footplate for better adhesion.

narrow (0.4 mm) stem. Irrespective of the side, an incus hook is taken in the left hand and a strut guide in the right. The hands are steadied against the speculum holder. The hook is placed anterior to and beneath the incus but no attempt made to pull it laterally. The strut guide engages the prosthesis and is used to manipulate it beneath the incus. As the prosthesis approaches the lenticular process, the hook is used to steady and minutely lift the incus (Fig. 15–13). Once underneath the lenticular process, the incus hook is released and the prosthesis tends to snap onto the lenticular process. In case of difficulty, the positioning of the prosthesis can be done with one hand, but this disturbs the vestibule more than is desirable.

COMPLETION

The bucket handle is flipped over the long process and the mechanical action of the prosthesis checked by gentle palpation (Fig. 15–14). If it is difficult to fit the bucket handle, it should be left alone. It should not be forced onto the incus. Too tight a fit prevents the prosthesis from centering. Blood is gently suctioned away and the tympanic membrane replaced. An intraoperative air threshold audiogram is obtained. This is a qualitative test only. The patient is expected to hear better, but not at the final level. It is

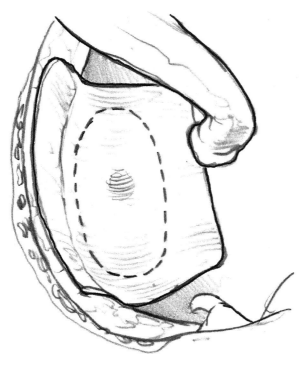

FIGURE 15–11 Place the 4 × 4 areolar fascia graft.

incus and the vestibule. The distance is very consistent in many anatomic studies done over many years. The prosthesis is a Robinson, 4.0-mm length overall, with a large well (1.0-mm bucket) and a

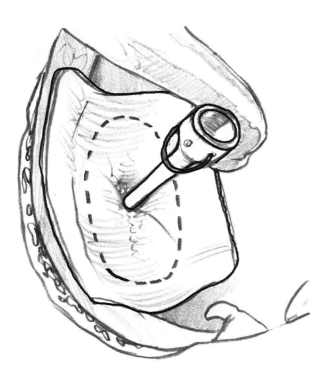

FIGURE 15–12 The Robinson prosthesis is placed in the depression in the graft over the opening in the stapes footplate and rested against the incus.

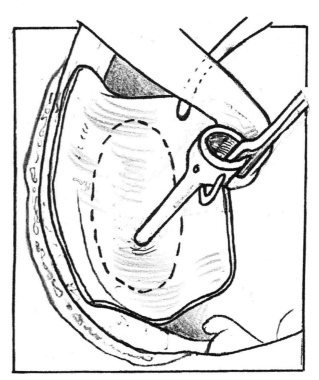

FIGURE 15–13 An incus hook is bent and placed under and behind the incus, to steady it and to lift it ever so gently.

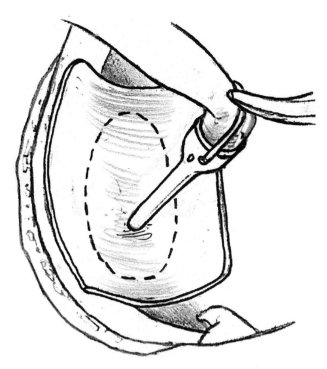

FIGURE 15–14 The bucket handle is placed over the incus if possible. The mobility of the whole assembly is checked using a blunt instrument.

important not to expect too much of this test. Ideally, the hearing should be within 15 dB of the preoperative bony threshold. If it is not improved, the drum is lifted and a cause sought for the failure to improve. Antibiotic ointment is used to fill the external canal and the patient returned to the recovery room.

COMPLICATIONS OF STAPEDECTOMY

DIZZINESS

The three most common causes for vertigo, unsteadiness, and disequilibrium are vestibular end organ damage and an overlong prosthesis. In years past, when the oval window was not closed with a seal, perilymphatic fistulas occurred regularly. They are fortunately now rare. Vestibular symptoms occur in the immediate postoperative period in up to 96% of cases. These symptoms seem to be less when the vestibule is manipulated to a lesser degree. Most persist for only 24 to 48 hours, but 5% may last for up to a week. Patients with evidence of balance problems in the first week should be started on labyrinthine compensatory exercises. Those who do not respond after 2 to 3 weeks should be suspected of an overlong prosthesis. Computed tomography (CT) scanning may assist in the decision to revise the case.

HEARING LOSS

Delayed sensorineural hearing loss may occur in cases of stapedectomy as they do in the general population. These cases should be treated similarly to those cases with high-dose oral steroids, antiviral agents, and inhalational carbogen. Unfortunately, some of these cases do not recover hearing and unfortunately go on to regain little or no hearing. It is the role of the physician to assist the unfortunate patient in working through the phases of loss that accompany such a terrible outcome. Further, the physician should assist the patient in making accommodations to the new reality of the hearing loss.

TYMPANIC MEMBRANE PERFORATION AND FLAP TEARS

The majority of torn flaps heal with simple reapposition of the edges. Any significant tissue defect, or injury to the tympanic membrane, can be repaired in an underlay fashion with a fascia graft. A generous graft should always be taken in case a repair is required.

THE CHORDA TYMPANI

It is often preferable to section a stretched chorda to prevent prolonged taste disturbance. In the majority (>98%) of cases, adequate surgical access can be gained without sacrificing the chorda. When operating on a second ear, every effort should be made to preserve the chorda if it was damaged in the opposite ear. If the original first ear was operated elsewhere, you must assume it was damaged. If the chorda tympani nerve is stretched or cut on both sides, there may be a permanent dry taste disturbance, but more importantly, a permanent dry mouth may result.

OSSICULAR DISLOCATION

The incus may be inadvertently injured while curetting. If only subluxed, a rigid stapes prosthesis may assist in fixing it in position. As the joint capsule heals and fibroses, a surprisingly good hearing result may ensue in most of the cases. A more severe injury may require revision or management with a different ossicular reconstruction.

MALLEUS OR INCUS FIXATION

When either the malleus or the incus is fixed, the situation can be handled in the same fashion.

Reduced malleus mobility on pneumatic otoscopy may provide a preoperative clue to this diagnosis. If necessary, the malleus can be palpated during an office visit. Phenol is placed on the umbo for anesthesia, and a rigid instrument is used to touch the manubrium under microscopic control. At surgery, once the middle ear is entered, the malleus should always be palpated under direct vision. An assessment is made of whether this is slight, moderate, or total. The operation should continue until an assessment of footplate mobility can be made. If otosclerosis coexists, a stapedectomy is indicated. In cases where malleus fixation is slight or moderate, the result will be as if there were no fixation. If the malleus is totally fixed, a large amount of oval window should be removed in the anticipation of a second procedure. In a series of 45 cases with both stapes and complete malleus fixation, 70% improved to within 10 dB and 84% to within 20 dB of the preoperative bone conduction level when treated with stapedectomy alone.[26]

INCUS NECROSIS

Incus necrosis is often evident preoperatively if secondary to retraction or may be noted during revision stapedectomy when the lenticular process is eroded or missing, or a Lippy modified Robinson prosthesis (usually 4.5 mm or longer depending on the extent of necrosis) is used.[27] Incus necrosis is most likely to occur in cases when the tympanic membrane is atrophic. In these cases the drum should be thickened by using a tissue graft on the underside.[28]

PERSISTENT STAPEDIAL ARTERY

The stapedial artery usually disappears during the embryologic development of the ear. Occasionally, it persists as a remnant that passes through the arch of the stapes. When vestigial, it can easily be cauterized and removed. When prominent, other techniques of management should be considered if a stapedectomy is to be attempted at all.[29]

FACIAL NERVE ANOMALIES

The facial nerve is frequently dehiscent and this rarely presents a problem. When overhanging and yet some footplate is visible, a number 26 suction is used to gently push the nerve aside. This may allow enough access to the footplate for the operation to proceed. Alternately, first a Hough hoe and then a microdrill may be used to drill off the inferior margin of the oval window and promontory. Place the drill on the footplate, push aside the facial nerve

with the suction, and gently sweep up several times. There will be no damage to the hearing nerve from the drill. Remove whatever footplate you can and blindly perforate the rest. Then place a vein graft and a prosthesis. Even though the prosthesis indents the facial nerve, there will be no damage or paralysis. It is unwise to attempt this technique, however, without experience. The nerve may exist as other anomalies that may prevent the completion of a stapedectomy.

The surgeon may want to contemplate the implications of the above situation. A facial nerve paralysis is a devastating consequence of stapes surgery. There are few to no consequences of closing a complicated ear and referring to another surgeon with more experience at handling such a complicated ear. One is seldom sorry for the operation that was not done.

OBLITERATIVE OTOSCLEROSIS

This extensive form of otosclerosis is dramatically less common than it was in the 1960s. The footplate is considered to be obliterated when the margins cannot be seen. Occasionally the footplate is partially or totally obliterated with only the top of the superstructure visible. A 0.7-mm diamond bur should be used to saucerize the footplate region, drilling gently and slowly. Irrigation should be used to minimize heat transfer. The vestibule should be blue-lined and the final layer of bone opened with a needle. Remove bone on a broad front and avoid a small opening into the footplate. On occasion the superior margin of the promontory may need to be drilled. A slightly longer prosthesis may be required to be sure that the prosthesis is below the edge of the annulus of the window, preventing regrowth. If the bone is well saucerized, prosthesis action should be near normal. Results, however, are not as good as in routine cases (80% within 10 dB).

FLOATING FOOTPLATE

The footplate may inadvertently mobilize while it is manipulated. Regardless of whether it is solid (white) or diffuse (blue), a graft should be placed over it and a 4-mm prosthesis inserted. Long-term success rates with this technique are 97% within 10 dB if there is a blue footplate. If this occurs with a white footplate, hearing success is only 52%. However, this situation can often be safely revised. Should the footplate mobilize again during revision, no future surgery should be advised. In a series of 8000 stapedectomies, there were no cases of sensorineural loss in 147 cases of floating footplate treated in this fashion.[30] An inadvertently mobilized footplate treated in this manner is a fortuitous event, not a disaster.

POSTOPERATIVE COURSE

After the completion of stapedectomy, no matter what technique is used, the patient lies in bed with the operated ear up toward the ceiling for 2 hours. This permits the ear to settle into its former position. Better, it allows dizzy patients to recuperate, and allows the blood in the middle ear to coagulate, holding the prosthesis and the drum in position.

After the stay in the surgery center, patients are slowly ambulated, and when stable, are discharged. Instructions during the home interval include no heavy lifting (> 20 lb), no blowing of the nose, and no vigorous activities for 3 weeks. Patients are permitted to fly after 1 week. They return to the office for removal of the ointment in 4 to 6 weeks.

When patients come from a distance, a routine for follow-up makes it much easier to manage them. The staff knows exactly what to tell the patients, and the patients know what to expect. Thus, education is enhanced, and quality and consistent results are assured. Further, when all the staff members involved in the care of the patient know just what to expect, the patient achieves a much more relaxed and comfortable state of mind. Thus, practice guidelines and care plans can significantly improve the entire course of care.

PROGNOSIS

The natural history of otosclerosis is a gradually progressive hearing loss. Individuals with a long-standing hearing loss may present with a profound hearing loss. Because of the limits of audiometry, it may not be possible to determine whether there is a reserve of hearing present. Occasionally, placing a tuning fork on the incisors will be met with eye widening and a look of excitement. In these cases, a stapedectomy may bring the hearing back to an aidable level of 60 dB. Others, however, will require a cochlear implant for rehabilitation. In these select cases, the surgeon should attend to the CT scan to be sure that the otosclerosis has not obliterated the interior of the basal turn.

After the operation, the prognosis for patients is quite good. Excellent hearing results are obtained and are durable for the life of the patient in the vast majority of cases. The progression of the sensorineural component of otosclerosis seems to slow down after stapedectomy. Therefore, the long-term outcome is stabilization of hearing. Patients often experience no more hearing loss over the years. In several long-term studies, patients lost a maximum of one-half decibel per year over a period of 30 years. This makes for a very positive and stable experience for the stapedectomy patient.

REFERENCES

1. Bonnafont S. *Traite Theoretique et Pratique des Maladies de l'Oreille*. Paris: Bailliere; 1860.
2. Lempert J. Improvement of hearing in cases of otosclerosis: new one stage surgical technique. *Arch Otolaryngol* 1938;28:42–44.
3. Rosen S. Palpation of the stapes for fixation. *Arch Otolaryngol* 1952;56:610–612.
4. Shea JJ Jr. Fenestration of the oval window. *Ann Otol Rhinol Laryngol* 1958;67:932–935.
5. Sheehy JL. Controversies in otosclerosis. *Am J Otol* 1983;4:273–275.
6. Robinson M. Juvenile otosclerosis: a 20-year study. *Ann Otol Rhinol Laryngol* 1983;92:561–565.
7. Nager FR. Zur Klinik und pathologischen Anatomie der Otosklerose. *Acta Otolaryngol* 1939;27:542–551.
8. Shambaugh GE. Clinical diagnosis of cochlear (labyrinthine) otosclerosis. *Laryngoscope* 1965;75:1558–1562.
9. Larsson A. Otosclerosis, a genetic and clinical study. *Acta Otolaryngol Suppl* 1960;154:1–86.
10. Friedmann I. *Pathology of the Ear*. Oxford: Blackwell Scientific; 1974.
11. McKenna JM, Kristiansen AG, Barley ML, et al. Association of COL1A1 and otosclerosis: evidence for a shared genetic etiology with mild osteogenesis imperfecta. *Am J Otol* 1998;19:604–610.
12. McKenna MJ, Mills BG. Ultrastructural and immunohistochemical evidence of measles virus in active otosclerosis. *Acta Otolaryngol Suppl* 1990;470:130–139.
13. Carhart R. Clinical application of bone conduction audiometry. *Arch Otolaryngol* 1950;51:798.
14. Terkildsen K, Osterhammel P, Bretlau P. Acoustic middle ear muscle reflexes in patients with otosclerosis, *Arch Otolaryngol* 1973;98:152–155.
15. Lippy WH, Burkey JW, Fucci MJ, Schuring AG, Rizer FM. Stapedectomy in the elderly. *Am J Otol* 1996;17:831–834.
16. Lippy WH, Burkey JW, Schuring AG, Rizer FM. Short and long term results of stapedectomy in children. *Laryngoscope* 1998;108:569–572.
17. Lippy WH, Battista RA, Schuring AG, Rizer FM. Far-advanced otosclerosis. *Am J Otol* 1994;15:225–228.
18. Causse J, Causse JB. Eighteen year report on stapedectomy. II: postoperative therapy. *Clin Otolaryngol* 1980;5:329–337.
19. Lundy LB. "Ethics" of stapedectomy. *Am J Otol* 1999;20:137–138.
20. Sismanis A, Hughes GB, Abedi E. Coexisting otosclerosis and Meniere's disease: a diagnostic dilemma. *Laryngoscope* 1986;96:9–13.

21. Katzav J, Lippy WH, Shamiss A, Davidson BZ. Stapedectomy in combat pilots. *Am J Otol* 1996;17:847–849.

22. Lippy WH, Schuring AG, Rizer FM. Intraoperative audiometry. *Laryngoscope* 1995;105:214–216.

23. Patterson ME, Lockwood RW, Sheehy JL. Temporalis fascia in tympanic membrane grafting: tissue culture and animal studies. *Arch Otolaryngol* 1967;85:287–291.

24. Moon CN Jr. Loose areolar connective tissue: a graft for otologic surgery. *Laryngoscope* 1973;83:771–777.

25. Lippy WH, Berenholz LP, Burkey JM. Otosclerosis in the 1960s, 1970s, 1980s and the 1990s. *Laryngoscope* 1999;109:1307–1309.

26. Lippy WH, Schuring AG, Ziv M. Stapedectomy for otosclerosis with malleus fixation. *Arch Otolaryngol* 1978;104:388–389.

27. Krieger LW, Lippy WH, Schuring AG, Rizer FM. Revision stapedectomy for incus erosion: long-term hearing. *Otolaryngol Head Neck Surg* 1998;119:370–373.

28. Lippy WH, Schuring AG. Prosthesis for the problem incus in stapedectomy. *Arch Otolarygnol* 1974;100:237–239.

29. Tien HC, Linthicum FH Jr. Persistent stapedial artery. *Otol Neurotol* 2001;22:975–976.

30. Lippy WH, Schuring AG. Treatment of the inadvertently mobilized footplate. *Arch Otolaryngol* 1973;98:80–81.

Chapter 16

REVISION STAPES SURGERY

William J. Garvis and Gary E. Garvis

"Revision stapes surgery offers an entirely different challenge to primary stapes surgery."[1]

Although still the crown jewel of otology, stapes surgery is no longer performed with the breadth and wealth of experience once enjoyed; the "golden era" of otologic surgery has passed. Over the last 35 years there has been a decline in the number of stapes surgeries performed, with the depletion of back-logged older otosclerotic patients partly to blame.[2] By 1970, the number of stapes surgeries performed yearly had dropped to about one third of the peak number done in 1964.[2] With the vanishing numbers of these surgeries has come the loss of the broader technical proficiency enjoyed by those who trained during the earlier era. Nowadays fewer and fewer ears suitable for stapes surgery are available for teaching; so senior residents finish their training with little hands-on experience and feel ill-at-ease performing this technically demanding surgery.[3] Not uncommonly, as they may encounter only a few potential stapes cases yearly, they may feel compelled to refer these either to those with a larger otologic practice or to specific centers of excellence.[1]

Perhaps because of the noted diminution of primary surgical cases, the advent of the "occasional" stapes surgeon, the various kinds of prosthesis failures, or the variable results seen even in the hands of the most experienced surgeons, revision stapes surgery has emerged as an important component to modern otology. Since the description of oval window fenestration by Shea[4] in 1958, there has been both the opportunity and need to correct postoperative failures following stapes surgery. Sheehy and House,[5] in 1962, were the first to report the need for revision surgery. Since then, the literature has been replete with articles detailing the growing experience with revision stapes procedures as the "relative frequency of revision operations is increasing."[1] Initially the reported results of revision surgery were much worse than those of primary surgery, calling into question the safety and efficacy of this approach. With the introduction of the laser to primary stapes surgery[6] and its subsequent expansion to revision surgery, however, the results encountered in the revision cases have markedly improved. Presently, as it parallels the record of primary surgical procedures, revision stapes surgery represents a safe, effective option for failures.

Admittedly, although primary otosclerotic surgery may be technically demanding, revision stapes procedures are often some of the most challenging otology cases to be encountered. Whereas a virgin otosclerotic ear may have pathology centered near the oval window, the revision's surgeon often encounters various other problems outside of the typical one centered within the fossa ovalis. Veil-like adhesions, which may extend from the tympanic membrane, the incus, the prosthesis, and the scutum, are often found obscuring one's vision upon elevating the flap. And it is just behind, or through, these concealing investments that more potential pathology exists. Typically, the findings are characterized by one or more of the following problems: prosthesis dysfunction (displaced, loose-wire, too-short, or too-long prosthesis); ossicular resorptive osteitis (incus necrosis); oval window pathology (lateralized neomembrane, adhesions, regrowth of obliterative otosclerosis, or a perilymphatic fistula); or lateral ossicular chain fixation (adhesions, attic ankylosis, or ossification of the anterior malleal ligament). The surgeon should also be cognizant that a failure may also reflect obliterative otosclerosis at the *round* window. Therefore, a surgeon performing revision stapes surgery should be prepared to encounter and address any of these various findings at surgery.[7]

PRESENTATION

During the nearly 50 years of stapes surgery, the development of different prostheses, both with respect to design and material, has afforded better and more consistent long-term results. The type of oval window fenestration, which includes the complete stapedectomy, the platinectomy, and the small-fenestra stapedotomy, has changed in accordance with the evolution of the prosthesis and with a desire to diminish the risk of complications.[8,9] Currently, with the different techniques and prostheses, primary stapes surgery results in closure of the air–bone gap to less than 10 dB in nearly 85% of the cases, with an approximate 1% risk of sensorineural hearing loss.

Despite acknowledging that the vast majority of primary stapes surgeries are successful, a small percentage fails. Either the patient or the surgeon recognizes a suboptimal outcome. Problems may present shortly after surgery or many years later. Common problems likely to prompt early assessment include symptoms of dizziness or vertigo or a marked drop in hearing. Presenting signs and symptoms later can include a delayed but progressive hearing loss, dizziness, dysequilibrium, vertigo, or hearing that fluctuates.

Even with an uncomplicated and successful surgery it is not uncommon to have mild postoperative dizziness when perforating the footplate.[10] The frequency of this occurrence has dropped with the development and use of the fenestration (stapedotomy) technique. Nonetheless, short-term dysequilibrium can occur but usually requires little more than tempered observation, rest, and occasionally medications, such as oral steroids, vestibular suppressants, or antiemetics. The dizziness or dysequilibrium is usually secondary to a serous labyrinthitis (secondary to either blood or displaced proteolytic enzymes in the vestibule),[11] infrequently benign paroxysmal positional vertigo,[12] or rarely a pneumolabyrinth.[13] The persistence of severe vertigo, lasting more than a week and not responding to conservative measures, however, requires a more attentive assessment and raises concern for the presence of a perilymphatic fistula, an overly long prosthesis, or a reparative granuloma.

Shortly after surgery, depending on the approach, technique, and postoperative course, most patients experience an appreciation of improved audition. If they judge diminished or equivocal hearing, however, then further assessment is warranted at that

time. Typically this is done not only to assuage general concerns but also to assess the retention of the preoperative cochlear function. If there has been a drop in the bone curve, then attention should focus on the possibility of saccular injury (as from a too-long prosthesis), a perilymphatic fistula, or a reparative granuloma.

Delayed hearing problems can occur at any time following the operative procedure. The loss of hearing acuity may reflect lenticular process erosion, obliterative otosclerotic regrowth at the fossa ovalis, lateral ossicular fixation, adhesions causing prosthesis fixation or displacement, or a perilymphatic fistula. Other pathologies can coexist, though, and may include suppurative labyrinthitis, endolymphatic hydrops, or retrocochlear disease.[10]

EVALUATION

As with any otologic evaluation, obtaining a good history is very important. What was done, as well as when and under what circumstances, can help direct the assessment and possible intervention. Signs and symptoms presenting early are more likely to indicate more serious problems, for example a perilymphatic fistula, whereas those presenting years later are more likely to reflect a loss of lenticular process integrity or the propagation of adhesions with prosthesis displacement.

Otomicroscopy should be performed to evaluate the appearance, position, and integrity of the tympanic membrane. Other problems such as perforations, retraction pockets, and cholesteatomas may coexist within an otosclerotic ear, and if unrecognized, substantially alter the surgical approach and outcome. Furthermore, a dull and erythematous tympanic membrane, in the face of vertigo and sensorineural hearing loss, may be indicative of a reparative granuloma.[14]

Microscopic evaluation of membrane mobility, or otomicropneumotoscopy, should also be done in the office examination. Adhesive otitis media localized to the epitympanic recess, or a subtle retraction pocket into Prussak's space, may be demonstrated by this exam. Ear insufflation is also important in evaluating two other causes of surgical failure. A temporary shift in auditory acuity with positive- or negative-pressure insufflation suggests a loose prosthetic wire. In a similar manner, but with the addition of Frenzel glasses, a perilymphatic fistula is implicated when ear insufflation produces ocular deviation and/or nystagmus (positive fistula test).

Perhaps lost on some otolaryngologists is the invaluable information obtained from a careful tuning-fork evaluation. The audiologist's assessment of hearing acuity should not preclude this examination, especially when there is concern regarding anacusis in an operated ear or when there is a coexisting bilateral moderately severe sensorineural hearing loss. The use of a tuning fork with a Bárány box masker can be invaluable.

The patient must unabashedly have a full audiologic assessment. Establishment of both air and bone curves is essential. The audiologist can assist in objectifying the degree and type of hearing loss, aspects of cochlear insult, and even fluctuating hearing levels.

In cases of vertigo that last beyond the immediate postoperative period, one should consider obtaining multiplanar fine-cut temporal bone computed tomography (CT).[15] Prosthesis subluxation into the vestibule, an overly long prosthesis, perisaccular bone fragments, reparative granuloma, and pneumolabyrinth have all been adequately visualized and identified with this imaging modality.[13,16,17]

SURGICAL FINDINGS

"Prior to undertaking revision stapes surgery, it is helpful for the otologic surgeon to know what problems he may encounter."[18]

The most common finding at revision surgery is related to prosthesis dysfunction, which is reported to occur in perhaps up to 80% of the cases. The most common intraoperative findings, as cited in the literature, are summarized in Table 16–1. But prosthesis dysfunction, like the other findings noted below, is unlikely to be the only problem detected at surgery. In more than 50% of the cases, it is typical to find more than one cause of failure.[7] Within the category of prosthesis dysfunction are the reported findings of slipped, loose, too-long, too-short, bent, fractured, and displaced prostheses. Of these, a displaced prosthesis is most commonly found, and is often seen with other problems including oval window adhesions, obliterative regrowth of otosclerosis, a lateralized neomembrane, and incus necrosis (Fig. 16–1).

The finding of a deficient incus is encountered in between 5 and 30% of revision surgeries.[19] The spiculated, atrophic, or even absent long process has, at best, only limited contiguity with the stapes prosthesis (Fig. 16–2). Nadol[20] notes in his series, though, that it is the *only* finding on histopathology in just 7% of the cases. There exist many theories as to the etiopathogenesis of this problem. The loss of incus integrity is thought to result from the disruption of an already tenuous vascularity, and can occur

TABLE 16–1 FINDINGS AT REVISION SURGERY: CAUSES OF FAILURE

Author(s) and Published Year (No. of Cases)	Prosthesis Dysfunction (%)	Incus Necrosis (%)	Adhesions (%)	Obliterative Regrowth (%)	Oval Window Fistula (%)	Lateral Ossicular Chain Fixation (%)
Sheehy et al 1981[24] (n = 258)	48	17	5	9	16	2
Derlacki 1985[18] (n = 217)	82	30	8	10	10	0.5
Glasscock et al 1987[25] (n = 79)	38	19	—	8	9	4
Farrior and Sutherland 1991[26] (n = 109)	43	28	—	8	12	3
Langman and Lindeman 1993[27] (n = 66)	49	41	—	9	6	6
McGee et al 1993[22] (n = 185)	20	5	9	6	—	1
Cokkeser et al 1994[28] (n = 52)	32	34	23	16	10	14
Silverstein et al 1994[7] (n = 76)	53	29	29	13	12	6
Peter 1995[29] (n = 39)	67	8	—	13	—	5
Pedersen 1996[30] (n = 186)	38	11	19	16	0.3	—
Han et al 1997[31] (n = 74)	58	43	18	24	5	1
Somers et al 1997[1] (n = 332)	33	28	13	5	7	2
Hammerschlag et al 1998[32] (n = 250)	39	14	14	5	2	0.8
De La Cruz and Fayad 2000[33] (n = 356)	53	26	—	14	2	0.8

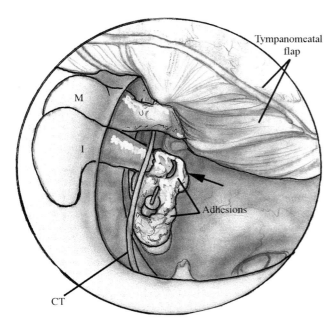

FIGURE 16–1 Appearance of the middle ear. Upon elevating the tympanomeatal flap, it is common to find the long and lenticular processes of the incus (I), along with the stapes prosthesis, engulfed in scar tissue. The region of the lenticular process is indicated by the arrow. M, malleus.

with any type of prosthesis.[19,20] Medial fixation of the prosthesis, a loose crimping, postoperative inflammation, and fixation of the prosthesis (i.e., from adhesions or otosclerotic regrowth) creating friction at the point of incudal-prosthetic contact are postulated causes of the avascular necrosis and resorptive osteitis.[20] Management of this problem may be accomplished with recrimping more proximally on the long process (which is associated with a high rate of re-erosion[19]) or as discussed below.

Patients may present with fluctuant hearing, especially evident with changes in middle ear aeration. The loose-wire syndrome occurs in cases where the attachment of the prosthesis to the incus is via a crimped wire. It consists of a triad of one or more symptoms that are improved with middle ear insufflation. These symptoms include an increase in auditory acuity, an improvement in sound distortion, or an improvement in speech discrimination.[21,22] With middle ear insufflation, the tympanic membrane is displaced laterally, tensing the prosthesis wire crimp against the similarly lateralized ossicular chain, and thereby improving mechanical sound conduction. During middle ear exploration, the wire crimp is typically found somewhat loosely secured around the long process rather than solidly connected. The wire may be recrimped or the prosthesis replaced.

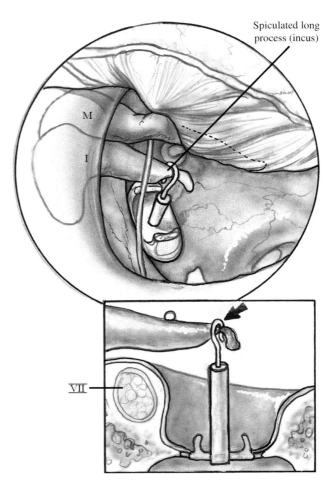

FIGURE 16–2 Resorptive osteitis of the incus (I). The loss of incus integrity can often be recognized, as in this illustration, by a spiculated long process with the loop of the prosthesis nearly free. The arrow points to the limited area of contact between the prosthesis and the long process of incus. M, malleus.

Although quite rare nowadays, the presence of a reparative granuloma still must be considered a cause when sensorineural hearing loss and dizziness occur shortly after stapes surgery. Hearing loss, vertigo, and a dull, erythematous, tympanic membrane typically herald the occurrence of a reparative granuloma. It may occur with any type of prosthesis or grafting material but is seen to occur less frequently with the stapedotomy–blood sealant technique.[14] Upon entering the middle ear, the surgeon commonly finds a brawny-red mass of granulation tissue that engulfs the prosthesis and incus and extends from the tympanic membrane down into the fossa ovalis. The prosthesis must be removed, the granuloma vaporized or removed, and a tissue sealant placed over the oval window fenestration.

An important cause for middle ear exploration following stapes surgery is the persistence of a perilymphatic leak. A perilymphatic fistula may account for up to 10% of all stapedectomy failures.[23] The association of a fluctuant sensorineural hearing level, typically within the low frequencies, along with vertigo often implicates a perilymphatic fistula. However, the symptoms may be quite variable and instead consist of mixed or purely conductive hearing losses, dysequilibrium, and/or tinnitus.[23] Fistulas have been identified radiographically by an aggregate of tiny air bubbles at the end of the prosthesis on high-resolution thin-cut CT.[16] The presence of a perilymphatic fistula may be confirmed at surgery by the accumulation of clear fluid within or around the oval window during a Valsalva maneuver. To close a fistula the adjacent mucosa should be gently scored. Then either small pledgets of adipose tissue or a larger pressed piece of fat or fascia may be widely laid over the fistula site and this seal augmented with a drop of fibrin glue.

INDICATIONS FOR RE-EXPLORATION

There are three occurrences that typically prompt re-exploration: dizziness, progressive sensorineural hearing loss, and a widened air–bone gap. Sheehy et al[24] believe that if "a persistent balance disturbance ... incapacitates the patient, or [if] there is a progressive sensorineural hearing impairment, exploration of the middle ear may be indicated." Mann et al[34] cite suspicion of a perilymphatic fistula or demonstration of an overly long prosthesis penetrating too deeply into the vestibule (as seen on CT) as the only absolute indications for revision surgery. To this list, however, should be added the clinical suspicion or evidence of a reparative granuloma as discussed previously. Han et al[31] cite a persistent conductive hearing loss as reason enough to consider raising a tympanomeatal flap and evaluating the middle ear mechanics.

SURGICAL APPROACH

"Nowhere is the laser more appropriate than in revision stapes surgery."[22]

In preparing to approach a failed stapes surgery, the availability of a laser is extremely important. A large meta-analysis demonstrated the significant benefit to outcome with the use of lasers as compared to conventional techniques in revision surgery. Wiet et al[35] showed that a successful (<10 dB) result occurred in 69% of cases treated with a laser, whereas only 51% attained the same result when conventional techniques were used ($p = 0.002$).[35] Of the available lasers, the fiberoptic handpiece probes are uniquely advantageous compared to the micromanipulator controls found with CO_2 lasers. Horn et al[36] and Nissen[37] extolled the virtues of the argon laser for these cases.

Although some patients may not prefer local anesthesia with sedation, performing revision stapes surgery in this manner affords greater assurance and safety. Patients under general anesthesia cannot react to vestibular irritation nor can they be queried intraoperatively about hearing acuity. Unless there are extenuating circumstances, or significant patient concerns, the surgeon should plan to do the cases under local anesthesia with sedation.

Fisch et al[38] proposed that all revision cases be performed via an endaural approach. In their experience, the view, orientation, and greater ability to assess the ossicular mobility dictate this approach. Farrior and Temple[9] also cited the advantage of this approach if the prosthesis must be attached to the malleus instead of the incus. There is indeed an advantage to placement of the prosthesis via the endaural approach. But with an adequate external auditory canal that can accommodate at least a 6-mm surgical ear speculum and visualization of the tympanic annulus and tympanic membrane anterior to the short process of the malleus, it is not essential. Nevertheless, the endaural approach should be within the armamentarium of the surgeon, as it is invaluable in the most difficult cases and when performing a malleostapedotomy.

After the patient has been given medication for sedation, along with intravenous steroids, an antibiotic, and an antiemetic, a periauricular block is performed. The ear canal is then injected in quadratic fashion until light blanching of the tympanic membrane occurs.

After the ear is prepped, the ear canal is suctioned of any residual fluids. After examining the meatus and ear canal, the largest speculum to be accommodated just medial to the hair-bearing line in the canal is chosen. A wide apex is positioned posterior to the scutum, and a generous triangular-shaped tympanomeatal flap is incised and raised. The incision must extend anterior and lateral to the short process of the malleus, so when the flap is raised the anterior malleal process and ligament are visualized as well as the posterosuperior quadrant (Fig. 16–3). Often the tympanomeatal flap is quite thick. It may be thinned sharply on its medial surface to facilitate mobilizing and reflecting the flap forward. Quite commonly there are multiple adhesions in the posterosuperior quadrant, so the tympanum is

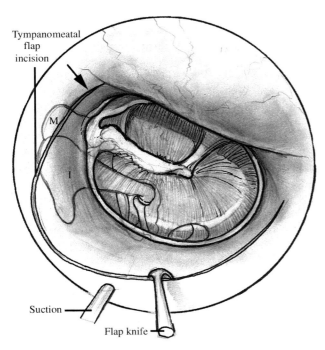

FIGURE 16–3 Raising the tympanomeatal flap. A generous triangularly shaped flap should be elevated. The incision, as indicated by the arrow, must extend anterior and lateral to the short process of the malleus.

entered inferiorly and the drum elevated from there. All adhesions not encasing the prosthesis are lysed using the laser with 1 to 2 W of power and a 0.1-second-duration pulse.

It is imperative in revision stapes surgery to palpate and determine the mobility of the lateral ossicular chain. Fisch et al noted[38] that although "complete fixation of the incus and malleus is easily detected … partial fixation of these ossicles may defy years of experience." Incus-malleus fixation or ankylosis is more frequent in ears with otosclerosis and represents a significant cause of revision stapes surgery. This type of ossicular fixation may be evident in between 3 and 13.5% of revision stapes surgeries.[39] To correctly assess and correct malleus ankylosis, it is important to both visualize and directly inspect the anterior malleal process and ligament[38] (for cases of malleal ankylosis, see below).

The fallopian canal is inspected to determine any areas of bony dehiscence or prolapse of the nerve itself. Then the promontory is followed posteriorly to the round window. The lip and niche of the round window are inspected. If there is obliterative involvement by otosclerosis, then the surgery is terminated and the patient should be fitted with a hearing aid.

Horn et al[36] stated, "The most difficult problem of revision stapedectomy is management of the soft tissue and prosthesis in the oval window." Understandably, if there does not appear to be lateral ossicular fixation, if the facial nerve does not obscure the well of the oval window, and there is no obvious obliteration of the round window, the surgeon must now deal with the likely pathology extending from or involving the incus to the oval window.

The incus is examined first, and in particular the attachment of the prosthesis to the long process. Adhesions may be easily lysed, with the laser exposing the wire or ribbon loops or the handle of the Robinson prosthesis. Then the laser is used to undress the prosthesis of its investing bands or adhesions down to the lip of the fossa ovalis (Fig. 16–4).

One must explore the oval window neomembrane; otherwise the depth to the fenestration cannot be ascertained, nor can one determine the presence of obstructing footplate parts or otosclerotic regrowth.[22] This is most easily accomplished with a 20- or 24-gauge suction stabilizing the prosthesis and working with the laser probe to dissect the adhesions of the neomembrane away.

Usually it is difficult to ascertain the depth of the prosthesis and whether it is positioned favorably within the fenestration or oval window. Therefore, as advocated by Prasad and Kamerer[40] and Langman and Lindeman,[27] the prosthesis should be removed. (Even in cases where the findings point to a loose prosthesis, the prosthesis should be removed because it has often been displaced outside of the oval window fenestration.) To remove it, the prosthesis must be released from its attachment to the incus. The incus is stabilized either with a suction or alligator. Then the loop or bucket handle can be

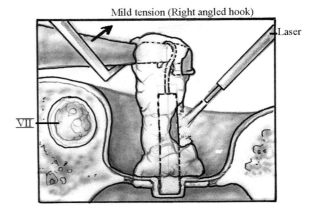

FIGURE 16–4 Dissection within the fossa ovalis. Dissection around the prosthesis and incus may be facilitated with gentle distraction using a right-angle pick. The laser allows safe vaporization of adhesive tissue and scar engulfing the incus and prosthesis.

lifted away using a 1-mm right-angle pick, and, without suctioning within the oval window, the prosthesis may be gently removed from the middle ear.

Although an initial response would be to replace the prosthesis with one measured against the one removed, further exploration and removal of scar and adhesions must be performed within the oval window. Once the footplate or fenestration is visualized, a new prosthesis may be placed. A measurement from the undersurface of the long process to the footplate or annulus is made, adding 0.2 mm of length to allow for the thickness of the footplate and sufficient penetration into the vestibule. A custom piston prosthesis is made from a 6-mm-long Fisch Teflon piston-platinum wire prosthesis (Smith-Nephew Richards, Memphis, TN).

Utilizing the 1-mm-long, right-angle pick to center and place the prosthesis, high field magnification ensures placement into the oval window. Proper crimping around the long process may be accentuated with a pressed piece of fibroareolar material applied over the wire and around the incus at that point. Promontory mucosa may be gently scraped to prompt a bit of bleeding that, along with a single drop of fibrin glue, acts as the sealant.

If, during the elevation of the tympanomeatal flap, ossification of the anterior malleal ligament and process is recognized, there are two paths one can follow to address this problem. If the ligament and process are not too rigidly fixed, then one can proceed with either mechanical or laser separation in this area, protecting the underlying chorda tympani nerve. When the region anterior to the lateral process is narrowed, however, it is common to find the ligament and process more densely ossified and the fixation to be greater. These cases are better addressed with resection of the head of the malleus and attached process and ligament followed by the malleostapedotomy (see below).

When there is not sufficient incus length, or there is lateral ossicular fixation or severe subluxation and disassociation at the incudomalleal joint, then a malleostapedotomy may be performed. Originally described as an incus-replacement prosthesis by Shuknecht,[41] the ability to circumvent an incus deficiency or attic ossicular fixation has gone through various iterations. Fisch[38] presents a simple and compelling approach to this problem. (An alternative to the malleostapedotomy for a deficient incus has been detailed. Tange[42] describes using ionomeric cement to lengthen the long process to accept placement of a new prosthesis.)

The incus is removed when performing a malleostapedotomy. Once this is complete, if the tympanic membrane has not been released from the short process of the malleus, this is done. As the malleus is stabilized with the suction, a sickle knife can lift the cartilaginous cap and then be dragged along the superior surface of the malleus, dividing the plica mallearis.

The head of the malleus is removed, either with a malleus nipper or high-speed otology drill, just superior to the attachment of the tensor tympani tendon. The malleus is notched and this is contoured to accept a secure crimping of a wire loop (Fig. 16–5). A Fisch Teflon piston-platinum wire prosthesis is obtained and the wire loop carefully opened. This may be done by hanging it on the tapered end of the right-angled pick and carefully moving along toward the wider portion with a jeweler's forceps. Then, in a similar fashion to work with an intact incus, the ribbon wire loop may be secured to the neck of the malleus just below the offshoot of the short process. Typically the length of the prosthesis is between 5.5 and 6.0 mm.

When the wire ribbon loop has been secured and a blood-fibrin glue patch applied to seal the oval window, the tympanomeatal flap may be reflected back into position. A whisper into the operative ear is done to confirm audition. Finally, moistened and pressed pieces of Gelfoam are placed to secure the edges of the flap, and the medial canal is filled with antibiotic ointment.

OUTCOME

"Perhaps the single most important factor in stapes surgery is surgical experience."[30]

A review of 10 published series on revision stapes surgery demonstrates that the successful rate of air–bone gap to 10 dB or less may vary from approximately 20 to 81%[33] (Table 16–2). These results are good, but do not equal the outcomes typical of primary stapes surgery. Moreover, the incidence of postoperative sensorineural hearing loss and anacusis are slightly greater than with primary stapes surgery. De La Cruz and Fayad[33] found postoperative partial sensorineural hearing loss occurred in 7.7% of the patients, and dead ears in 1.4%.

Certainly, technique may affect the outcome. Results reported by Wiet et al[35] in a meta-analysis of laser and nonlaser revision stapes surgeries from 1970 to 1995 demonstrate this. For those cases revised using conventional methods, there was a 1.5% incidence of postoperative partial sensorineural hearing loss and 1.4% incidence of anacusis. For the revisions performed with a laser, utilizing either the visible [argon or potassium titanyl phosphate (KTP)]

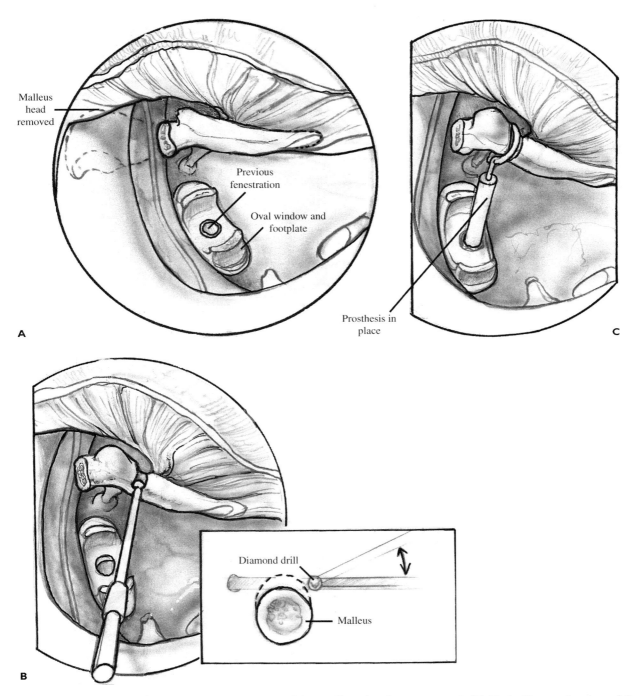

FIGURE 16–5   Malleostapedotomy. (A) The head of the malleus has been removed. (B) To facilitate crimping of the wire loop, a 1-mm diamond bur is used to notch the malleus. The notching should be done to create a rounded contour by changing the angle of the drill over the malleus. (C) The prosthesis is in place.

or infrared-invisible (CO_2) lasers available, no patient had postoperative partial sensorineural hearing loss, and there was a 0.6% occurrence of a dead ear.

Beyond the variance attributable to technique and technology, outcomes in revision surgery also depend on the pathology prompting the revision. Cokkeser et al[28] pointed out that the best results

are most often found when the reason for the revision surgery is not within the oval window. A dislocated prosthesis repair yielded the best hearing results in their series. Furthermore, in patients with vestibular symptoms, it is best to preoperatively counsel the patients that the goal is the relief from the vertigo and the prevention of further sensori-

TABLE 16–2 HEARING RESULTS AFTER REVISION SURGERY

Author(s) and Published Year (No. of Cases)	<10 dB Gap (%)	<20 dB Gap (%)	SNHL (%)	Dead Ear (%)
Sheehy et al 1981[24] (n = 258)	44	71	7	3
Derlacki 1985[18] (n = 217)	60	72	4	1
Glasscock et al 1987[25] (n = 79)	39	64	3	1
Farrior and Sutherland 1991[26] (n = 102)	57	84	—	—
Langman and Lindeman 1993[27] (n = 66)	61	84	3	0
McGee et al 1993[22] (n = 77)	81	92	2	0
Cokkeser et al 1994[28] (n = 49)	17	60	14	4
Silverstein et al 1994[7] (n = 61)	47	62	10	4
Peter 1995[29] (n = 39)	44	77	—	—
Pedersen 1996[30] (n = 186)	—	25[a]	—	—
Han et al 1997[31] (n = 60)	52	82	4	1
Somers et al 1997[1] (n = 332)	40	64	3	—
Hammerschlag et al 1998[32] (n = 250)	80	93[b]	4	1
De La Cruz and Fayad 2000[33] (n = 356)	60	78	8	1

[a]Results reported in postoperative speech reception threshold format.
[b]Gap closure within 30 dB.
SNHL, sensorineural hearing loss.

neural hearing loss, rather then the closure of an air–bone gap.[28]

To undertake revision stapes surgery requires an appreciation of the potential problems one is likely to encounter and a wide armamentarium of techniques with which to deal with them. The surgeries are technically demanding, with a smaller margin of error compared to a primary stapes procedure. Nonetheless, as the number of otolaryngologists comfortable and proficient in primary surgery diminishes, there will be an ever-greater demand for those able to capably undertake the challenge of the revision case.

REFERENCES

1. Somers T, Govaerts P, de Varebeke SJ, Offeciers E. Revision stapes surgery. *J Laryngol Otol* 1997; 111:233–239.
2. Belluci RJ. Trends and profiles in stapes surgery. *Ann Otol Rhinol Laryngol* 1979;88:708–713.
3. Harris JP, Osborne E. A survey of otologic training in U.S. residency programs. *Arch Otolaryngol Head Neck Surg* 1990;116:342–345.
4. Shea JJ Jr. Fenestration of the oval window. *Ann Otol Rhinol Laryngol* 1958;67:932–951.
5. Sheehy JL, House HP. Causes of failure in stapes surgery. *Laryngoscope* 1962;72:10–31.
6. Perkins RC. Laser stapedotomy for otosclerosis. *Laryngoscope* 1980;90:228–241.
7. Silverstein H, Bendet E, Rosenberg S, Nichols M. Revision stapes surgery with and without laser: a comparison. *Laryngoscope* 1994;104:1431–1438.
8. Lippy WH, Berenholz LP, Burkey JM. Otosclerosis in the 1960s, 1970s, 1980s, and 1990s. *Laryngoscope* 1999;109:1307–1309.
9. Farrior JB, Temple AE. Teflon-wire piston or stainless-steel bucket stapes prosthesis: does it make a difference? *Ear Nose Throat J* 1999;78:252–253,257–260.
10. Belal A, Ylikoski J. Poststapedectomy dizziness: a histopathologic report. *Am J Otol* 1982;3:187–191.
11. Causse JB, Causse JR, Cezard R, et al. Vertigo in postoperative follow-up of otosclerosis. *Am J Otol* 1988;9:246–255.
12. Atacan E, Sennaroglu L, Genc A, Kaya S. Benign paroxysmal positional vertigo after stapedectomy. *Laryngoscope* 2001;111:1257–1259.
13. Isaacson JE, Laine F, Williams GH. Pneumolabyrinth as a computed tomography finding. *Ann Otol Rhinol Laryngol* 1995;104:974–976.
14. Seicshnaydre MA, Sismanis A, Hughes GB. Update of reparative granuloma: survey of the American Otological Society and the American Neurotology Society. *Am J Otol* 1994;15:155–160.
15. Woldag K, Meister EF, Kosling S. Diagnostik bei persistierenden Gleichgewichtsstorungen nach Operationen am Stapes. *Laryngol Rhinol Otol* 1995; 74:403–407.
16. Pickuth D, Brandt S, Berghaus A, Speilmann RP, Heywang-Kobrunner SH. Vertigo after stapes surgery: the role of high resolution CT. *Br J Radiol* 2000;73:1021–1023.
17. Swartz JD, Lansman AK, Berger AS, et al. Stapes prosthesis: evaluation with CT. *Radiology* 1986; 158:179–182.

18. Derlacki EL. Revision stapes surgery: problems with some solutions. *Laryngoscope* 1985;95:1047–1053.

19. Krieger LW, Lippy WH, Schuring AD, Rizer FM. Revision stapedectomy for incus erosion: long-term hearing. *Otolaryngol Head Neck Surg* 1998;119:370–373.

20. Nadol JB. Histopathology of residual and recurrent conductive hearing loss after stapedectomy. *Otol Neurotol* 2001;22:162–169.

21. McGee TM. The loose wire syndrome. *Laryngoscope* 1981;91:1478–1483.

22. McGee TM, Diaz-Ordaz EA, Kartush JM. The role of KTP laser in revision stapedectomy. *Otolaryngol Head Neck Surg* 1993;109:839–843.

23. Wiet RJ, Harvey SA, Bauer GP. Complications in stapes surgery: options for prevention and management. *Otolaryngol Clin North Am* 1993;26:471–490.

24. Sheehy JL, Nelson RA, House HP. Revision stapedectomy: a review of 258 cases. *Laryngoscope* 1981;91:43–51.

25. Glasscock ME, McKennan KX, Levine, SC. Revision stapedectomy surgery. *Otolaryngol Head Neck Surg* 1987;96:141–148.

26. Farrior J, Sutherland A. Revision stapes surgery. *Laryngoscope* 1991;101:1155–1161.

27. Langman AW, Lindeman RC. Revision stapedectomy. *Laryngoscope* 1993;103:954–958.

28. Cokkeser Y, Naguib M, Aristegui M, et al. Revision stapes surgery: a critical evaluation. *Otolaryngol Head Neck Surg* 1994;111:473–477.

29. Peter B, Grossenbacher R. Stapesrevisionen: Befunde und Resultate. *Laryngol Rhinol Otol* 1995;74:399–402.

30. Pedersen CB. Revision surgery in otosclerosis: an investigation of the factors which influence the hearing result. *Clin Otolaryngol* 1996;21:385–388.

31. Han WW, Incesulu A, McKenna MJ, Rauch SD, Nadol JB Jr, Glynn RJ. Revision stapedectomy: intraoperative findings, results, and review of the literature. *Laryngoscope* 1997;107:1185–1192.

32. Hammerschlag PE, Fishman A, Scheer AA. A review of 308 cases of revision stapedectomy. *Laryngoscope* 1998;108:1794–1800.

33. De La Cruz A, Fayad JN. Revision stapedectomy. *Otolaryngol Head Neck Surg* 2000;123:728–732.

34. Mann WJ, Amedee RG, Fuerst G, Tabb HG. Hearing loss as a complication of stapes surgery. *Otolaryngol Head Neck Surg* 1996;115:324–328.

35. Wiet RJ, Kubek DC, Lemberg P, Byskosh AT. A meta-analysis review of revision stapes surgery with argon laser: effectiveness and safety. *Am J Otol* 1997;18:166–171.

36. Horn KL, Gherini SG, Franz DC. Argon laser revision stapedectomy. *Am J Otol* 1994;15:383–388.

37. Nissen RL. Argon laser in difficult stapedotomy cases. *Laryngoscope* 1998;108:1669–1673.

38. Fisch U, Acar GO, Huber A. Malleostapedotomy in revision surgery for otosclerosis. *Otol Neurotol* 2001;22:776–785.

39. Vincent R, Lopez A, Sperling NM. Malleus ankylosis: a clinical, audiometric, histologic, and surgical study of 123 cases. *Am J Otol* 1999;20:717–725.

40. Prasad S, Kamerer DB. Results of revision stapedectomy for conductive hearing loss. *Otolaryngol Head Neck Surg* 1993;109:742–747.

41. Sheehy JL. Stapedectomy: incus bypass procedures: a report of 203 operations. *Laryngoscope* 1982;92:258–262.

42. Tange RA. Repair of the ossicular chain with an ionomer cement by an inadequate incus after prior stapes surgery for otosclerosis. *Eur Arch Otorhinolaryngol* 1996;253:313–315.

LASER STAPEDOTOMY MINUS PROSTHESIS (LASER STAMP) AND OTHER MINIMALLY INVASIVE OTOLOGIC PROCEDURES

Seth I. Rosenberg

Over the past decade the emphasis on surgery has been to find ways of performing minimally invasive techniques using lasers and endoscopes. Many otologic procedures already fit the category of minimally invasive, or are already being done in the surgeon's office operating room, thus avoiding hospitalization and all the associated costs that accompany it.

The advantages of minimally invasive procedures are many and include the fact that procedures can be performed safely in an office operating room or surgery center. Patients especially like procedures that are done in the office, because both patient and surgeon time is minimized, the large expense of in-hospital surgery is saved, all procedures are performed using topical or infiltrative local anesthesia, and the results are as good as those of more extensive procedures.

Starting with laser stapedotomy minus prosthesis (laser STAMP), a variety of minimally invasive procedures including laser-assisted tympanostomy (LAT), endoscopic middle ear exploration, inner ear perfusion, and fat myringoplasty are described here, and the necessary equipment and anesthesia are presented. Minimally invasive surgical procedures can be an enormous addition to the otologist's armamentarium.

PROCEDURE ROOM SETUP AND EQUIPMENT

The minimum size of the minor surgery room should be 150 square feet, although a larger room is preferable. Two instruments that are not standard to all otologic offices but contribute tremendously to the success of office-based otologic surgery are the CO_2 laser and the 1.7-mm rigid otoendoscope

(Smith-Nephew Richards, Memphis, TN). The laser is instrumental in creating an instant, bloodless, and nearly painless myringotomy for middle ear aeration or other procedures. The otoendoscope provides near microscope-quality images of the middle ear, allowing the surgeon to see areas not visualized by the operating microscope. The Lumenis CO_2 laser (Lumenis Ltd., Yokneam, Israel) is used with a Microslad optical delivery system (Lumenis Ltd.,Yokneam, Israel) attached to the microscope. A remote foot pedal allows the surgeon to fire the laser with precise control. The laser allows variable spot size (0.65 to 3.4 mm), power (5 to 30 W), and pulse duration (0.05 seconds to continuous). The Surgi-Touch CO_2 flash scanner (Lumenis Ltd.) is used to make a circular opening in the tympanic membrane. The flash scanner beam moves in a spiral pattern at a constant velocity and must be in sharp focus. The laser beam never lingers at any given point longer than the thermal relaxation time of the tissue, resulting in char-free ablation and minimal depth of laser energy penetration. This provides the advantage of creating a controlled tympanostomy of a predictable size and depth with a single burst of focused laser energy. Pulse duration of 0.15 seconds and a power of 10 to 20 W are typically used to penetrate the tympanic membrane. Note that laser safety precautions must be followed at all times when using any laser. All persons in the procedure room (including the patient) are required to wear eye protection in the form of laser safety goggles when the laser is being fired.

Two different-angled otoendoscopes are used, with 0-degree and 30-degree views. The 30-degree angled scope is the most commonly used scope and provides visual perspectives of the middle ear not seen with direct microscopic visualization. These scopes are shorter and narrower than standard nasal rigid endoscopes usually seen in an otolaryngology office, with a length of 10 cm and a diameter of 1.7 mm. The 2.7-mm endoscopes are too large to be useful. The otoendoscopes have excellent optics and produce images of superior quality comparable to the operating microscope.

An Olympus camera is attached to the otoendoscope (Olympus America Inc., Melville, NY). The camera is connected to color monitors, which allows the surgeon, assistants, patient, and patient's family members to view the procedure. The procedure can be documented with video and/or photos; the authors employ a super-VHS recorder and a color video printer. Multiple copies of the still photos can be immediately produced for placement in the office chart, for explaining the procedure to the patient, and for the patient's personal medical records. The otoendoscope can also be used without the camera if the surgeon prefers to look directly through the eyepiece of the endoscope.

An essential component of almost all forms of otologic surgery is the operating microscope. It is preferable to use a standard wall-mounted microscope that is stable and frees both of the surgeon's hands for operating. The microscope has a 300-mm objective lens and adjustable magnification. The speculum holder can be very useful at stabilizing the speculum while freeing both of the surgeon's hands for the procedure. A standard foot-pedal–operated suction is also essential for otologic surgery.

Instruments that are usually found in a minor surgical procedure set are frequently needed, including No. 15 blades and handles, skin scissors, skin hooks, forceps, and so on. Standard otologic instruments should be available and sterile if needed. These instruments include various-sized speculums and a full range of hand-held suction tips, picks, hooks, curettes, cup forceps, alligator forceps, Bellucci scissors, sharpened sickle knives, round knives, and so forth.

ANESTHESIA

Anesthetic options for minimally invasive office-based otologic surgery include topical anesthesia or local (injected) anesthesia. These options are usually sufficient to keep almost all adults and many pediatric patients comfortable and relaxed during otologic surgery.

In 1968, Silverstein developed a technique of anesthetizing the tympanic membrane utilizing topical tetracaine without the use of injections.[1] Since that time, over 3000 cases have been successfully performed using this topical anesthesia. The method is well tolerated by patients because needle injections are avoided. It also allows the anesthetization of younger children who otherwise would not cooperate with conventional injections.[1]

The topical tetracaine adequately anesthetizes the tympanic membrane, and the effects last for approximately 1 hour after removal of the liquid from the ear canal. The surgeon must be aware that the ear canal and middle ear mucosa are not anesthetized. Consequently, topical tetracaine anesthesia should be used for procedures involving the tympanic membrane only, such as LAT, ventilation tube insertion, and minor middle ear exploration where the mucosa is not traumatized. To avoid pain during the procedure, instrumentation of the ear canal must be avoided. More extensive middle ear work, including exploration of the middle ear using otoendoscopes or chemical perfusion of the inner ear, generally requires additional anesthesia in the form of injections.

The technique of topical anesthesia using tetracaine solution is as follows. A single-use vial is created by measuring 160 mg of tetracaine powder and placing it into a 1-cc vial. The greatest efficacy is obtained when the solution is prepared just prior to use. Isopropyl alcohol (0.2 cc) is added to the vial, and the contents are shaken until the tetracaine powder is completely dissolved, producing an 80% solution.

The patient's ear is inspected with an otoscope or microscope to ensure that the tympanic membrane is unobstructed and that no perforation of the tympanic membrane exists. Any defect in the tympanic membrane precludes the use of topical tetracaine solution. Cerumen and other debris are removed if necessary.

The patient is placed on his or her side on the procedure table with the affected ear facing upward. Using a 27-gauge needle on a tuberculin syringe to direct the flow, the surgeon places 0.2 cc of tetracaine solution into the ear canal to be anesthetized. Do not inject! It is best to visualize the tympanic membrane to ensure that the medicine has covered the drum.

The patient is then instructed to remain in the lateral decubitus position for a minimum of 8 minutes. No ill effects are encountered if the medication is left in place longer than this minimum allotted time period.

The patient is then instructed to turn his or her head to drain the ear of the medication by gravity. The surgeon then aspirates any remaining solution from the ear canal and tympanic membrane with a suction tip. It is imperative that no tetracaine is left behind that could enter the middle ear and diffuse into the inner ear, causing transient violent vertigo lasting several hours. At the same time, the surgeon can verify adequate anesthesia by touching the tympanic membrane with the suction tip and assessing for residual sensation. The surgeon is free to perform the procedure within 1 hour of the medication's removal.

For younger children who cannot remain still in the lateral decubitus position for a full 8 minutes, an alternate technique is used. A few drops of tetracaine are instilled in the ear canal as above. Then a 9 × 15 mm Merocel Pope ear wick (Medtronic Xomed Inc., Jacksonville, FL) is gently inserted into the canal so that it nearly touches the tympanic membrane. The remainder of the solution is used to expand the wick so that it touches the tympanic membrane and fills the canal. The child is then free to move about for 10 minutes until the wick is removed for the procedure.

Laser Stapedotomy Minus Prosthesis (Laser STAMP)

History

It is important first to review the history of surgery for otosclerosis, which is marked with major breakthroughs by a number of pioneering otologists. In the 1950s, Rosen[2] developed the stapes mobilization procedure. In patients with stapes fixation due to otosclerosis, the stapes footplate was fractured with chisels or picks. Hearing was improved, though only temporarily. Refixation of the stapes usually occurred after several months. Fowler[3] introduced the anterior crurotomy technique of stapes mobilization in 1956 with results similar to those of Rosen. In 1958, Shea[4] developed the stapedectomy procedure, which produced long-lasting results. Since that time, Shea's procedure or modifications of the technique have remained the most popular method for improving hearing in patients with otosclerosis and stapes fixation. In 1980, Perkins[5] introduced the laser for stapes surgery, which allowed the surgeon to vaporize the stapes footplate without instrumentation. Stapedotomy could be performed on a mobilized footplate, reducing the danger of a floating footplate.

Stapes mobilization procedures have been largely abandoned because of the possibility of refixation of the stapes. In 1969, Rosen and Siegal[6] studied the long-term results of 154 patients who had undergone a stapes mobilization procedure, yielding a 42% complete closure of the air–bone gap and 32% closure within 10 dB at 4 years. Myers et al's[7] report of a 50-year-old man who had a mobilization procedure done 7 years before his death supports the theory that the footplate does not refix. On histologic examination, a fibrous union to a normal and mobile footplate was noted without evidence of otosclerosis, despite extensive otosclerosis elsewhere.[7] Thus, it can be assumed that even if there is a significant amount of otosclerosis at the fissula ante fenestram, a linear defect across an uninvolved footplate should heal with a fibrous union. In 1998, Silverstein[8] reintroduced the concept of partial stapedotomy surgery for otosclerosis without the use of a prosthesis. It can be performed when stapes fixation is localized to a focus of otosclerosis at the fissula ante fenestram. A linear laser stapedotomy at the anterior one third of the footplate with vaporization of the anterior stapes crus allows the stapes to become mobile while allowing stapes and stapedius tendon preservation with avoidance of the need for a prosthesis.

Indications

The success of the laser STAMP procedure depends on the proper selection of patients. A candidate should have a blue footplate free of otosclerosis, except for the area adjacent to and involving the fissula ante fenestram. These characteristics can be assessed only at the time of surgery after entering the middle ear. Interestingly, it is difficult to predict candidacy based solely on preoperative audiogram. Rather, the patient is prepared for the possibility of laser STAMP versus conventional stapedotomy with prosthesis insertion. The surgeon should be prepared to do a stapedotomy with prosthesis, if the stapes is not completely mobilized after isolating the posterior two thirds of the stapes. If hearing should deteriorate in the future, the patient should be informed that a stapedotomy with prosthesis can be performed.

Surgical Technique

Standard stapes surgery setup and patient positioning is used. One percent lidocaine with adrenaline 1:100,000 is injected subcutaneously into the external auditory canal. A tympanomeatal flap is elevated in the standard fashion. A portion of the scutum is removed with a diamond bur while preserving the chorda tympani nerve, thus providing a good view of the horizontal facial nerve and stapes. The stapes is inspected and palpated to determine if the otosclerosis is localized to the fissula ante fenestram. If the patient is confirmed to be a laser STAMP procedure candidate, the laser endoprobe hand piece with the HGM argon laser (Lumenis Ltd., Yokneam, Israel) is used to vaporize the anterior crus of the stapes using 2.0 W at 0.2-second duration. Routinely, the metal laser probe tip is bent to a 30-degree angle using a

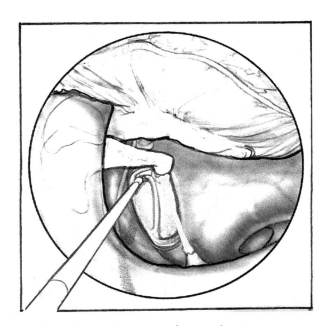

FIGURE 17–1   Vaporizing the anterior crus.

small hemostat without breaking the laser fiberoptic cable, to create the proper angle for vaporizing the anterior crus (Fig. 17–1). By direct vision, palpation with the tip of the laser probe, or visualization with a 30-degree, 1.7-mm-diameter otoendoscope, the anterior crus is cut by placing the laser probe tip against the crus (Fig. 17–2). A 1.5-mm right-angle pick or the fiberoptic laser tip is passed through the area of the anterior crus to document complete transection of the crus.

Next, the thin blue footplate is vaporized in a linear fashion across the anterior one third of the footplate (Fig. 17–3). The laser is set from 0.8 to 1.0 W at 0.2-second duration with at least 3-second pauses between laser bursts to prevent overheating the perilymph, which can cause transient vertigo for up to several days after the surgery. Small picks are

used to be sure there is complete transection of the footplate and that the posterior two thirds of the footplate is completely mobile. If fixation has occurred because of otosclerosis at the fissula ante fenestram, and there is a blue footplate free of otosclerosis, the stapes should become completely mobile. After laser vaporization of the linear stapedotomy, there should be a half-millimeter separation between the fixed anterior one third and movable posterior two thirds of the footplate. A 2×3 mm piece of ear lobe adipose tissue is placed over the footplate to seal the perilymph space (Fig. 17–4).

The most difficult part of the procedure is the transection of the anterior crus when it cannot be directly visualized with a microscope. Use of a 20-gauge CeramOptic probe (Ceramoptics, Naas, Ireland) with a 200-μm fiber that is bent to a 30-degree angle by the surgeon makes this part of the procedure easier. More bony exposure may be needed than with a traditional stapedotomy to manipulate the probe tip onto the anterior crus. One should be able to visualize the tympanic portion of the facial nerve and the pyramidal eminence prior to attempting to laser. Before vaporization, the anterior crus should be palpated with the laser probe. The probe tip can be inserted between the incus and the malleus handle over the horizontal portion of the facial nerve, or from inferiorly over the promontory of the cochlea.

CLINICAL OUTCOMES

In a review of 137 patients who underwent surgery for otosclerosis, in 46 patients (33.6%) a laser STAMP procedure was performed.[9] In all of these cases, there was a blue footplate with fixation confined to the anterior portion. Intraoperative success was determined by verifying mobility of the posterior footplate with palpation of the ossicles.[9] Of these 46

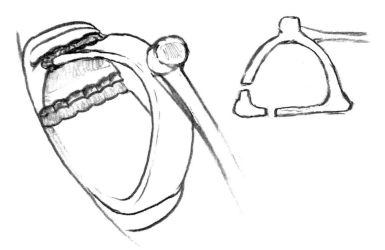

FIGURE 17–2   Cut the anterior crus.

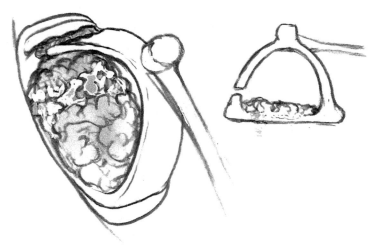

FIGURE 17–3 The footplate is vaporized in a linear fashion.

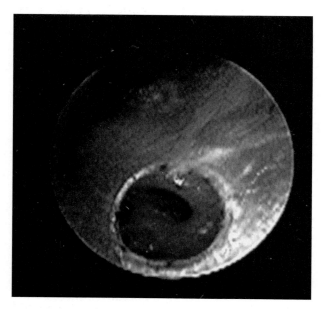

FIGURE 17–4 The footplate is sealed with adipose tissue.

patients, only three have required reoperation for conversion from a laser STAMP procedure to a traditional stapedotomy procedure with use of a prosthesis. Sixteen patients (11.7%) were initially thought to be laser STAMP candidates and underwent attempted laser STAMP procedures, but were converted intraoperatively to a stapedotomy with prosthesis insertion.[9] The most common cause of failure was unrecognized fixation of the posterior footplate, which became evident intraoperatively when the stapes remained fixed following the laser STAMP procedure. In 57 patients (41.6%), a laser STAMP procedure was not attempted secondary to extensive otosclerosis.[9]

A review of clinical outcomes in 46 patients with greater than a 4-month follow-up shows the average 6-week postoperative air–bone gap was closed from 22 dB [standard deviation (SD) 10 dB, range 8 to 49 dB] to 6 dB (SD 4 dB, range 0 to 14 dB).[9] For the most recent audiograms, the average long-term air–bone gap observed was 5 dB (SD 6 dB, range 0 to 23 dB, average follow-up 25 months). The average discrimination score remained stable at 95% preoperative, 95% at 6 weeks, and 96% for the latest audiograms.[9]

COMPLICATIONS

Few complications have been seen with the laser STAMP procedure. One patient experienced profound hearing loss after the procedure. Three patients eventually required conversion from a laser STAMP procedure to a stapedotomy with prosthesis.[9] Finally, one patient had postoperative labyrinthitis and sensorineural hearing loss. Aggressive treatment with antibiotics, steroids, and hospitalization yielded a nearly perfect hearing result.[9]

CONCLUSIONS

The laser STAMP technique is a procedure that allows the surgeon to do minimal surgery for minimal otosclerotic disease and achieve lasting results. The key to successful laser STAMP surgery is the proper selection of patients whose otosclerosis is localized to the anterior portion of the footplate. In almost one third of primary stapes procedures, a successful laser STAMP procedure is possible. Thus far the follow-up data suggest that patients maintain excellent hearing with reduced surgical risk and without evidence of refixation.

LASER-ASSISTED TYMPANOSTOMY (LAT)

INDICATIONS

LAT is offered to adult patients with serous otitis media (SOM) for whom medical management has failed or to those patients requiring immediate relief of symptoms of SOM (e.g., SOM in an only hearing ear).[10] The majority of these patients present with middle ear effusions following upper respiratory tract infections or recent air travel. It is imperative to visualize the nasopharynx and eustachian tube orifice in adult patients with new-onset SOM to rule out neoplasms blocking the eustachian tube. Patulous eustachian tube is another indication for the LAT procedure, to determine whether middle ear aeration will be effective in relieving the associated symptoms. Cooperative children with persistent SOM are also candidates for the procedure. Middle ear ventilation is achieved without the risk of general anesthesia, hospitalization, or associated costs. LAT also provides middle ear ventilation prior to air travel for patients susceptible to barotrauma during descent. Finally, LAT is performed to create a controlled bloodless opening for laser-assisted otoendoscopy or inner ear perfusion.

SURGICAL TECHNIQUE

The adult patient or older child is placed in the supine position wearing laser-approved safety goggles. The tympanic membrane is viewed through an operative microscope using a 300-mm objective lens. The microscope is adapted for the model 1030 Lumenis CO_2 laser using a microslad optical delivery system.

A defocused beam technique is employed to achieve the tympanostomy with only a few laser bursts. This is especially useful when there is fluid in the middle ear, or when performing the technique on children. Often, a 1.5- to 2.0-mm opening can be created with one laser burst. The microslad is defocused to three units (a 1.64-mm spot) or four units (a 2.12-mm spot), and the laser is set at 10 to 15 W with a pulse duration of 0.1 second. The wattage selection depends on the apparent thickness of the tympanic membrane and whether or not middle ear fluid is present. A thicker tympanic membrane requires higher power. Middle ear effusion absorbs laser energy and allows a higher power to be directed at the tympanic membrane without inadvertently striking the promontory and causing pain.

Occasionally, two or three bursts are necessary to penetrate the drum. This occurs when the laser beam is not focused sharply or the drum is thickened. When repeating the laser vaporization, the power setting should be reduced. Laser hits to the promontory are not dangerous and do not cause hearing loss, but can cause discomfort if the middle ear has not been anesthetized. The black char looks ominous but is innocuous. The most recent evolution of the technique employs the SurgiTouch ENT flash scanner. The scanner enables the surgeon to create a controlled tympanostomy of a predictable size and depth with a single burst of focused laser energy. The beam moves in a spiral pattern at a constant velocity resulting in char-free ablation and minimal depth of laser energy penetration. The power settings are similar to those used in the defocused technique, and a second burst of laser energy is rarely required. With the pulse duration set at 0.15 second, 15 to 20 W is used to penetrate the tympanic membrane when middle ear effusion is present. When no effusion is present, 10 W is used. Lower-power settings are used when the tympanic membrane appears thin, and increased when the drum is thickened. Repeat vaporization should be done with reduced wattage. The advantage of using this technique in a dry middle ear is that the laser energy penetrates minimally (i.e., a circular opening is created with less risk of laser energy touching the promontory).

The tympanostomy is placed anterior to the malleus when treating SOM. The site is identical to that traditionally used for the placement of pressure equalizing (PE) tubes. At this site, the laser beam encounters the surface of the tympanic membrane in an almost perpendicular plane, and the promontory is relatively far away. Laser energy occasionally strikes the promontory bone; however, no sensorineural hearing loss has been demonstrated. The tympanostomy site is made over the round window niche when performing inner ear perfusion and over the incus when conductive hearing loss is being evaluated.

If children do not tolerate lying supine and still underneath the microscope, then the OtoLAM (Lumenis Ltd., Yokneam, Israel) is utilized. The device is similar to an otoscope with a laser and TV camera attached. The procedure can be performed with the child sitting up, even sitting in the parent's lap, and is generally well tolerated. The child and parents can watch the procedure on the TV monitor. The procedure is painless after the topical tetracaine anesthesia has been applied to the drum for 10 minutes. The drum is visualized while the surgeon positions the OtoLAM and watches the TV monitor. When the circulating beam is brought into sharp focus, the laser is fired using settings of 15 to 20 W at 0.15 second. Sometimes the loud noise of the laser frightens children; however, the procedure can be performed on any cooperative child. Children are not restrained during the procedure because it is thought to be too traumatic psychologically.

POSTOPERATIVE CARE

Very little care is required in the postoperative period. The majority of patients experience immediate relief of their symptoms. Patients are counseled to avoid water exposure to the operated ear, and are followed until the opening completely heals. Often patients are placed on topical eardrops for 5 days after LAT. Prior to tympanostomy closure, they are encouraged to use cotton coated with a petroleum-based ointment or a commercially available water-proof earplug in the ear canal when bathing or swimming.

RESULTS

Over 1000 LAT procedures have been performed in the author's practice. LAT size has been correlated to patency time. LATs less than 1.0 mm in diameter heal within 2 weeks, LATs that are 1.5 mm heal within 3 weeks, and LATs that are 2.0 mm heal within 4 weeks. LAT successfully resolves persistent SOM in 80% of adult cases without the need for PE tube placement.[10] Children of all ages tolerate the procedure well, and placement of PE tubes is avoided in almost half (46%) of these patients.

COMPLICATIONS

Creating a laser opening in the drum of an atrophic membrane may result in no postoperative healing and permanent perforation. This has occurred in one case. Otorrhea is rare (<1%) and is treated with antibiotic eardrops. Recurrent serous otitis can be treated with a repeat LAT. If two sequential LATs do not resolve the problem, then a PE tube is used with the third procedure.

EXPLORATION OF THE MIDDLE EAR: LASER-ASSISTED OTOENDOSCOPY

INDICATIONS

The technique of otoendoscopy has multiple applications in the office-based setting.[11] It also has multiple intraoperative applications. It is useful in evaluating the etiology of unexplained conductive hearing losses, examining the round window membrane prior to inserting the Silverstein MicroWick

(Micromedics, Eagan, MN), evaluating tympanic cavity masses, checking the status of the middle ear and ossicular chain prior to mastoid-tympanoplasty, and evaluating the patency of the eustachian tube in cases of recurrent SOM or patulous eustachian tube. When there is an obvious history of trauma or surgical manipulation, office endoscopy is used to evaluate the round and oval windows for perilymph fistula.

SURGICAL TECHNIQUE

The patient is placed in the supine position, and tetracaine anesthesia is achieved. A 2.0-mm LAT is performed. This creates a round bloodless opening for placement of the endoscope. The posteroinferior portion of the tympanic membrane allows for the best visualization of the round window and middle ear. Cadaver studies have indicated that the round window niche lies 3.14 mm posterior from the umbo of the malleus at a 113-degree angle.[12] The round window niche usually can be seen as a dark shadow beneath the normal tympanic membrane (Figs. 17–5 and 17–6). This posteroinferior LAT also provides visual access to the oval window and the incudostapedial joint, as well as the eustachian tube and undersurface of the tympanic membrane.

Once the LAT is created, the 1.7-mm-diameter, 10-cm-length otoendoscope of 0 or 30 degrees is inserted to examine the tympanic cavity. The otoendoscope is held in the surgeon's nondominant hand

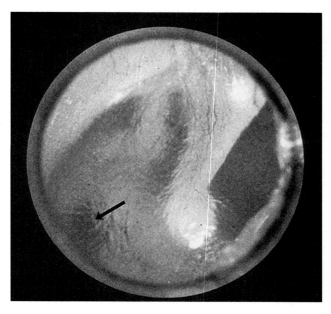

FIGURE 17–5 The arrow points to the round window under tympanic membrane.

Right ear

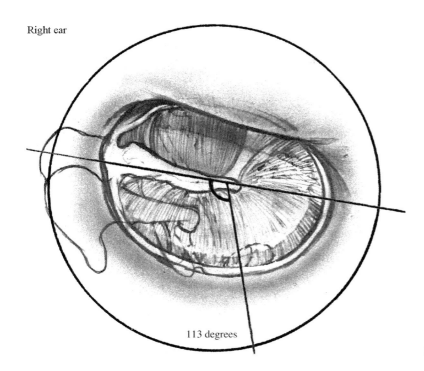

113 degrees

FIGURE 17–6   Posterior inferior quadrant.

and steadied by placing it against the speculum. The 30-degree otoendoscope is most commonly used and provides better visualization of the round and oval widows than does the 0-degree otoendoscope. The dominant hand is left free to focus the lens and handle any instrumentation required during the procedure.

The superior optics of these rigid endoscopes makes them far more useful than similarly sized flexible endoscopes. The images provided are nearly equivalent to those of the operating microscope, whereas the angled lenses provide visual perspectives and access to the middle ear not obtainable with the microscope. A camera is attached to the otoendoscope, and the procedure is viewed on a color monitor. The physician, assisting personnel, and patient can all view the procedure on the monitor. Pictures are taken of the tympanic membrane and middle ear at appropriate moments. Four views are usually photographed on one print. Depending on the procedure being performed, these four views could include a view of the tympanostomy site, the round window niche, the round window membrane, and the incudostapedial joint. Other views may be photographed depending on the diagnosis and procedure.

The otoendoscope is then removed, and the LAT is either patched with Gelfilm covered in antibiotic ointment or allowed to heal spontaneously. Water precautions are followed until the tympanic membrane is healed.

COMPLICATIONS

Complications can occur during otoendoscopy, such as iatrogenic fracture of the lenticular process of the incus, nonhealing of a thin atrophic tympanic membrane, and nonhealing of a previous tympanoplasty graft. It is not recommended to do laser-assisted otoendoscopy through a tympanoplasty graft because it may result in nonhealing of the drum after the procedure.

CHEMICAL PERFUSION OF THE INNER EAR

INDICATIONS

Inner ear perfusion through the round window is indicated for patients with vertigo related to Meniere's disease that is unresponsive to initial medical therapy.[12,13] Consideration must be given to the possibility of further hearing loss in the perfused ear when gentamicin is utilized. Patients must be counseled that hearing loss is a common side effect, and that other treatments for Meniere's disease may pose less risk to their hearing. Other candidates for inner ear perfusion include patients with autoimmune inner ear disease and idiopathic sudden sensorineural deafness. Steroid perfusion using dexamethasone drops is particularly useful in patients unresponsive to oral steroids, or in those with medical contraindications to oral steroids, such as diabetes or peptic ulcer disease.

Additional supplies are required for chemical perfusion of the inner ear. These include the Micro-Wick, which is a patented cylindrical polyvinyl acetate material measuring 1×9 mm long and compressed into a polyethylene tube for storage. The Silverstein silicone ventilation tube (Micromedics) with a 1.42-mm inner diameter and a 3.25-mm flange is also needed. The larger inner diameter allows the round window to be well visualized through the tube and is also an ideal conduit for the MicroWick. The lumen of the ventilation tube can be directed with an instrument to visualize the round window niche, and the MicroWick is easily guided through the tube down to the round window membrane. Then the patient can self-administer medications for prolonged and near-continuous inner ear perfusion, thus obtaining high perilymph concentrations while minimizing systemic side effects.

SURGICAL TECHNIQUE

The patient's ear is anesthetized with 1 to 2 cc of a solution of 1% Xylocaine and 1:100,000 epinephrine. The CO_2 laser is used to create a bloodless 2-mm opening in the posterior quadrant of the tympanic membrane over the area of the round window membrane (Figs. 17–5 and 17–6). A vertical myringotomy incision posterior to the malleus handle can also be used. An otoedoscope 1.7 mm in diameter is introduced into the middle ear to visualize the round window membrane. If membranes are obstructing the round window membrane, they are removed with a micropick. This allows the medication to directly reach the round window membrane.[12,13] The vent tube is inserted through the tympanostomy over the round window niche. Adjusting the vent tube with an instrument to visualize the round window membrane allows proper placement of the wick into the round window niche (Fig. 17–7). Once the niche is seen through the vent tube, the MicroWick is inserted through the tube until resistance is met, and medication is also injected into the middle ear. Medication is placed on the MicroWick, which diffuses into the middle ear and down to the round window. Patients continue to instill medication in the ear three times a day while lying on their side for 15 minutes with the treated ear facing upward.

The MicroWick is simple and easy to use. The advantage of using the laser to make the opening in the tympanic membrane is that it makes a bloodless opening, with less chance of blood touching either the wick or the endoscope. Any fluid that touches the MicroWick will cause it to swell immediately and prevent its proper placement into the round

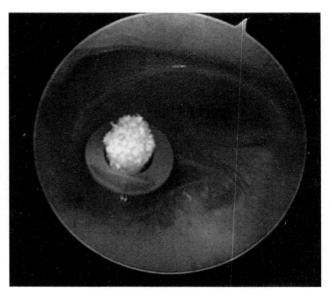

FIGURE 17–7 MicroWick in place.

window niche. If there is blood or fluid in an area where it cannot be removed, the procedure can be terminated after endoscopic viewing of the middle ear and insertion of the ventilation tube. The Micro-Wick can then be placed in a delayed fashion when the ear is dry. The advantage of looking into the round window niche with the endoscope is that obstructing membranes (present in 20%) can be visualized and removed.[12] The round window niche should be completely unobstructed for the Micro-Wick to work optimally.

The MicroWick can be placed without using the laser and the endoscope if they are not available. Phenol or tetracaine base solution can be used to anesthetize the tympanic membrane after which a vertical myringotomy 3 mm in length and 1 mm from the annulus is made over the round window area. The ventilation tube can be inserted directly over the round window niche. The placement of the incision in the tympanic membrane is critical to successful placement of the ventilation tube and MicroWick into the round window niche. The round window niche lies posterior (3.44 mm, SD $\pm$ 0.68 mm) and slightly inferior to the umbo of the malleus (113 degrees, SD $\pm$ 9.80 degrees).[12] Usually the round window niche can be seen through a normal tympanic membrane as a dark shadow beneath the tympanic membrane. When there is scarring of the tympanic membrane from previous infection, it can be difficult to determine the exact location of the round window beneath the tympanic membrane. With the laser, a small opening can be made in the tympanic membrane over the suspected site, and the location of the 2-mm opening can be adjusted so that the opening is placed directly over the round window niche.

The surgeon installs the first drops of medication onto the MicroWick using a 27-gauge, ½-inch needle on a tuberculin syringe and injects the remainder of the 0.2 cc into the middle ear through the tympanic membrane. Depending on the disease process, the patient is then given a prescription for the medication, which can be filled at a compounding pharmacy. The patient is instructed to self-administer three drops, three times daily into the ear canal and return to the office weekly for evaluation.

After 4 weeks, the MicroWick and tube are removed as one unit without the use of anesthesia. Removal is performed using either a right-angle pick placed under the flange or a cup forceps to grab the tab of the vent tube. The tympanostomy will heal spontaneously or can be patched with a 3-mm circular piece of Gelfilm soaked in antibiotic solution. The tympanic membrane usually heals rapidly in 1 to 2 weeks. If the MicroWick is left in for extended periods of time (i.e., over 6 weeks), the polyvinyl acetate may become adherent to the mucosa of the round window niche. This may make removal of the MicroWick more difficult and can result in its breaking, thus leaving a piece of polyvinyl acetate in the middle ear. If this occurs, the ear is injected with a buffered 1% Xylocaine and adrenaline solution, and a pick is used to tease the MicroWick from the mucosa. This procedure has been done in 5% of cases, and no MicroWick material has been left knowingly inside the middle ear.

USE OF GENTAMICIN TO TREAT VERTIGO OF MENIERE'S DISEASE

In a compounding pharmacy, sterile techniques are used to prepare a 10-cc dilute solution of gentamicin otic solution. Five, 10, or 20 mg/cc is prepared and then transferred into a sterile dropper bottle. The usual concentration used is 10 mg/cc. The patient is instructed to lie in the supine position for 15 minutes with the treated ear up, and to administer three drops of this medication into the ear canal three times daily. At the end of each week, hearing is evaluated using audiometric testing of air, bone, and discrimination score. Also, electrocochleography is completed, and balance function is tested using warm and ice-air caloric electronystagmography (ENG). Depending on the test results, treatment is either continued or discontinued. The ideal goal of this treatment is to obtain a 100% reduced vestibular response (RVR) to both warm and ice-air caloric ENG testing without producing a hearing loss. The usual length of treatment is 2 to 3 weeks (range 1 to 6).

During the treatment period, if the hearing significantly decreases but vestibular function is still present, oral prednisone 60 mg/day is prescribed for 2 weeks with a rapid taper to help preserve or improve hearing while the gentamicin drops are continued. If the patient cannot take oral steroids for medical reasons such as hypertension, diabetes, or gastric ulceration, dexamethasone eardrops (4 mg/cc) are used. When the vestibular function reaches 100% RVR, or remains stable and does not decrease after several weeks of treatment, the gentamicin treatment is discontinued.

USE OF DEXAMETHASONE

A solution of dexamethasone 4 mg/cc is prepared at a compounding pharmacy and placed in a sterile dropper bottle. Originally, the dosage used was 24 mg/cc, but this appeared to cause delayed healing; 20% required a fat graft myringoplasty to repair the nonhealing perforation. The patient is given instructions to lie in the supine position with the head turned for 15 minutes and to instill three drops three times daily. In addition, antibiotic eardrops (Vasocidin ophthalmic) are instilled once daily to prevent infection. Hearing is measured at 2 weeks, at which time it is determined whether to continue or terminate the treatment.

RESULTS OF MICROWICK USAGE

Since August 1998, over 200 patients in our clinic have been treated using the polyvinyl acetate MicroWick.[14] When retrospectively reviewing the first 114 patients, the majority of the patients (92) were treated for Meniere's disease. The remaining 22 had a diagnosis of sudden deafness or autoimmune inner ear disease. Not all patients have complete follow-up data, so results include patients for whom long-term follow-up data are available. Patient acceptance of the procedure has been excellent.

MENIERE'S DISEASE TREATMENT RESULTS

Vertigo symptoms were relieved in 74 (85%) patients responding to a questionnaire. Seven patients (8%) needed further treatment for Meniere's disease: two patients had retreatment with the MicroWick and gentamicin drops; two patients had a labyrinthectomy; two patients had a combined retrosigmoid/retrolabyrinthine vestibular neurectomy; and one patient had transtympanic injections of gentamicin performed elsewhere. Pressure in the ear was improved or relieved in 67% responding, whereas tinnitus was relieved or improved in 57% of patients. The average length of treatment was 3 weeks (range 1 to 6 weeks).

Hearing results were evaluated using the 1995 American Academy of Otolaryngoloy criteria for Meniere's disease [i.e., a 10-dB change of pure tone average (PTA) or a 15% change in discrimination] in 37 patients who had hearing better than or equal to 50 dB PTA. In these patients, profound hearing loss occurred in two patients. One of these patients failed to return to the office, used the drops continually for 5.5 weeks, and developed sudden deafness. This resulted in a total chemical labyrinthectomy. The PTA remained the same in 54% (20/37) patients, was improved in 11% (4/37) patients, and worsened in 35% (13/37) patients. The discrimination score remained the same in 70% (26/37), was better in 5% (2/37), and was worse in 24% (9/37). The average hearing loss for all patients in this group was 9 dB PTA and 9% discrimination score. For just the 11 patients with a loss of hearing, the average drop was 26 dB PTA and 24% discrimination score.

SUDDEN DEAFNESS AND AUTOIMMUNE INNER EAR DISEASE TREATMENT RESULTS

Nineteen patients were treated for sudden deafness. Five of the patients had a positive response to the self-administered dexamethasone. It appeared that patients treated early in the disease had better results, although one patient had a good response after more than 1 year. There was no statistically significant difference between patients treated in less than 4 weeks after their hearing loss and those who had a more than 4-week delay before treatment. Only three patients were treated for autoimmune inner ear disease and the results were inconclusive.

COMPLICATIONS

Complications using the self-treatment technique with the MicroWick were infrequent. Two patients had a permanent tympanic membrane perforation after the MicroWick and dexamethasone infusion that was repaired using an adipose tissue graft as an office procedure. Two patients developed acute otitis media, which responded to local treatment with antibiotic eardrops. Two patients had the MicroWick and tube spontaneously extrude from the eardrum during treatment. Two patients had severe unsteadiness after the MicroWick and gentamicin treatment that did not quickly respond to vestibular rehabilitation therapy.

ADIPOSE TISSUE MYRINGOPLASTY

INDICATIONS

Fat graft myringoplasty is offered to patients with benign-appearing perforations of the tympanic membrane that are 3 mm or smaller in size (≥30% of the tympanic membrane). The mucosa of the middle ear should be normal in appearance, and the perforation should be dry for at least the preceding 6 months. Small defects that occur soon after tympanoplasty can be repaired successfully. If the conductive hearing loss appears out of proportion to the size of the perforation, a paper patch is placed over the perforation, and the audiogram is repeated. If the conductive loss remains, a problem with the ossicular conductive mechanism is suspected, and a standard tympanoplasty is performed in a certified outpatient operating room setting. The office myringoplasty procedure is not offered to patients with perforations exhibiting a growth of squamous epithelium around the edges and onto the undersurface of the tympanic membrane. Prior to surgery, aspirin and other known anticoagulating medications are stopped for the appropriate time period preoperatively.

SURGICAL TECHNIQUE

The patient is placed in a supine position. The posterior surface of the earlobe is injected with 0.5 cc of buffered 1% lidocaine with epinephrine 1:100,000. The external auditory canal is injected similar to stapes surgery.

The ear lobe is prepped and draped in a sterile fashion. A 5- to 10-mm incision is made in the ear lobe skin down to the subcutaneous fat. It is easier to remove the fat if the incision is placed along the edge of the ear lobe. In women, it is preferable to make the incision behind the ear lobe to help hide the scar. Care is taken to avoid entering an earring tract if one is nearby. The skin is undermined and fat is removed using a No. 15 blade or sharp dissecting scissors, making sure not to "button hole" the anterior ear lobe skin. The diameter of the harvested fat should be about twice the size of the perforation. The fat is set aside in sterile saline. The incision is closed with simple interrupted 5-0 plain gut sutures and coated with a mild antibiotic ointment. The sutures fall out after several weeks.

The speculum holder is assembled and used to hold the largest speculum possible in the ear canal. The 30-degree, 1.7-mm-diameter otoendoscope is passed through the perforation, and the middle ear and undersurface of the tympanic membrane are carefully viewed. If skin is seen growing around the edges of the perforation and onto the undersurface of the tympanic membrane for a significant distance, the procedure is aborted and a formal tympanoplasty is scheduled in a certified outpatient surgery center. If skin is not seen, the otoendoscope is removed, and using the operating microscope the edges of the perforation are freshened with a small right-angled pick. It is important to produce bleeding from the edge of the perforation with this maneuver.

Directly medial to the perforation, the middle ear is filled with Gelfoam soaked in antibiotic solution. The oversized piece of fat is placed through the perforation in a dumbbell fashion. Most of the graft should be medial to the level of the tympanic membrane, but some fat should be lateral to it. The edges of the perforation are elevated with a small pick to ensure that fat is tucked beneath the skin and that growth of the skin edges is directed over the lateral surface of the fat graft. Polyester packing strips (Medtronic Xomed Inc.) are placed over the drum and graft, and held in place for 2 weeks with cottonoid packing dots (Medtronic Xomed Inc.).

POSTOPERATIVE CARE

The patient is cautioned to avoid any Valsalva maneuvers. Routine water precautions are given with instructions to continue until the perforation is healed. The packing is removed 2 weeks postoperatively. The tympanic membrane is inspected weekly until it completely heals (usually 3 to 4 weeks), and a postoperative audiogram is obtained following healing. Patients are permitted to Valsalva a few times daily after 3 weeks. If patients hear an air leak, they are instructed to stop the Valsalva maneuver.

REFERENCES

1. Silverstein H, Call D. Tetracaine base: an effective surface anesthetic for the tympanic membrane. *Arch Otolaryngol* 1969:90:150–151.
2. Rosen S. Mobilization of the stapes to restore hearing in otosclerosis. *N Y State J Med* 1953;53:2650–2653.
3. Fowler EP. Anterior crurotomy and mobilization of the ankylosed stapes footplate: introduction to motion picture demonstration. *Acta Otolaryngol* 1956:46:319–322.
4. Shea JJ Jr. Fenestration of the oval window. *Ann Otol Rhinol Laryngol* 1958:67:932–951.
5. Perkins RC. Laser stapedotomy for otosclerosis. *Laryngoscope* 1980;90:228–240.
6. Rosen S, Siegal K. Rosen mobilization and stapedectomy: long-term results with special reference to high frequencies. *Arch Otolaryngol* 1969;89:425–428.
7. Myers EN, Ishiyama E, Heisse JW. Histology of a successful stapes mobilization. *Ann Otol Rhinol Laryngol* 1970;79:321–330.
8. Silverstein H. Laser stapedotomy minus prosthesis (laser STAMP): a minimally invasive procedure. *Am J Otol* 1998;19:277–282.
9. Silverstein H, Jackson LE, Conlon S, Rosenberg SI, Thompson JH. Laser stapedotomy minus prosthesis (Laser STAMP): absence of refixation. *Otol Neurotol* 2002;22:152–157.
10. Silverstein H, Kuhn J, Choo D, Krespi YJ, Rosenberg SI, Rowan PT. Laser-assisted tympanostomy. *Laryngoscope* 1996;106:1067–1074.
11. Rosenberg SI. Endoscopic otologic surgery. *Otolaryngol Clin North Am* 1996;29:291–300.
12. Silverstein H, Arruda J, Rosenberg SI, Deems D. Direct round window membrane application of gentamicin in the treatment of Meniere's disease. *Otolaryngol Head Neck Surg* 1999;120:649–656.
13. Rosenberg SI. Vestibular surgery for Ménière's disease in the elderly: a review of techniques and indications. *Ear Nose Throat J* 1999;78:443–446.
14. Silverstein H. The MicroWick to deliver medication to the inner ear. *Ear Nose Throat J* 1999;78:595–600.

Chapter 18

SURGERY FOR TRAUMATIC MIDDLE EAR CONDITIONS

Bassem M. Said and Gordon B. Hughes

Trauma to the middle ear can present as an isolated injury or may be associated with severe trauma to the skull base with resultant neurologic sequelae. The cause of injury varies from motor vehicle collisions and industrial accidents to recreationally related mishaps, falls, and assault. In all cases the structures embedded in the temporal bone are at risk for significant injury. Temporal bone injuries can present with facial paralysis, conductive hearing loss, sensorineural hearing loss, vertigo, and/or cerebrospinal fluid (CSF) leak (otorrhea or rhinorrhea).

CLASSIFICATION OF TEMPORAL BONE FRACTURES

Middle ear injuries can occur with or without fracture of the temporal bone. When a fracture is present, however, its configuration may help predict the resultant injury. Temporal bone fractures have been classified as longitudinal or transverse. Longitudinal fractures account for 70 to 90% of temporal bone fractures and usually result from direct blunt injury to the temporal region. The fracture line extends from the squamous portion of the temporal bone, bypassing the dense bone of the otic capsule, and travels toward the foramen lacerum and the jugular foramen. The middle ear space and the posterosuperior external auditory canal are often involved in the path of the fracture. As a result, the clinical presentation of longitudinal fractures often includes conductive hearing loss caused by hemotympanum, tympanic membrane perforation, or ossicular discontinuity. Sensorineural hearing loss, facial nerve injury, and CSF leak occur less frequently with this type of fracture, and are usually less severe.

Transverse fractures account for 20 to 30% of temporal bone injuries. These fractures most frequently occur after a severe blow to the occipital or frontal region. The fracture line crosses the petrous apex, extending from the jugular foramen to the foramen lacerum or spinosum. The otic capsule often is violated, resulting in a sensorineural hearing loss. Vertigo often accompanies traumatic sensorineural hearing loss. Immediate facial paralysis is common, occurring in up to 50% of these injuries. CSF leaks are relatively common, resulting in otorrhea or, if the tympanic membrane is intact, rhinorrhea.

Although the classification of temporal bone fractures into longitudinal and transverse is a useful guide in delineating the clinical features and prognosis of patients presenting with these injuries, many patients present with a mixed fracture. In fact, as was shown by Ghorayeb and Yeakley,[1] most fractures are oblique. The clinical findings in these patients are dependent on the path of the fracture line and the specific structures involved.

Despite the myriad mechanisms leading to middle ear injury, generally four clinical presentations may require surgical intervention: facial paralysis, conductive hearing loss, CSF otorrhea or rhinorrhea, and (rarely) persistent vertigo. In all cases, prior to addressing issues dealing with the temporal bone, patients should be assessed for cervical spine, hemodynamic, and neurologic stability.

FACIAL PARALYSIS

Overall, temporal bone trauma results in facial nerve injury approximately 7% of the time.[2] Posttraumatic facial paralysis may present immediately after the injury or may be delayed for several hours or days.

Patients experiencing paralysis immediately after trauma are relatively more likely to have nerve transection, whereas those presenting in a delayed fashion do not have transection. Immediate paralysis is more common with transverse fractures of the temporal bone and is generally associated with more serious closed head injuries.

Every effort should be made in the emergency room to determine facial nerve function. Painful stimuli to evoke a grimace should be sought of comatose patients prior to the use of a muscle relaxant. During the physical examination, the clinician should note if paralysis is complete and if all branches of the facial nerve are involved. This may be difficult if multiple facial injuries are present. Intratemporal facial nerve injuries usually affect the entire distribution of the facial nerve. Radiographic evidence of facial nerve injury, such as temporal bone comminution, transverse fracture of a temporal bone, or fracture through the geniculate area of the facial nerve, also can help determine the need for surgery. A high-resolution computed tomography (CT) scan of the temporal bone should be obtained.

Although management of traumatic paralysis remains controversial, a systematic approach that accumulates all of the available clinical and electrodiagnostic data is best. The important issues that need to be considered include the following:

1. Which patients are most likely to recover facial nerve function spontaneously?
2. Which patients should undergo facial nerve exploration and when should the intervention be carried out?
3. Which surgical approach should be used?
4. Which nerve repair should be carried out once the pathology is identified?

WHICH PATIENTS ARE MOST LIKELY TO RECOVER SPONTANEOUSLY?

As Turner[3] demonstrated, 84% of patients presenting with facial nerve dysfunction resulting from temporal bone injury recover to full function spontaneously. With this in mind, the challenge is to identify the minority of patients who require surgery for nerve decompression or repair. Stratification based on clinical presentation and electroneurography (ENoG) helps determine prognosis and timing of surgery. Patients who present with delayed facial nerve paresis or paralysis have a 94 to 100% chance of spontaneous recovery to House-Brackmann (HB) grade 1 or 2 and therefore should be treated conservatively.[2-4] Brodie and Thompson[2] found that the latency to recovery could vary from 1 day to 1 year, but that 88% had recovered by 3 months.

WHICH PATIENTS SHOULD UNDERGO FACIAL NERVE EXPLORATION, AND WHEN?

In general, patients presenting with immediate-onset complete facial paralysis are most likely to need surgery. Some authors argue that ENoG should be the primary method of determining which patients should be explored because it is more objective than historic information.[5,6] Nosan et al[5] found that all patients presenting with temporal bone trauma with facial paralysis who demonstrated ENoG > 90% degeneration had significant facial nerve pathology at time of exploration, regardless of time of onset of paralysis.

Fisch[7] demonstrated the utility of ENoG in assessing facial nerve function and prognosticating likelihood of recovery. He noted that patients who had undergone deliberate facial nerve transection for tumors resulted in 100% degeneration on ENoG in 3 to 5 days. Fisch also presented three patients with delayed facial paralysis occurring 3 to 7 days after vestibular nerve section. ENoG showed progressive denervation that became complete after 14 to 21 days, and all three patients had nearly complete return of facial function. Therefore, if ENoG demonstrates > 90% degeneration in the first 6 days, one can infer that significant facial nerve injury has occurred and surgical exploration should be carried out. On the other hand, if > 90% degeneration does not occur until 14 days, then good recovery is expected without surgical intervention.

The group of patients who obtain > 90 to 95% degeneration between 6 and 14 days have various degrees of intermediate nerve injury. Facial nerve exploration in these patients can benefit those few who would otherwise have poor spontaneous recovery. Patients who present several months after the initial injury can be followed with electromyography (EMG) to detect subclinical return of facial nerve function. If no return of function is detected within 6 to 12 months, facial nerve exploration is warranted. Delayed exploration should be performed within 1 year, as nerve-grafting results tend to deteriorate after this interval.

WHICH SURGICAL APPROACH SHOULD BE USED?

The surgical approach for facial nerve exploration depends on the site of the lesion and the status of hearing on the affected side. Several authors have observed that the perigeniculate region is the site of injury in 80 to 90% of traumatically induced facial nerve lesions.[6,8] Furthermore, as Felix et al[9] demonstrated, traumatic injury at the geniculum induces retrograde degeneration through the labyrinthine and distal meatal segments of the facial nerve. Therefore, the surgical approach to facial nerve exploration should provide access to these areas. In addition, the surgical field should be prepped for exposure of the entire facial nerve from the brainstem to the pes anserinus, and should include the neck for a great auricular nerve graft, even if more limited exposure and repair are likely.

Initial exposure of the facial nerve is accomplished using a transmastoid approach. This allows for visualization of vertical and horizontal segments of the facial nerve, as well as the opportunity to repair ossicular discontinuity transcanal.[10,11] If hearing is good, then the transmastoid approach is combined with a middle cranial fossa approach to allow visualization of the nerve proximally. If hearing is not useful, then a translabyrinthine dissection following a transmastoid approach provides adequate visualization of the facial nerve.

WHICH NERVE REPAIR SHOULD BE CARRIED OUT ONCE THE PATHOLOGY IS IDENTIFIED?

Once the facial nerve has been exposed and the location, type, and severity of pathology have been discovered, surgical repair can be performed. Findings at the time of facial nerve exploration include intraneural hematoma or contusion, bony impingement, and nerve transection. If hematoma is found, then facial nerve decompression should be carried out along the path of the nerve above and below the site of injury. Bony impingement should be removed, again followed by decompression.

Should the epineurium be incised following decompression? May,[10] Fisch,[12] and Yanagihara[13] advocated opening the nerve sheath to allow the nerve fascicles to expand and relieve edema. However, animal experimental data by Greer et al[14] and Boyle[15] suggest that widely incising the nerve sheath may inadvertently damage some of the axons and result in poorer outcomes. We do not recommend incising the nerve sheath.

Facial nerve transection is found in 30 to 64% of explored facial nerves.[4,16] Regardless of the method used for nerve repair, recovery to HB grade 1 or 2 has not been reported. Instead, HB grade 3 or 4 is the result in 75 to 100% of patients.[17,18] With this in mind, facial nerve resection and repair should be undertaken only when transection is evident. Because the degree of transection is usually worse than it appears, if 50% or more of the nerve appears transected, resection of the injured segment and repair should be performed.

The two main options for repair are primary end-to-end anastomosis and interposition grafting. The decision to choose one technique over the other is based on whether a tension-free repair can be accomplished with primary anastomosis. Primary anastomosis is known to result in superior results over interposition grafting,[19] perhaps due to better matching of neural fascicles. If the nerve defect is 1 cm or less, mobilization of the cut ends can be accomplished by subtotal parotidectomy, release from the second genu, or release from the geniculate ganglion (by transecting the greater superficial petrosal nerve), with tension-free primary repair.

If a tension-free primary repair cannot be carried out, then interposition grafting is required. The greater auricular nerve is the preferred graft because of its proximity to the operative field, as well as its close match in size to the facial nerve.[19] Nerve anastomosis using 9-0 or 10-0 monofilament sutures provides adequate strength using two or three sutures. Although Fisch[20] and others advocate perineurial repair with resection of the epineurium at the anastomotic site, improved functional results have not been demonstrated over standard epineurial repair. In addition to suture technique, nonsuture techniques have been applied to facial nerve repair. In particular, the use of fibrin glue in the internal auditory canal and the labyrinthine segment can provide nerve repair in the areas that are not easily amenable to suture technique.

If for some reason nerve grafting cannot be performed in the first 12 to 18 months, then a hypoglossal/facial end-to-side neurorrhaphy should be carried out. This technique results in return of facial tone, symmetry, and some voluntary motion, while preserving tongue function.

Although May et al[21] used an interposition graft between the facial nerve trunk and the partially transected hypoglossal nerve, Atlas and Lowinger[22] and Yoleri et al[23] recommended more extensive facial nerve and hypoglossal mobilization resulting in direct attachment between the two nerves.

SURGICAL TECHNIQUE

Because the exact site and extent of lesion and the method of repair are difficult to anticipate, the patient should be prepped and draped for middle fossa craniotomy (if hearing is good), mastoidectomy, parotidectomy, great auricular nerve graft, and even hypoglossal nerve dissection—virtually the entire side of the head and neck. Extensive exploration at multiple sites and mobilization or nerve grafting can require considerable time; most patients should have a Foley catheter placed that can be removed at the end of the procedure. A facial nerve monitor/stimulator is unnecessary because the nerve will not respond, since several days or longer often are required to evaluate and stabilize neurolo-

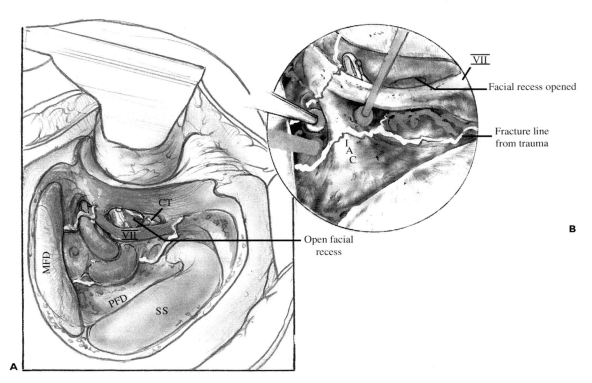

FIGURE 18–1   (A) Facial recess approach to the facial nerve. (B) Skeletonized fallopian canal and internal auditory canal (IAC). MFD, middle fossa dura; PFD, posterior fossa dura; SS, sigmoid sinus; CT, chorda tympani; VII, facial nerve.

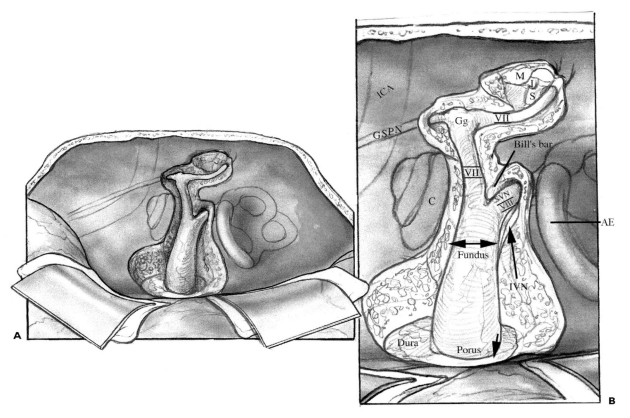

FIGURE 18–2   Middle cranial fossa approach to the facial nerve. (A) Orientation. (B) Close-up view. GSPN, greater superficial petrosal nerve; Gg, geniculate ganglion; M, malleus; I, incus; S, stapes; VII, facial nerve; SVN, superior vestibular nerve; IVN, inferior vestibular nerve; ICA, internal carotid artery; C, cochlea; AE, arcuate eminence.

gic and other injuries. We routinely ask a neurosurgeon and a head and neck surgeon to stand by in case they are needed.

A mastoidectomy is performed first, and the nerve from the geniculate to the stylomastoid foramen is examined through the facial recess (Fig. 18–1). If perigeniculate trauma extends proximally and hearing is good, a middle fossa craniotomy is performed and the canalicular and labyrinthine segments are examined (Fig. 18–2). If hearing is poor, a translabyrinthine approach suffices (Fig. 18–3). If the nerve is sheared off at the stylomastoid foramen, the mastoid tip is removed and a superficial parotidectomy performed. By this time the traumatized nerve has been decompressed and bone spicules have been removed.

If the nerve is transected, the surgeon then decides whether proximal and distal segments can be mobilized for primary anastomosis; otherwise, a great auricular nerve graft is obtained. An imaginary line drawn inferior and perpendicular to a second line that connects the mastoid tip and angle of the mandible will lie in the location and direction of this nerve (Fig. 18–4). A separate incision is used to obtain a 2- or 3-cm graft, as needed. The traumatized ends of the facial nerve are freshened, and two or three 9-0 or 10-0 monofilament sutures are used for anastomosis. If the injury lies in the tympanic fallopian canal or labyrinthine canal, the graft can be laid in the canal in an S shape and held against the facial nerve ends with connective tissue or fibrin glue (Fig. 18–5). If the defect is large and suturing in

the cerebellopontine angle is not possible, a hypoglossal-facial anastomosis can be performed at the same time or as a separate procedure.

Nerve recovery following primary repair or grafting requires at least 3 months for injuries at the stylomastoid foramen, 6 months for the second genu, 9 months for the geniculate ganglion, and 12 months for the internal auditory canal. Depending on the estimated time for recovery, a gold weight can be placed in the upper eyelid at the time of nerve repair to assist eyelid closure. The weight is removed when recovery is complete.

Drains are left in any parotid and neck incisions and a large bulky dressing is applied to the craniotomy and mastoid sites. Drains are removed when 24-hour drainage is less than 30 cc and the dressing is removed at 3 days or sooner if the patient is ready for discharge.

CONDUCTIVE HEARING LOSS

Conductive hearing loss can result from injury to the middle ear with or without temporal bone fracture. Often the injury causes bleeding from the external auditory canal skin. If CSF otorrhea also is present, the clot should be left alone to form a natural biologic dressing as the CSF leak usually stops spontaneously (see below). If no leak is present, under appropriate magnification blood can be gently cleaned in an attempt to delineate if the source of bleeding is the external or middle ear. Debris,

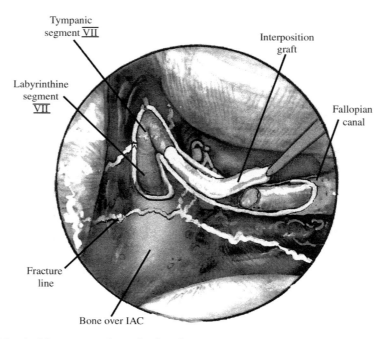

Tympanic segment VII

Labyrinthine segment VII

Interposition graft

Fallopian canal

Fracture line

Bone over IAC

FIGURE 18–3 Translabyrinthine approach to the facial nerve. IAC, internal auditory canal.

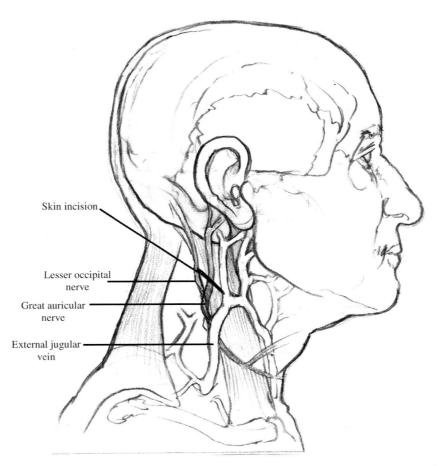

Skin incision

Lesser occipital
nerve

Great auricular
nerve

External jugular
vein

FIGURE 18–4   Skin incision and anatomic relationships in obtaining a graft of the greater auricular nerve.

cerumen, keratin, and hair should be removed. The membrane may be perforated, or it may be intact with blood accumulation in the middle ear (hemotympanum). Within the middle ear, ossicular discontinuity or fracture occurs in 30% of patients with tympanic membrane lacerations.[24] Even if the tympanic membrane is torn, the majority of tympanic membrane perforations will heal spontaneously, most within 6 weeks and nearly all the rest within 12 weeks. If hemotympanum is noted on examination, it is left to resolve spontaneously over 4 to 6 weeks. Alternatively, hemotympanum can be evacuated after myringotomy, although some authors have noted a potential risk of infection. Patients should undergo serial audiometric assessment to follow recovery of the conductive hearing loss.

If a conductive hearing loss persists after hemotympanum resolves or after the drum heals, then ossicular discontinuity is suspected. Surgical exploration is recommended for a persistent conductive hearing loss of 25 dB or greater. A period of 3 to 4 months is advised prior to exploration to allow for a decrease in posttraumatic edema, as well as to allow for spontaneous recovery. Patients should be informed that a hearing aid is a viable alternative to exploration and ossicular reconstruction.

Incudostapedial joint separation accounts for up to 82% of ossicular causes of a conductive hearing loss discovered at exploration.[25,26] Other findings can include incudomallear disarticulation, incus dislocation, and fracture of the stapes crura or footplate. Fracture of the footplate mainly occurs secondary to transverse fractures passing through the oval window.[27] A fracture of the footplate (with or without displacement of the fragments) may cause a perilymph fistula with pneumolabyrinth.[28]

SURGICAL TECHNIQUE

Surgical reconstruction can be carried out as dictated by the injury and the surgeon's preference. Techniques for ossicular reconstruction and stapedectomy are covered in Chapters 19 and 20.

CEREBROSPINAL FLUID LEAK

Cerebrospinal fluid leaks occur in 1.4% of injuries involving the temporal bone.[29] The great majority

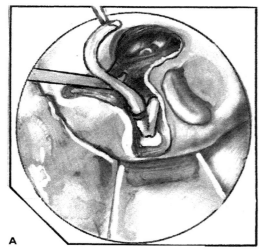

A

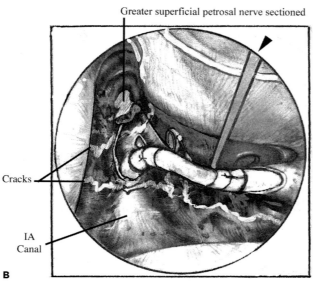

Greater superficial petrosal nerve sectioned

Cracks

IA
Canal

B

Extensive loss, tympanic and proximal vertical segment

▶ Pointer to interposition graft

FIGURE 18–5 (A) Donor graft in place through the middle fossa approach. (B) Graft through the translabyrinthine approach.

resolve spontaneously with conservative measures within a few days. Patients present with rhinorrhea or, if the tympanic membrane has been perforated, otorrhea. In addition, patients may complain of associated headaches. Meningitis represents the primary risk in persistent CSF leak. In a series of 1800 patients, Canniff[29] found that 20% of patients with CSF leak resulting from temporal bone trauma developed meningitis.

Generally, head elevation and placement of a lumbar subarachnoid drain suffice. Prophylactic use of antibiotics is controversial. Although some argue that antibiotics in this setting decrease the

instance of meningitis, others believe that they may mask the progression of meningitis, resulting in a worse neurologic outcome. Nonetheless, antibiotic administration is recommended if a subarachnoid drain is to be placed. To minimize risk of contamination, usually from *Staphylococcus aureus*, the drain is removed at 5 days. By this time the leak usually has sealed. If CSF leak recurs after removal of the subarachnoid drain, then a new drain is placed and surgery can be carried out when the patient is neurologically stable.

SURGICAL TECHNIQUE

If a subarachnoid drain has been removed and CSF leak persists, a new one is replaced now under general anesthesia. A Foley catheter and facial nerve stimulator are not needed. Because it is difficult to anticipate whether a middle cranial fossa approach is required or a transmastoid approach will suffice, the patient must be informed in advance and prepped for both middle fossa and mastoid surgery. We routinely ask a neurosurgeon to stand by. The lower left quadrant of the abdomen is prepped for a fat graft (lower left, so the scar will not be confused with an appendectomy scar later on).

If a pressure equalizing (PE) tube has been placed previously for any reason, it is removed now. A complete mastoidectomy is performed and the tegmen and perilabyrinthine air cells carefully examined for CSF leakage. The extent of surgical exposure depends on the location and size of the dural defect and the status of hearing. If the leak occurs in a deaf ear, it is repaired through a transmastoid approach by direct reinforcement with fascia or other connective tissue, and by obliteration of the mastoid with abdominal fat, and of the middle ear and eustachian tube with temporalis muscle. Removing the incus, opening the facial recess, and transecting the tensor tympani tendon facilitate exposure of the eustachian tube.

If hearing is good, the initial approach is again transmastoid. If the dural defect is less than 1 cm and posteriorly located along the mastoid tegmen or posterior fossa, it can be sealed with fascia, the mastoid can be obliterated with abdominal fat in a similar fashion, and the mesotympanum and ossicles can be left alone. If the defect is more than 1 cm, or anteriorly located so that packing would immobilize the ossicles, a middle fossa approach is carried out and the dural defect repaired intra- or extradurally with suture or connective tissue.

No drain is placed. A large bulky dressing is applied to the ear and side of the head as needed and is left in place for 3 days. On the third day, both dressing and subarachnoid drain are removed. The patient is observed for CSF rhinorrhea; if none occurs, the patient is discharged later that day or the next morning. The patient refrains from strenuous activity for 6 weeks; light work is permitted after 2 weeks.

VERTIGO

Vertigo occurring after temporal bone or middle ear trauma most often results from benign paroxysmal positioning vertigo (BPPV).[30] Onset is immediately following the injury. The usual course is spontaneous resolution within 3 months.[31] Other types of traumatic inner ear vertigo usually resolve within 6 months. Surgery is indicated if symptoms are severe, if vestibular tests confirm unilateral inner ear origin with incomplete compensation, and if 6 to 12 months have elapsed to allow for spontaneous recovery. Unfortunately, when severe posttraumatic vertigo persists, it is often accompanied by central vestibular dysfunction from brain injury, which limits the potential benefit of inner ear surgery.

Patients presenting with vertigo associated with fluctuating sensorineural hearing loss may have traumatic perilymph fistula. Associated findings may include tinnitus and aural fullness. Surgical exploration is indicated if vertigo is immediate and severe, if vertigo fails to resolve, or if bone conduction deteriorates on serial audiograms. The defect is found in the oval or round window.

SURGICAL TECHNIQUE

The surgical approach for intractable vertigo is dictated by the status of hearing. If hearing is not serviceable, then a transmastoid labyrinthectomy is used. If hearing is preserved, a retrosigmoid (suboccipital) vestibular nerve section is performed. These techniques are described fully in the chapters on labyrinthectomy and other neurotologic procedures.

Perilymph fistula exploration is performed transcanal under intravenous sedation and local anesthesia, or can be combined with ossicular reconstruction under general anesthesia if desired. A posterior tympanomeatal flap is raised and the oval window observed under high magnification. Serum and other fluids are carefully removed with a No. 22 suction tube. The patient is placed in the Trendelenburg position and is asked to bear down to increase intracranial pressure. Any increase in local fluid accumulation, however slight, is noted. Even a shift in light reflex across the footplate can be diagnostic.

Whether a fistula is found or not, tragal perichondrium is obtained, cut into very small strips, and placed through and around the crura to fill the niche with connective tissue. Alternatively, in more severe fractures of the crura and footplate, a stapedectomy can be performed with connective tissue seal of the oval window held in place by a prosthesis.

Exploration and repair are repeated in the round window niche. Very often mucosal folds must be dissected away to reveal the true membrane. Even if no fistula is found, the niche also is packed with tragal perichondrium. Packing both the oval and round windows regardless of fistula resolves this management dilemma in case dizziness persists.

CONCLUSION

Temporal bone and middle ear trauma often is associated with neurologic, cervical, or vital organ injury, which takes priority in management. When the patient becomes stable, surgical exploration and treatment of facial paralysis, conductive hearing loss, CSF leak, or vertigo can be performed. Particularly with facial nerve injury and CSF leak, the exact site and extent of injury usually are not known until exploration; therefore, the patient must be informed of all possible procedures and the head and neck prepped and draped accordingly. If perilymph fistula is suspected, the oval and round windows should be packed, even if no fistula is seen.

REFERENCES

1. Ghorayeb BY, Yeakley JW. Temporal bone fractures: longitudinal or oblique? The case for oblique temporal bone fractures. *Laryngoscope* 1992;102:129–134.
2. Brodie HA, Thompson TC. Management of complications from 820 temporal bone fractures. *Am J Otol* 1997;18:188–197.
3. Turner JWA. Facial palsy in closed head injuries: prognosis. *Lancet* 1944;1:756–757.
4. McKennan KX, Chole RA, Facial paralysis in temporal bone trauma. *Am J Otol* 1992;13:167–172.
5. Nosan DK, Benecke JE Jr, Murr AH. Current perspective on temporal bone trauma. *Otolaryngol Head Neck Surg* 1997;117:67–71.
6. Lambert PR, Brackmann DE. Facial paralysis in longitudinal temporal bone fractures: a review of 26 cases. *Laryngoscope* 1984;94:1022–1026.
7. Fisch U. Prognostic value of electrical tests in acute facial paralysis. *Am J Otol* 1984;5:494–498.
8. Fisch U. Facial paralysis in fractures of the petrous bone. *Laryngoscope* 1974;84:2141–2154.
9. Felix H, Eby TL, Fisch U. New aspects of facial nerve pathology in temporal bone fractures. *Acta Otolaryngol* 1991;111:332–336.

10. May M. Total facial nerve exploration: transmastoid, extralabyrinthine, and subtemporal indications and results. *Laryngoscope* 1979;89:906–917.

11. Yanagihara N. Transmastoid decompression of the facial nerve in temporal bone fracture. *Otolaryngol Head Neck Surg* 1982;90:616–621.

12. Fisch U. Surgery for Bell's palsy. *Arch Otolaryngol* 1981;107:1–11.

13. Yanagihara N. Transmastoid decompression of the facial nerve using supralabyrinthine approach. In: Portmann M, ed. *Facial Nerve*. New York: Masson; 1984:479–481.

14. Greer JA, Cody DJ, Lambert EH, Weiland LH. Experimental facial nerve paralysis: influence of decompression. *Ann Otol Rhinol Laryngol* 1974;83:582–595.

15. Boyle WF. Evaluation of facial nerve decompression in experimental facial nerve paralysis in monkeys. *Laryngoscope* 1967;77:1168–1178.

16. Fisch U. Current surgical treatment of intratemporal facial palsy. *Clin Plast Surg* 1979;6:377–388.

17. Kamerer DB. Intratemporal facial nerve injuries. *Otolaryngol Head Neck Surg* 1982;90:612–615.

18. Green JD, Shelton C, Brackmann DE. Surgical management of iatrogenic facial nerve injuries. *Otolaryngol Head Neck Surg* 1994;111:606–610.

19. May M. Facial reanimation after skull base trauma. In: May M, ed. *The Facial Nerve*. New York: Thieme; 1986:421–440.

20. Fisch U. Facial nerve grafting. *Otolaryngol Clin North Am* 1974;7:517–529.

21. May M, Sobol SM, Mester SJ. Hypoglossal-facial nerve interposition-jump graft for facial reanimation without tongue atrophy. *Otolaryngol Head Neck Surg* 1991;104:818–825.

22. Atlas MD, Lowinger DS. A new technique for hypoglossal-facial nerve repair. *Laryngoscope* 1997;107:984–991.

23. Yoleri L, Songur E, Yoleri O, Vural T, Cagdas A. Reanimation of early facial paralysis with hypoglossal/facial end-to-side neurorrhaphy: a new approach. *J Reconstr Microsurg* 2000;16:347–356.

24. Silverstein H, Fabian RL, Stool SE, Hong SW. Penetrating wounds of the tympanic membrane and ossicular chain. *Trans Am Acad Ophthalmol Otolaryngol* 1973;77:125–135.

25. Hasso AN, Ledington JA. Traumatic injuries of the temporal bone. *Otolaryngol Clin North Am* 1988;21:295–316.

26. Hough JV, Stuart WD. Middle ear injury in skull trauma. *Laryngoscope* 1968;78:899–937.

27. Meriot P, Veillon F, Garcia JF, et al. CT Appearance of ossicular injuries. *Radiographics* 1997;17:1445–1454.

28. Mafee MF, Valvassori GE, Kumar A, Yannias DA, Marcus RE. Pneumolabyrinth: a new radiologic sign for fracture of the stapes footplate. *Am J Otol* 1984;5:374–375.

29. Canniff JP. Otorrhoea in head injuries. *Br J Oral Surg* 1971;8:203–210.

30. Griffiths MV. The incidence of auditory and vestibular concussion following minor head injury. *J Laryngol Otol* 1979;9:253–265.

31. Gordon N. Post-traumatic vertigo with special reference to positional nystagmus. *Lancet* 1954;1:1216–1218.

Chapter 19

OSSICULOPLASTY I

Dennis I. Bojrab and Seilesh C. Babu

Wullstein[1] and Zollner[2] first introduced the term *tympanoplasty* in 1951 to describe surgical reconstruction of the middle ear hearing mechanism that had been impaired or destroyed by disease. Successful tympanoplasty requires a mobile tympanic membrane or graft and a secure sound-conducting mechanism between this mobile membrane and the inner ear fluids. Since the introduction of the concept of hearing restoration in surgery for chronic otitis media, numerous materials have been used to recreate the sound-conducting mechanism. Aeration of a mucosal-lined middle ear is essential for sound conduction. If this can be accomplished, then the most biocompatible implant material with appropriate design and weight must be used for the optimal hearing restoration.

This chapter reviews the mechanics of hearing and the history of ossicular chain reconstruction and implant design, and focuses on the authors' preferred material, prostheses design, and evolution of technique.

ACOUSTIC MECHANICS

The middle ear functions to convey sound pressures from the air into the fluids of the inner ear via the ossicular chain. It is an impedance-matching system that ensures that energy is not lost. The normal human middle ear couples sound from the low-impedance sound energy in the ear canal through the tympanic membrane and ossicles to the relatively high impedance of fluid within the cochlea. The acoustic transformation theory states that this occurs via three lever systems: the tympanic membrane lever, the ossicular lever, and the hydraulic lever.[3] As a result of these three lever systems, the acoustic

transformer theory predicts a middle ear gain of approximately 27 to 34 dB.[4]

Implied in this transformer theory is the expectation that this gain is independent of frequency. Further investigations indicate that the acoustic transformer theory should be modified, proposing that middle ear sound transmission is actually frequency dependent.[5] Three areas account for this: ossicular coupling, acoustic coupling, and stapes-cochlear input impedance.

TYMPANIC MEMBRANE LEVER

The anatomy of the tympanic membrane and bony tympanic annulus provide a mechanical advantage. The tympanic membrane is a tense surface formed by the fibers of the tympanic membrane, which are tightly stretched over the malleus. Sound energy is directed toward the center of the tympanic membrane so that the manubrium receives the greatest amount. This creates amplification of the energy and provides at least a twofold gain in sound pressure at the malleus.[6]

OSSICULAR LEVER

The anatomy of the ossicles lends itself to another mechanical advantage. The malleus and incus work as a unit, but the manubrium is 1.3 times longer than the long process of the incus. This provides a lever action ratio of 1.3 to 1 as sound energy is transferred.[7]

HYDRAULIC LEVER

The anatomy of the middle ear also lends itself to the third lever, the hydraulic lever. The area of the tympanic membrane is considerably larger than the area of the stapes footplate. Sound pressure collected over the area of the tympanic membrane and transmitted to the area of the smaller footplate results in an increase in force proportional to the ratio of the areas. The average ratio has been calculated to be 20.8 to 1.[2]

OSSICULAR COUPLING

Ossicular coupling refers to the sound pressure gain that occurs through the actions of the tympanic membrane and the ossicular chain. The pressure gain provided by the normal middle ear with ossicular coupling, however, is frequency dependent. The mean middle ear gain is approximately 20 dB at 250 to 500 Hz, reaches a maximum of about 25 dB around 1 kHz, and then decreases at about 6 dB per octave at frequencies above 1 kHz.[8]

Certain portions of the tympanic membrane move differently depending on the frequency of vibration presented. At low frequencies, the entire tympanic membrane moves in one phase. At higher frequencies, the tympanic membrane divides into smaller vibrating portions that vibrate at different phases. Another factor for the change in gain above 1 kHz is slippage of the ossicular chain, especially at frequencies above 1 to 2 kHz.[4] Slippage is due to the translational movement in the rotational axis of the ossicles or flexion in the ossicular joints. In addition, some energy is lost because of the forces needed to overcome the stiffness and mass of the tympanic membrane and ossicular chain.[4]

Loss of the tympanic membrane and ossicular chain can cause a hearing loss that exceeds 30 dB, because sound now has access to both the round and oval windows, which can decrease the movement of cochlear fluids.

ACOUSTIC COUPLING

Movement of the tympanic membrane produces a sound pressure in the middle ear that is transmitted to the oval and round windows. Acoustic coupling is due to the difference in sound pressures acting on these areas. The pressure at each window is different because of the small distance between windows and the different orientation of each window relative to the tympanic membrane. In normal ears, the difference in pressures between the oval and round windows (acoustic coupling) is negligible.

In some diseased and reconstructed ears, the difference becomes significant and can greatly affect hearing. Specifically, when the ossicular chain is interrupted or absent, shielding of the round win-

dow results in redirection of all sound energy into the oval window.[9] When this is performed, acoustic coupling plays a significant role in sound pressure conduction for cochlear stimulation.

IMPEDANCE AT THE OVAL WINDOW

At the oval window, sound impedance occurs by several structures, including the annular ligament, the viscosity of the cochlear fluids, and the round window membrane. The round window impedance contribution is negligible in the normal ear. When the round window niche is filled with fluid or fibrous tissue, the round window impedance increases, resulting in a conductive hearing loss.

MIDDLE EAR AERATION

The middle ear space must be well aerated to facilitate ossicular function and tympanic membrane motion. Middle ear air pressure is less than the external canal air pressure in normal conditions, providing an environment conducive to ossicular coupling. If middle ear aeration is poor and the space is reduced, the pressure of the middle ear increases relative to the external canal pressure as the impedance increases. The pressure difference leads to a reduction in ossicular and tympanic membrane motion. The minimal amount of air required to maintain ossicular coupling within 10 dB of normal has been estimated to be 0.5 mL.[3]

IMPLANT CHARACTERISTICS

Many materials have been used for ossicular substitution or reconstruction. The ideal prosthesis for ossicular reconstruction should be made of material that maintains its shape, rigidity, and acoustic properties, as well as being cost-effective. This material should also be biocompatible, safe, and easily inserted and modified (Table 19–1).

TABLE 19–1 CONSIDERATIONS FOR THE IDEAL PROSTHESIS

Shape

Size

Material

Weight

Cost

Easily modified

TABLE 19–2   SUMMARY OF DIFFERENT TYPES OF MATERIALS FOR MIDDLE EAR IMPLANTS

	Autograft	Hydroxyapatite	Plastipore	HAPEX/Flex H/A	Titanium
Advantages	Biocompatible	Biocompatible, osteoconductive	Easily trimmed	Easily trimmed, biocompatible	Rigid, lightweight
Disadvantages	May not be present, may have residual disease	Not easily trimmed	Not biocompatible, high extrusions	Cost	Reactivity? Cost

Ossicular reconstruction materials are categorized as autografts, homografts, and alloplastic prosthetics. Each of these materials has advantages and disadvantages for use in the middle ear (Table 19–2).

AUTOGRAFTS

Autograft material, such as cartilage and bone, was one of the first materials used for ossiculoplasty. Studies have shown that cartilage was unstable, loses rigidity, and resorption occurs.[10] This loss of stiffness, due to ingrowth of blood vessels with subsequent chondritis, led to the conclusion that cartilage struts are unsatisfactory as long-term implants.[11,12]

Schuknecht and Shi[13] discussed the fate of bone middle ear implants. Incus and malleus grafts demonstrated no evidence of bone erosion and little resorption. Autologous incus grafts have been used for many years for middle ear reconstruction by modifying them to fit between the manubrium of the malleus and the stapes capitulum. These grafts may be used as a repositioned incus strut or as a total prosthesis. These bone implants maintain their contour, shape, size, and physical integrity for at least 11 years.[9,10] Today the preferred material for ossicular chain reconstruction when appropriate is the autograft biologic ossicle, if available, reshaped to fit the reconstruction needs of the surgery. In a series of 2200 cases, allograft and homograft prostheses yielded better hearing results than even the most biocompatible allograft prostheses.[14]

Autografts have several disadvantages, including prolonged operative time to obtain and shape the material, possible lack of availability in chronically diseased ears and revision cases, possible resorption, and loss of rigidity. These grafts may lose their blood supply and become nonviable. Sculpting with a high-power drill may create a thermal injury that leads to this loss of blood supply. Another disadvantage is that new bone formation and remodeling occur, characterized by a slow creeping substitution of revascularized bone. This neo-osteogenesis may serve as a hindrance to the transmission of sound. In addition, there may be osteitis within the ossicles and an increased risk of residual cholesteatoma in patients with cholesteatoma.

HOMOGRAFTS

To overcome some of the disadvantages of autografts, irradiated homograft ossicles and cartilage were introduced in the 1960s. Homograft ossicles or cartilage are either presculpted by the manufacturer or sculpted during surgery. Since 1986, homograft materials have been rarely used because of the risk of disease transmission (e.g., AIDS; Creutzfeldt-Jakob disease).[15]

ALLOPLASTS

Because of the disadvantages of autograft and homograft implants, synthetic materials, or alloplasts, have been investigated and have recently become the most commonly used materials for ossicular reconstruction. They are presculpted, readily available, and free from infectious disease. Alloplastic materials that have been used include polyethylene tubing, Teflon, Silastic tubing, stainless steel, titanium, gold, high-density polyethylene sponge (HDPS), bioglasses, and bioceramics.

By the 1960s, biocompatible solid polymeric materials, such as polyethylene, Teflon, and Proplast, were being used for ossicular reconstruction. Use of those materials is limited today because of high rates of migration, extrusion, and reactivity causing fibrosis.

In the 1970s, the HDPS was developed that had nonreactive properties and sufficient porosity to encourage tissue ingrowth. The original form was a machine-tooled prosthesis (Plastipore) and then a more versatile manufactured thermal-fused HDPS (Polycel). This later form permitted coupling with other materials such as stainless steel, thus lending itself to a wide variety of prosthetic designs.[16]

The major disadvantage of Plastipore is its lack of biocompatibility, which can lead to a high incidence of extrusion when in contact with the tympanic membrane, especially in the presence of infection or eustachian tube dysfunction.[17] Extrusion rates have averaged 3 to 5% in large series with 5 to 10 years of follow-up.[18] Extrusion is reduced considerably when cartilage is placed between the prosthesis and the tympanic membrane.

To improve biocompatibility, bioactive materials such as bioceramics were developed. This material is composed of calcium phosphate, resembling the mineral matrix of human bone, and becomes incorporated with human tissue. Hydroxylapatite (HA) is a type of bioceramics that is used in the middle ear. HA has many of the ideal characteristics required to be a good prosthesis. It is extremely biocompatible, exhibits a very low extrusion rate, has no transmittal of disease, and provides good sound transmission.

Over time, a large proportion of HA implants are completely covered with an epithelial layer, containing all cell types characteristic of the middle ear, indicating good biocompatibility.[19] HA forms a chemical bond with living bone that is osteoconductive with little biodegradation.[20] HA can be placed directly against the tympanic membrane or tympanic membrane graft without the need for any cartilage. If it is placed next to the scutum, however, osseointegration can occur, with subsequent conductive hearing loss.

Grote[21] was the first to report the clinical use of HA in middle ear reconstruction and has reported excellent long-term hearing results. Goldenberg's[22] study of 157 consecutive cases found a very low extrusion rate for hydroxyapatite 2.6% when compared to Plastipore at 6.5%. Even in the face of eustachian tube dysfunction with an atelectatic tympanic membrane, low extrusion rates were noted.

A disadvantage of HA is that it is technically difficult to sculpt intraoperatively, because it is brittle and shatters easily when drilled or trimmed with a sharp instrument.

To deal with this disadvantage, composite materials were devised that combine HA with other materials, such as Silastic or polyethylene. One design, termed Flex H/A, uses a 50/50 mixture of medical-grade Silastic rubber with HA. This composite material is easier to trim and sculpt in the operating room than pure HA. By combining a Flex H/A shaft with an HA head, many disadvantages are overcome. This implant can be easily trimmed and still maintains the advantages of pure HA in terms of biocompatibility. Because of easy trimming, implants made of this material can be easily converted from a total ossicular replacement prosthesis (TORP) to a partial ossicular replacement prosthesis (PORP) by simple cutting.

Another composite material blends HA with polyethylene and is called HAPEX. The HA stiffens the polyethylene, and the polyethylene toughens the composite. This composite mimics bone, itself a composite of HA and collagen. These composite implants blend the benefits of both substances, including easy trimming ability with the biocompatibility of HA. The histopathology of HAPEX implants at revision surgery revealed overgrown fibrous tissue without evidence of macrophages or foreign body giant cells associated with foreign body reaction.[23]

Titanium is another alloplastic material that has become increasingly popular for use in the middle ear implants. The properties of titanium make it possible to manufacture an extremely fine and light prosthesis with substantial rigidity in the shaft. Titanium forms a biostable titanium oxide layer when combined with oxygen, which has shown significant biostability in the middle ear for the past decade.[22] Studies in rabbits have shown that within 28 days after implantation, a thin, noninflamed layer of epithelium forms over the inserted implant.[24] Similar results in human studies have shown the same type of reactivity. Furthermore, differential processing of the material surfaces triggers various tissue reactions. For example, if titanium implants are rough milled, their contact points are increased. Rough-milled surfaces are most appropriate in areas that contact cartilage or the stapes head or footplate. Conversely, the smoother the surface, the less connective tissue reaction occurs, and the epithelial covering is minimized.[25]

IMPLANT DESIGN

Design of the prosthesis requires understanding of the acoustic mechanisms involved in the middle ear, as well as the anatomic and acoustic changes that occur with reconstruction. Reconstructing a defect in the ossicular chain requires adequate conduction of sound energy from the tympanic membrane to the stapes footplate. This must take advantage of the lever mechanisms inherent in the middle ear and transmitting the energy in a piston-like manner from the manubrium of the malleus to the footplate. Many designs have been developed that accomplish this goal (Fig. 19–1).

Adequate function of this design depends on maintaining contact with the stapes superstructure or footplate, as well as over the surface area in contact with the tympanic membrane. Poor outcomes result from movement at the lateral attachment of the prosthesis, movement at the medial

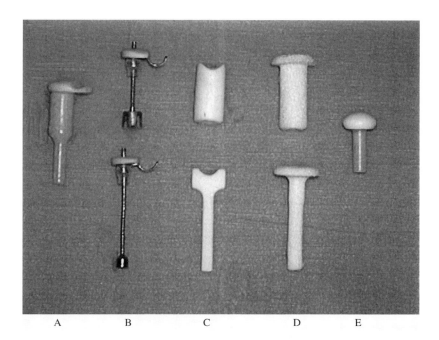

FIGURE 19–1 Prosthesis designs: (A) Bojrab universal; (B) Grace titanium adjustable designed by Bojrab; (C) hydroxyapatite incus strut and incus-stapes strut designed by Kartush; (D) Polycel PORP and TORP designed by Sheehy; (E) Micro-PORP designed by Bojrab.

attachment, extrusion of the prosthesis, or from poor eustachian tube function.[26]

Failure of ossicular chain reconstruction arises from two main causes: extrusion, and movement of the prosthesis (Table 19–3). To overcome this, the design of the prosthesis should decrease these risks (Table 19–4). Many implant designs have been developed with myriad materials, shapes, sizes, and weights to be used in the middle ear. Success seems comparable among many of these. Other factors contribute to the success of ossicular chain reconstruction, such as eustachian tube function and aeration of the middle ear. The principles applied to improving tympanoplasties can contribute to ossiculoplasty success by preventing atelectasis or lateralization. These include proper graft placement, grommet insertion when needed to ventilate middle

ear, using Silastic sheeting to maintain middle ear, and staging the reconstruction when necessary.

BOJRAB UNIVERSAL PROSTHESIS DESIGN

The ideal prosthesis must be biocompatible, able to optimize sound conduction based on material and weight, and easily trimmed. The prosthesis must not extrude or move once placed. Failures with reconstruction occur from movement at either the lateral

TABLE 19–3 REASONS FOR OSSICULAR RECONSTRUCTION FAILURES

Disease	Recurrent or residual middle ear disease
	Eustachian tube dysfunction
Prosthesis failure	Extrusion
	Improper size
	Design flaw
	Movement
	At lateral connection
	At medial connection

TABLE 19–4 ANATOMIC VARIANTS THAT MAY BE ENCOUNTERED IN THE MIDDLE EAR AND SOLUTIONS TO THE PROBLEM: STABILIZATION OF PROSTHESIS

Location	Solution
Lateral	
Malleus	Notch
Tympanic membrane	Slightly rounded head
	Cartilage cap
	Middle ear glue
Medial	
Stapes capitulum	Prosthesis stem hole
Stapes no capitulum	Alter stem size
Footplate normal	Small with tissue ingrowth
Footplate abnormal	Small with tissue stabilization
Narrow	
Center ridge	
Tilted	

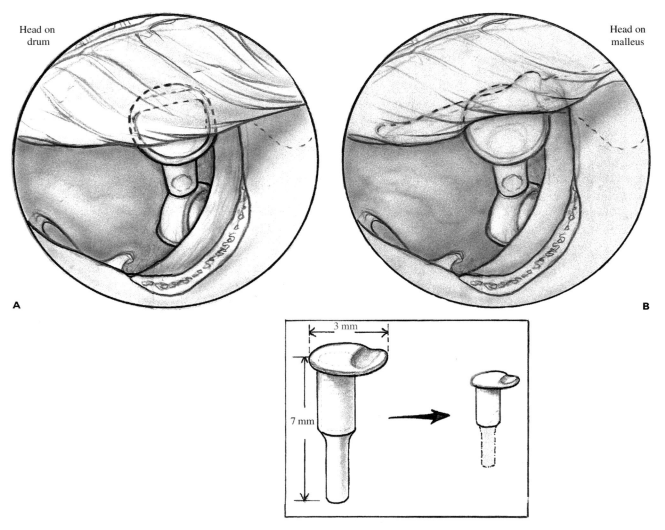

FIGURE 19–2 (A,B) The use of the Bojrab universal prosthesis design.

or medial connection. Dense HA has the advantage of being bioactive, allowing epithelial covering, and being osteoconductive. To allow for variations in size intraoperatively, the original composite Bojrab universal prosthesis has a stem that can be trimmed with a head design that is biocompatible against the tympanic membrane (Fig. 19–2). The design of this prosthesis allows use in multiple situations: as an incus-interposition, as a PORP, and as a TORP, depending on the ossicles present (Table 19–5).

HEAD DESIGN

This prosthesis has an HA head that is slightly rounded with a notch to allow lateral stabilization under the long process of the malleus. If there is no

TABLE 19–5 RECONSTRUCTIVE OPTIONS BASED ON STATUS OF OSSICLES IN MIDDLE EAR

Incus (Superstructure)	Stapes	Malleus (Long Process)	Reconstruction
Absent	Present	Present	Sculpted incus, PORP
Absent	Absent	Present	TORP
Absent	Absent	Absent	TORP + HA or cartilage
Absent	Present	Absent	PORP + HA or cartilage

PORP, partial ossicular replacement prosthesis; TORP, total ossicular replacement prosthesis.

malleus present, then the slightly rounded head design should be able to be placed under the tympanic membrane, allowing the bioactive HA to bond to the undersurface of the tympanic membrane with some stabilization during normal tympanic membrane movement.

STEM DESIGN

The stem of the prosthesis should be able to be altered at the time of surgery to fit the various pathologies that may be encountered. The variables include the lateral distance of the middle ear space and presence of stapes superstructure.

The stem material is made of either porous polyethylene or a composite of HA, such as HAPEX and Flex H/A. These materials are rigid enough for transmission of sound, yet may be trimmed as necessary for a better fit of the prosthesis.

The stem has two distinct areas—a thick area near the HA head, and a center hole that narrows to a solid stem. If the superstructure of the stapes is present with a capitulum, then the thicker stem with the center hole may be cut or machined to fit onto the capitulum (Fig. 19–2). If there is an abnormally large capitulum, then the center hole may be enlarged to the necessary size with a small drill bur or scalpel. If the stapes superstructure is not present, the stem is designed to be used in its entirety with the narrow portion of the stem fitting onto the center of the footplate. If abnormal footplate

pathologies are present, then the stem may be secured into place with fascia, perichondrium, or small cartilage blocks.

Titanium is a lightweight, malleable material that has rigid properties. It has the ability to be altered at the time of surgery to the necessary length and shape by cutting it. Titanium may be bent to accommodate certain anatomic variations, such as an anterior lying malleus. If the stapes superstructure is present, a claw design at the end of the titanium prosthesis may be adjusted to fit over a normal, small, enlarged, or absent capitulum (Fig. 19–3). The titanium claw may be adjusted with an alligator forceps. If the reconstruction is to the footplate, then two of the four prongs of the claw may be removed or a titanium shoe with a hole is used. The hole allows more tissue invasion to occur for security of the prosthesis.

COMPLICATIONS

Immediate, intraoperative complications occur from using a prosthesis that is too long or using too much force in placement. This could result in fracture of the stapes superstructure, dislocation of the stapes or stapes footplate, tear of the annular ligament with a perilymphatic fistula, or severe or total sensorineural hearing loss. To prevent these complications, the prosthesis must be handled and positioned with great care and precision without undue force.

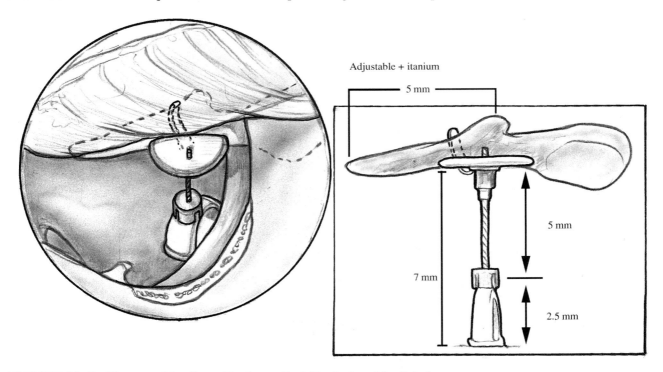

FIGURE 19–3 The use of the Grace titanium adjustable designed by Bojrab.

If a tear in the annular ligament or crack in the footplate occurs, a tissue seal of fat or fascia should be placed around the footplate. The ossicular reconstruction must be aborted at that time, with a second stage done at later date.

Immediate postoperative complications include vertigo that may be related to unrecognized oval window trauma or perilymph fistula. Exploration may be necessary if conservative therapy fails to resolve the symptoms.

Delayed postoperative complications include erosion or extrusion of the prosthesis. The cause may be recurrent middle ear cholesteatoma, poor healing, or graft failure. If this occurs and the hearing remains stable, the surgeon may elevate the tympanomeatal flap and carry the elevation over the prosthesis, leaving a perforation that can be fixed by conventional means. If hearing is poor, the prosthesis should be removed and replaced.

CONCLUSION

Ossicular chain problems are frequently encountered in otologic surgery and are amenable to reconstruction. Because various materials are used for ossiculoplasty, it is important to determine which type of prosthesis is appropriate. This decision is based on the status of the diseased ear and the surgeon's preference. Considerations must be made for the presence or absence of the malleus, the anatomic relationship of malleus to stapes, the severity of eustachian tube dysfunction, and tympanic membrane status. As newer materials are developed for use in the middle ear and implant design continues to be modified, the hearing results for patients will continue to improve as well.

REFERENCES

1. Wullstein H. The restoration of the function of the middle ear in chronic otitis media. *Ann Otol Rhinol Laryngol* 1971;80:210–217.
2. Zollner F. The principles of plastic surgery of the sound conducting apparatus. *J Laryngol Otol* 1955;69:637–652.
3. Gan RZ, Dyer RK, Wood MW, Dormer KJ. Mass loading on the ossicles and middle ear function. *Ann Otol Rhinol Laryngol* 2001;110:478–485.
4. Merchant SN, Ravicz ME, Puria S, et al. Analysis of middle ear mechanics and application to diseased and reconstructed ears. *Am J Otol* 1997;18:139–154.
5. Murakami S, Gyo K, Goode RL. Effect of increased inner ear pressure on middle ear mechanics. *Otolaryngol Head Neck Surg* 1998;118:703–708.
6. Goode RL, Killion M, Nakamura K, et al. New knowledge about the function of the human middle ear: development of an improved analog model. *Am J Otol* 1994;15:145–154.
7. Austin DF. Ossicular reconstruction. *Arch Otolaryngol* 1971;94:525–535.
8. Lesser TH. Mechanics and materials in middle ear reconstruction. *Clin Otolaryngol* 1991;16:29–32.
9. Mills RP, Wang ZG, Abel EW. In vitro study of a multi-layer piezoelectric crystal attic hearing implant. *J Laryngol Otol* 2001;115:359–362.
10. Smyth G. Long term results of middle ear reconstructive surgery. *J Laryngol Otol* 1971;85:1227–1230.
11. Merchant SN, Nadol JB Jr. Histopathology of ossicular implants. *Otolaryngol Clin North Am* 1994;27:813–833.
12. Merchant SN, Ravicz ME, Puria S, et al. Analysis of middle ear mechanics and application to diseased and reconstructed ears. *Am J Otol* 1997;18:139–154.
13. Schuknecht HF, Shi SR. Surgical pathology of middle ear implants. *Laryngoscope* 1985;95:249–258.
14. Portmann M. Results of middle ear reconstruction surgery. *Ann Acad Med Singapore* 1991;20:610–613.
15. Glasscock ME III, Jackson CG, Knox GW. Can acquired immunodeficiency syndrome and Creutzfeldt-Jakob disease be transmitted via otologic homografts? *Arch Otolaryngol Head Neck Surg* 1988;114:1252–1255.
16. Bayazit Y, Goksu N, Beder L. Functional results of Plastipore prostheses for middle ear ossicular chain reconstruction. *Laryngoscope* 1999;109:709–711.
17. Shinohara T, Gyo K, Saiki T, Yanagihara N. Ossiculoplasty using hydroxyapatite prostheses: long-term results. *Clin Otolaryngol* 2000;25:287–292.
18. Sheehy JL. TORPs and PORPs: causes of failure—a report on 446 operations. *Otolaryngol Head Neck Surg* 1984;92:583–587.
19. Bojrab DI, Causse JB, Battista RA, et al. Ossiculoplasty with composite prostheses. Overview and analysis. *Otolaryngol Clin North Am* 1994;27:759–776.
20. Horman K, Donath K. Is hydroxylapatite ceramic an adequate biomaterial in ossicular reconstruction? *Am J Otol* 1987;8:402–409.
21. Grote JJ. Reconstruction of the middle ear with hydroxyapatite implants: long-term results. *Ann Otol Rhinol Laryngol* 1990;99(suppl 144):12–16.
22. Goldenberg RA. Hydroxylapatite ossicular replacement prostheses: results in 157 consecutive cases. *Laryngoscope* 1992;102:1091–1096.
23. Meijer AG, Verheul J, Albers FW, Segenhout HM. Cartilage interposition in ossiculoplasty with hydroxylapatite prostheses: a histopathologic study in the guinea pig. *Ann Otol Rhinol Laryngol* 2002;111:364–369.
24. Dalchow CV, Grun D, Stupp HF. Reconstruction of the ossicular chain with titanium implants. *Otolaryngol Head Neck Surg* 2001;125:628–630.
25. Schwager K. Titanium as a biomaterial for ossicular replacement: results after implantation in the middle ear of the rabbit. *Eur Arch Otorhinolaryngol* 1998;255:396–401.
26. Bojrab DI. Alternatives in biocompatible ossicular implants. *Insights Otolaryngol* 1992;7.

Chapter 20

OSSICULOPLASTY II

Edward Gardner and John Dornhoffer

The goal of modern ossiculoplasty is the restoration of a stable sound transfer mechanism in the middle ear space. Typically this involves restoring the mechanical advantage of the tympanic membrane and the malleus without restoring the lever advantage of the incus. Unfortunately, published techniques and opinions on how to achieve this goal are numerous. With the exclusion of prostheses for stapes surgery, there are over 100 approved prostheses on the market. Additionally, there are multiple points of view regarding the preoperative evaluation of patients, the important anatomic landmarks of an ossiculoplasty, and the mechanisms to maintain the middle ear space postreconstruction. This chapter discusses the historical and current opinion on all of these issues.

The roots of ossiculoplasty began in Germany with Wullstein.[1] Despite the contemporary belief that any effort to reconstruct the hearing mechanism was doomed to failure, Wullstein was encouraged by results with Teflon prostheses in stapes surgery. His first ossiculoplasty attempts in 1951 utilized a vinyl acrylic prosthesis,[2] but, due to frequent extrusions, results with allografts were poor. Attention was then focused on the autograft incus, due to its widespread availability and inherent biocompatibility, and the extrusion rate decreased significantly. Based on results with the autograft incus, Wullstein published his now-famous work on the classification of tympanoplasty and established autograft incus as the standard in ossiculoplasty.[1]

As this technique gained rapid acceptance worldwide, it was soon discovered that a number of patients did not have an adequate incus for reconstruction. Because of this, utilization of homograft ossicles gained a great deal of popularity by the late 1960s. These ossicles could be banked for a period of time and presculpted for various situations. The first account of such a procedure is from Wehrs[3] in 1967. In this review, the homograft incus was used to replace the missing ossicular chain. Results over the next 20 years established the homograft incus as a reliable option for ossicular reconstruction.[4] In the mid-1980s, however, fears regarding the possible transmission of HIV or prions brought homograft use in the United States to a near halt. Newer sterilization techniques have emerged since that time,[5] and there is today a renewed interest in homografts as a source of reconstruction material.

Despite initial failures, interest in allograft sources for ossiculoplasty reappeared in 1956 with the work of Shea and Treace.[6] Like Wullstein's adaptation of stapes materials, Shea's first alloplastic implant was based on attempts by Treace to make a stapes implant from Teflon. This first implant was actually composed of Polyethylene 90 and, like Wullstein's implant, was fraught with complications from extrusion and migration in the middle ear. However, the risk of extrusion using alloplastic implants was reduced to the level obtained with autografts with the invention of Plastipore in 1976 and the addition of cartilage over the prosthesis.[6]

Given that allograft prostheses are easily stored and manipulated, the selection among this group of implants has continued to expand. The list of materials used for allograft prostheses includes hydroxylapatite (HA) (dense and porous), Plastipore, Ceravital (E. Leitz Wetzlar GmBh; Wetzlar, Germany), titanium, gold, or any combination of the above. Short-term hearing results with all of these materials have been universally acceptable, with only minor differences in published findings. In a recent review by Goldenberg and Emmet,[7] alloplastic implants were the most frequently utilized by otologic surgeons performing ossiculoplasty, with the HA prosthesis being the most popular.

Preoperative Evaluation of Patients

The Need for Patient Stratification

Unlike a number of surgical procedures in otolaryngology, there is no accepted form of preoperative staging for patients undergoing ossiculoplasty. Because of this, otologists must rely primarily on anecdotal information for evaluating a patient prior to ossicular reconstruction. Due to a lack of large-scale controlled analyses, variability in techniques, use of multiple prostheses, and variable diseases, it is not currently possible to evaluate a patient in the clinic and give a relatively accurate prognosis for an ossiculoplasty. Complicating the situation is the plethora of published results that lack patient stratification. As an example, a patient who requires a partial ossicular replacement prosthesis (PORP) has, by definition, less bone destruction than a patient receiving a total ossicular replacement prostheses (TORP). If one ignores other stratification factors, such as middle ear mucosal status, the presence or absence of preoperative drainage, or whether this is a primary or revision surgery, one could easily conclude that ossiculoplasty with a PORP offers a better outcome than that with a TORP. However, this represents a biased prediction due to the increased rate of middle ear fibrosis and revision surgery experienced by patients undergoing total prosthesis reconstruction. Therefore, to adequately evaluate and counsel patients preoperatively, we must first identify the aspects of a patient's ear that would have an impact on results and then stratify each patient accordingly for technique comparisons. Only then can we determine what is best for the patient.

Identifying Predictive Factors

The first attempt to stratify patients was performed by Wullstein.[1] His classification provided five groups of patients with essentially increasing disease severity based on the amount of ossicular chain remaining. Similarly emphasizing the role of the ossicular chain in predicting outcome, Austin[8] in 1985 revised Wullstein's classification to focus on the status of the malleus and stapes. Retrospective data to support his stratification of patients is included in this chapter. Another set of predictive factors was identified by Bellucci[9] in 1973. Over his many years of experience, Bellucci recognized preoperative drainage as a result of eustachian tube dysfunction and

therefore identified drainage as a likely predictor of ossiculoplasty failure. The Bellucci system graded the amount of drainage as none (I), occasional (II), continual (III), and drainage with craniofacial anomalies (IV).

The first attempt to tie multiple patient factors together to predict outcomes and group patients for analysis was that of Kartush.[10] His system examined multiple components of the patient history and surgical findings to stratify results. Although he incorporated the work of Austin and Bellucci, Kartush also included whether or not the surgery was a revision, the status of the middle ear mucosa, the presence of cholesteatoma, the presence of perforation, and the type of surgery performed. All of these factors were scored separately and then summed to produce a total patient score. Unfortunately, results supporting the validity of this scoring system have yet to be published.

Since the work of Kartush, a number of similar systems and multifactorial analyses have been proposed. In 1992, Black[11] examined 535 ossiculoplasties and produced what was called the SPITE (surgical, prosthetic, infection, tissue, eustachian) method. Significant factors in this review were the complexity of surgery, status of the malleus and stapes, presence of infection, status of the middle ear mucosa, and presence of eustachian tube dysfunction. In 1998, Albu et al[12] reviewed over 500 tympanoplasties and found a similar group of patient factors to be significant in predicting outcomes.

The Ossiculoplasty Outcome Parameter Staging (OOPS) Index

Uncertain of the statistical validity of previously proposed systems, we examined over 200 ossiculoplasties at our own institution, all of which had been performed by the same surgeon, to determine which factors best predicted outcome. These results were organized into the Ossiculoplasty Outcome Parameter Staging (OOPS) Index, as shown in Table 20–1.[13] Parameters examined included age, diagnosis, perforation, Bellucci classification score, Austin classification, middle ear mucosa status, preoperative audiogram, canal wall status, surgical procedure, revision status, ossicular status, type of prosthesis used (PORP or TORP), and presence or absence of drainage or fibrosis at the time of surgery. A multivariate analysis of variance was then performed to identify the factors to be most significant in predicting postoperative air–bone gaps. Pair-wise comparisons were made to identify the individual factors that were significant. These significant factors

TABLE 20–1 OSSICULOPLASTY OUTCOME PARAMETER STAGING (OOPS) INDEX

Risk Factor		Risk Value
Middle ear factors		
Drainage	None	0
	Present > 50% of time	1
Mucosa	Normal	0
	Fibrotic	2
Ossicles	Normal	0
	Malleus +	1
	Malleus −	2
Surgical factors		
Type of surgery	No mastoidectomy	0
	Canal-wall-up mastoidectomy	1
	Canal-wall-down mastoidectomy	2
Revision surgery	No	0
	Yes	2

Reprinted from Dornhoffer and Gardner,[13] with permission.

were then placed in a multiple linear regression to weigh each factor in its prediction of postoperative air–bone gaps. It is important to note that the multivariate analysis allowed all of the parameters to be examined for any significant correlation among them. As we had some concerns that patients with revision surgery might all have significant fibrosis, establishing these factors as independent variables was critical.

Factors found to be significant were the type of surgical procedure, whether the surgery was a revision, presence or absence of the malleus, presence or absence of drainage, and presence or absence of fibrosis in the middle ear.[13] Without question, the most heavily weighted of these factors was the presence of middle ear fibrosis at the time of surgery, defined as any mucosal disruption or adhesion between two adjacent structures. Based on these results, all attempts are now made at our institution to minimize fibrosis in the middle ear space, including minimal manipulation of the middle ear mucosa regardless of thickness, minimal use of Gelfoam, and the nearly exclusive use of free-standing prostheses. The least significant of the examined factors was the presence of occasional to severe drainage. As removal of the offending pathology and re-creation of an air-containing middle ear

space improves middle ear mucosa, it is to be expected that the effect of drainage on outcome would be minimized when compared to other factors. Our results showed that no two factors identified to be significant in our analysis also had significant multicollinearity.

Many factors considered to be significant by previously published reports were absent in our scoring system. The most notable of these was the status of the stapes in determining outcome. Because the superstructure presents no acoustical advantage, this result seems logical. Another factor noticeably absent from the OOPS index was the diagnosis that led to the surgical intervention. We listed cholesteatoma, chronic otitis, atelectasis, perforation, conductive hearing loss, and any combination of the above as diagnostic parameters. No single diagnosis predicted outcome, unlike the Austin/Kartush system. Another factor absent from the OOPS index was magnitude of the preoperative air–bone gap. Although common sense would dictate that a better hearing ear would have fewer comorbidities, and thus a better surgical outcome, than an ear with poorer hearing, there was no trend in the data to support this. As a number of patients undergoing ossiculoplasty have incus necrosis from previous insults or a slipped prosthesis from a previous surgery, outstanding results in the face of a maximal conductive hearing loss negate the preoperative air–bone gap as a factor.

The fourth parameter absent from our staging system was the presence of abnormally thickened mucosa. A number of studies to date include thickened or granular mucosa as a poor predictor in hearing outcomes.[10,12] However, all our patients with abnormally thickened mucosa had similar outcomes to those without thickened mucosa when all other factors were held constant. We believe that the status of middle ear mucosa is similar to that of nasal mucosa, which shows improvement after sinus surgery. Thus, we believe the middle ear mucosa reverts to normal once the pathology is removed.

Utilization of the OOPS index is simple and (similar to the other scoring systems) easy to apply to the individual patient. Prior to surgery, each of the risk factors in the index is discussed with the patient and scored, and the total score places a patient into an appropriate risk group. This allows us to predict the outcomes of the planned ossiculoplasty with a good deal of confidence. In our cohort of 200 patients, we were able to demonstrate a linear relationship between the postoperative air–bone gap and the OOPS index score, which ranged from 1 to 9.

ANATOMIC LANDMARKS

ANATOMY OF MIDDLE EAR RELATIONSHIPS

Prior to performing any ossiculoplasty, a clear understanding of the anatomic relationships of the middle ear is necessary. Despite well-accepted landmarks and the overall consistency of prosthesis length in stapes surgery, such consistency has not carried over into ossiculoplasty. Given a few simple and dependable landmarks, however, many of the complications and uncertainties regarding ossiculoplasty can be avoided.

The most critical of the middle ear landmarks is the proximal portion of the malleus manubrium (Fig. 20–1). Because the tensor tympani and the anterior malleolar ligament provide two-point fixation at this point, it represents a relatively stable location for reconstruction. A perfect example of the utility of this landmark is the case of the medially rotated manubrium, which results in the umbo resting on the promontory. As the axis of rotation is still about the anterior malleolar ligament, this common scenario can be easily managed by running the prosthesis to the neck of the manubrium, which has likely not been appreciably rotated. At times it is necessary to lift the umbo with a 1-mm hook to facilitate placement of the prosthesis under the manubrium after fixation over the superstructure or footplate (Fig. 20–2). The malleus is consistently 2 mm lateral and 3 to 4 mm anterior to the capitulum of the stapes. This standard distance allows a very predictable position for ossicular reconstruction, regardless of the make or model of the prosthesis.

Another critical portion of the anatomy is the stapes. Given that the capitulum is 1 mm in height and the crura is 2 to 3 mm in height, the height of a properly placed TORP should be 4 to 5 mm. With the

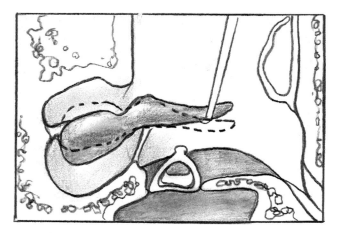

FIGURE 20–2 Lifting the umbo for prosthesis placement. The neck of the malleus is relatively stable.

additional 3 to 4 mm of anterior distance from the capitulum, this makes prosthesis design and positioning much more reliable in the stapes-absent situation (Fig. 20–3).

SPECIFIC SCENARIOS AND OPTIONS FOR RECONSTRUCTION

Although we typically prefer reconstruction to the stapes superstructure, this is not always the optimal procedure. The superstructure can be significantly rotated toward the promontory, as is typically the case with severe middle ear fibrosis. The resultant vector of any reconstruction placed on top of this superstructure will develop a significant degree of torque instead of a pure piston motion. Thus, we prefer to use a TORP to bypass the superstructure altogether when the oval window niche also allows room for the prosthesis. A previous review by Moretz[14] analyzed such reconstructions and found

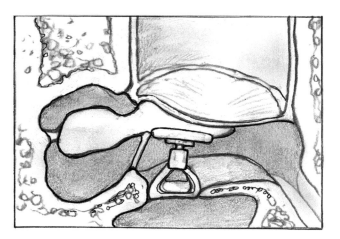

FIGURE 20–1 Properly placed prosthesis at neck of malleus. Note tilt of prosthesis head relative to shaft.

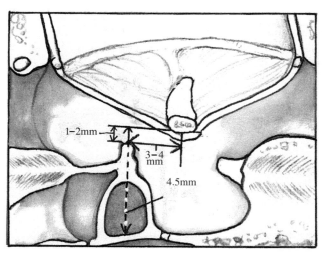

FIGURE 20–3 Critical distances for prosthesis design.

postoperative results to be stable and acceptable. When the oval window niche cannot accommodate the shaft of the prosthesis, one should consider removal of the superstructure altogether. Removal of the superstructure in the face of a mobile footplate is clearly difficult, however, and should not be undertaken lightly. The carbon dioxide laser appears to be the safest option for removing the superstructure as it theoretically displaces the footplate the least amount.

In the absence of a malleus for reconstruction, the most reliable anatomic relationship is the average height of the malleus above the stapes (2 mm) or the height of the malleus above the footplate when the stapes is absent (5 mm). Our own technique in this situation involves creating a neo-malleus for reconstruction, which also assists in establishment of adequate reconstruction length (see Chapter 6).

THE IDEAL PROSTHESIS

After evaluating the patient and understanding the appropriate anatomy, one must determine which prosthesis to use for the reconstruction. The ideal prosthesis should have the appropriate weight, provide an acoustically reliable mechanism for the transfer of sound while allowing the incorporation of existing ossicles, and be stable in the middle ear environment.

WEIGHT OF THE PROSTHESIS

The ideal weight of the prosthesis has been examined by a number of investigators. To date, the most compelling evidenced-based answer has been the result of laser vibrometer and finite element analysis studies at a number of institutions. Huttenbrink[15] and others in Germany have studied this question in depth utilizing a combination of mathematical models and temporal bone simulations. Their findings indicate that the ideal prosthesis should be lightweight and rigid. The lightweight prosthesis minimizes sound impedance, whereas rigidity maximizes the transfer function. Given these parameters, this group of otologists utilizes titanium prostheses, such as the Kurz prosthesis, almost exclusively. The weight of this prosthesis is 3 to 4 mg.

In a similar work, Goode and Nishihara[16] compared incus replacement prostheses of multiple weights and materials by measuring the stapes footplate displacement for each with a laser vibrometer. Their work concluded that the ideal prosthesis weight was 10 to 35 mg. Prostheses below this weight would cause low-frequency displacements to fall out of acceptable ranges, and prostheses above

this weight would lead to high-frequency losses. Interestingly, the human incus normally weighs 30 to 40 mg.

MECHANICS OF THE PROSTHESIS

Ideally, a prosthesis should have its center of gravity perpendicular to its intended movement. In the majority of cases, this would lead to a center of gravity located directly over the capitulum or the oval widow. Such a center of gravity would provide maximal resultant force in the intended direction of the hearing mechanism. This would also minimize any risk of the prosthesis slipping off the capitulum or oval widow. Only a minority of designs, however, have a center of gravity centered over the shaft of the prosthesis. Without this inherent balance, a surgeon relies on the tension generated by the malleus and stapes to stabilize a given prosthesis. All of our preferred prosthesis selections maintain their center of gravity over the intended vector.

Flexibility is another important benefit of an ideal prosthesis. Flexibility allows the head of the prosthesis to be altered relative to the shaft. This alteration allows the prosthesis head to conform to the conical shape of the tympanic membrane. We typically bend the prosthesis 30 degrees toward the promontory to accomplish this (Fig. 20–1).

The benefits gained by using any remaining ossicles in the reconstruction have been hotly debated. There has been ample evidence to support a theoretical acoustic benefit and a stability benefit from using any remaining malleus in the reconstruction. In work by Tonndorf and Khanna,[17] it was proposed that the malleus provided a focus point for any vibration of the tympanic membrane. Khanna theorized that the malleus was similar to a centrally placed tent pole in that any force placed on the tent would be focused to the centrally located pole supporting it. As an additional benefit, the stability provided by an intact malleus has been examined clinically. In work by Fisch[18] and others,[10,12] it has been clearly shown that the presence of the malleus led to reduced extrusion rates and overall improved postoperative air–bone gap closures. Unfortunately, separation of these two benefits has yet to be performed, and the importance of each one has yet to be determined. Our own analysis showed a clear and significant improvement in hearing when the malleus handle was present for reconstruction.[13] For this reason, and those listed above, we always endeavor to utilize the malleus in reconstruction.

The importance of incorporating the capitulum in reconstruction has been less clear. Although theoretically the crural arch provides no acoustical advantage, some reviews have shown improved results when the capitulum was incorporated.[10,12] The most compelling of these was that of Albu et al.[12] In their pair-wise comparison of over 500 tympanoplasties, a statistically significant benefit was identified in patients with an intact arch for reconstruction. However, because a multifactorial analysis was not performed, one cannot exclude confounding issues that might have occurred in an ear that had crural destruction versus one that did not. In our own evaluation using multifactorial analysis, we found that utilization of the stapes superstructure made no difference in postoperative air–bone gap closure.[13] Additional published data have shown no acoustical benefit in utilization of the stapes superstructure.[19] This stands to reason because, to our knowledge, the superstructure provides no acoustic benefit in any model of hearing.

PROSTHESIS MATERIALS

The ideal material for ossicular reconstruction should meet three principal criteria. First, the material must be stable in the middle ear environment. There should be minimal if any rejection phenomena to avoid any granulation tissue formation or subsequent degradation of the reconstruction. Second, the material should present no risk of interaction in the middle ear environment. In reference to this, the reconstruction should minimize the risk of infection or deleterious chemical reaction in the middle ear. Finally, the prosthetic material should allow stable coupling to the remaining ossicles to maximize sound transduction through the reconstructed chain. The options for prosthetic materials comprise autografts, homografts, and allografts.

The autograft incus is clearly well tolerated in the middle ear environment. Long-term results with this type of prosthesis abound in the literature and have proven its stable results over time.[20,21] Because of its nature as an autograft, there is no risk of rejection or transfer of nonhost disease in a reconstruction. The only caveats for using an autograft are the stability of the coupling and the risk of cholesteatoma within the haversian canals.[22] In a recent review by Goldenberg and Emmet,[7] the autograft prosthesis was shown to be in frequent use in the United States.

Homografts have similar benefits to autografts. These materials present no significant risk of rejection in the middle ear, and their use has been validated in numerous studies to date.[4] As with the autograft, homograft stability and effective coupling are dependent on the shape used in reconstruction. In contrast to autografts, however, homografts do bring an additional set of risks. Of particular concern is the risk of transmission of viruses or viral particles (prions). Although there are no reports in the literature of transmission of prions or HIV, the theoretical risk has greatly hampered use of homografts in the United States since the mid-1980s. Newer techniques of sterilization have been reviewed elsewhere[5] and might usher in a resurgence of homograft use in the middle ear.

Options for allografts include multiple plastics, ceramics, metals, and combinations of any of the above, with HA and titanium representing the most commonly used materials for allograft prostheses. Introduced in the 1980s by Grote,[23] HA is a calcium phosphate compound that comes in both dense and porous forms. The dense form is well tolerated by the tympanic membrane in terms of extrusion rates but is hard to shape or cut. The porous form is easier to cut and shape but induces more osteoblast activity and has a higher rate of extrusion when in contact with the tympanic membrane.[2] Because of its induction of osteoblastic activity, porous HA is considered bioreactive. As a totally synthetic material, HA carries no risk of disease transmission to the recipient site. Numerous studies regarding implants of this material have been published to date and have shown generally good results.[19,24] Although dense HA has been proven safe when placed directly against the tympanic membrane,[2] we espouse covering the prosthesis head with cartilage to prevent extrusion in the presence of continued poor eustachian tube function (Fig. 20–4). Placement of this firm and well-tolerated substance between the tympanic membrane and the prosthesis maximizes protection and controls the extrusion rate in even the most inhospitable middle ears.

The second allograft material worth mentioning is titanium. Used for years in Germany as the preferred material for reconstruction, titanium is gaining significant attention in the United States as an

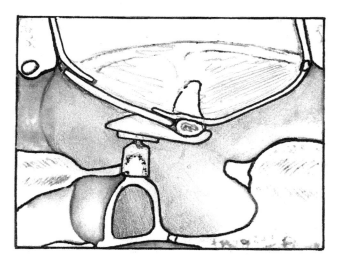

FIGURE 20–4 Correct cartilage placement over hydroxylapatite prosthesis.

implant material. Unlike HA, titanium is classified as a bioinert material. It poses little risk of rejection in the middle ear environment and has been clearly demonstrated to be of no risk for chemical reaction or degradation in the middle ear.[25] Unlike HA, use of titanium prostheses mandates the use of cartilage in any reconstruction. Because the titanium prosthesis is machined or pressed, its edges are much sharper than dense HA and, subsequently, pose a higher risk of extrusion. In addition to this caveat, the other issue with titanium is shaping and trimming the prosthesis. Many of the currently marketed products require separate cutting instruments when these prostheses are utilized.

To date, the senior author (J.D.) has implanted over 100 titanium prostheses and over 500 HA prostheses, and good results have been obtained from both. The authors have found both materials to be well tolerated in the middle ear and to result in very low extrusion rates; however, we espouse the copious use of cartilage and believe this helps account for our success with either type of prosthetic material. Although we prefer HA against the tympanic membrane, we appreciate the outstanding coupling of a titanium bell at the stapes superstructure. For this reason, the Dornhoffer titanium bell PORP (Gyrus ENT Division, Memphis, TN) is our choice for partial reconstructions (Fig. 20–5). For total reconstructions, we utilize the Dornhoffer HAPEX TORP (Gyrus ENT Division) when the malleus is present and the Kurz Tübingen type (TTP) aerial (Kurz Medical, Tübingen, Germany) when the malleus is not present or when the tympanic membrane is significantly lateralized. All of these prostheses have a center of gravity over the intended vector of the stapes and allow good coupling in the planned environment.

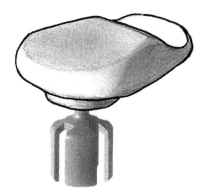

FIGURE 20–5   Dornhoffer titanium bell partial ossicular replacement prosthesis (PORP).

POSTOSSICULOPLASTY MANAGEMENT

MAINTAINING THE MIDDLE EAR SPACE

Once the reconstruction is complete, one must take the necessary steps to maintain a good reconstruction. The first step is the maintenance of an air-containing middle ear space during the immediate healing period. There are many options for maintaining this space. By far the most popular in the United States is the use of Gelfoam or Gelfilm.

Gelfoam is a cellulose-based foam that is thought to be enzymatically degraded in 50 to 60 days by the middle ear. Major benefits are its easy insertion into the middle ear, low cost, ability to be cut into any size, and relative stability over the first 3 to 4 weeks postreconstruction. The main drawback of Gelfoam is risk of fibrosis. Animal research utilizing multiple models has shown a propensity of Gelfoam to act as scaffolding for fibroblasts and adhesions when the mucosa is disrupted in the middle ear.[26–28]

Gelfilm, like Gelfoam, is also a cellulose-based product. Constructed into sheets, this very thin film allows coverage in areas of denuded mucosa to prevent fibrosis and maintain an adequate middle ear space. Unlike Gelfoam, animal studies using Gelfilm fail to show any propensity for fibrosis.[26] Unfortunately, this product conforms very poorly to the middle ear space and is not useful as a mechanism to maintain the entire space postoperatively.

Because of the shortcomings of both Gelfilm and Gelfoam, other products have recently been investigated. Currently, the most promising of these is sodium hyaluronate. Studies in both the orthopedic and ophthalmologic literature reveal this product to be a promoter of healing and, because of its natural occurrence in the body, to be well tolerated. In its esterified form, this chemical has been constructed into sheets and into an easily molded powder very similar to Avitene (CR Bard Inc., Murray Hill, NJ) in consistency. The hyaluronate products currently on the market are Epifilm (Medtronic Xomed Surgical Products Inc., Jacksonville, FL), Epidisc (Medtronic Xomed Surgical Products Inc.), Merogel (Medtronic Xomed Surgical Products Inc.), and SepraPak (Gyrus ENT Division). Epifilm and Merogel have been examined in animal models[29] and have been advertised to have results superior to those of Gelfoam. Particularly appealing is the fact that these products degrade more rapidly than Gelfoam, thus minimizing fibrosis. The principal drawback of hyaluronate is its inability to conform to the middle ear space, and the increased cost compared to Gelfoam or Gelfilm.

Another product that bears mention, which has been utilized for years to maintain the middle ear cleft, is Silastic sheeting. This biologically inert material can be placed into the middle ear to maintain the needed space until an adequate ossiculoplasty can be performed at a later date. The main drawback of Silastic sheeting is the lack of degradation of the product when placed into the ear. Because of this, the Silastic sheeting must be removed from the middle ear space at some point. Given the trend to avoid second-stage surgeries, use of this material has been increasingly limited.

Our current technique for the maintenance of the middle ear space is the sparing use of Gelfoam. Given the exceptional stability of the hybrid prosthesis, we typically use no additional material to support the middle ear space when utilizing this prosthesis. We utilize Gelfilm to cover areas of mucosa that have been totally denuded. As the sodium hyaluronate products continue to improve their middle ear conformability, we expect to eliminate our use of Gelfoam altogether.

Maintaining the Patency of the External Canal

Having stabilized the middle ear space and replaced the tympanic membrane, management of the patency of the external canal is the next issue. Due to the defined bony support, a number of options have proven of benefit, including Gelfoam, Pope Otowicks (Medtronic Xomed Surgical Products Inc.), and antibiotic ointment. As there has been little or no scientific investigation comparing techniques for this portion of an ossiculoplasty, no single recommendation can be made at this time. Our current approach is application of Gelfoam squares onto the tympanic membrane, followed by antibiotic ointment and a Pope Otowick for the most lateral portion of the external auditory canal.

Patient Follow-Up

Patients are typically seen 2 weeks following surgery. At this time, all packing is removed from the canal, the tympanic membrane is inspected, and the patient begins a regimen of steroid-containing antibiotic drops. At 6 to 8 weeks postossiculoplasty, an audiogram is performed. Depending on the mechanism to support the middle ear space, results at 6 to 8 weeks can vary. Given our recent results with the Dornhoffer titanium bell PORP, which requires no Gelfoam for support, we have found the 6- to 8-week audiogram to be representative of long-term results. In reconstructions that require more stabilization, audiograms may not be predictive of long-term results until 2 or 3 months postossiculoplasty.

Conclusion

There are numerous factors that determine a successful ossiculoplasty. The first and most critical is evaluation of the patient. This evaluation should be structured and complete. In our hands, the OOPS Index meets both of these criteria. One should also understand the anatomic relationships of the middle ear. The proximal manubrium of the malleus is a reliable landmark for ossicular reconstruction, regardless of the position of the umbo. The proper prosthesis should also be carefully chosen. The ideal prosthesis is free-standing, biologically inert or compatible, and incorporates the malleus when present. The final factor is maintenance of the middle ear space postoperatively. The ideal middle ear packing should be totally degradable over 10 to 21 days, should easily conform to the middle ear space, and should present no risk for postoperative fibrosis. Although the use of Gelfoam is currently popular in the United States, animal studies reveal a significant risk of fibrosis, which is the most significant factor for ossiculoplasty failure. The future of hyaluronate as a middle ear packing is a promising avenue to minimize this risk. It is important to highlight those questions that remain unanswered with regard to ossiculoplasty. These include the ideal tension of a prosthesis, the ideal weight of a prosthesis, and how to re-create the advantage of the incus in sound transmission. Additionally, further work maximizing prosthesis bio-integration and development of a biologically stable cement or glue needs to be performed. By continually pushing to improve current technology in ossiculoplasty through basic and clinical research, those patients beyond our help today will have hope for tomorrow.

References

1. Wullstein H. Theory and practice of tympanoplasty. *Laryngoscope* 1956;66:1076–1093.
2. Grote J. Biocompatible materials in chronic ear surgery. In: Brackmann D, Shelton C, Arriaga M, eds. *Otologic Surgery.* 2nd ed. Philadelphia: WB Saunders; 2001:141–154.
3. Wehrs R. The borrowed ossicle in tympanoplasty. *Arch Otolaryngol Head Neck Surg* 1967;85:371–379.
4. Wehrs RE. Homograft ossicles in tympanoplasty. *Laryngoscope* 1982;92:540–546.
5. Meylan P, Duscher A, Mudry A, Monnier P. Risk of transmission of human immunodeficiency virus infection during tympano-ossicular homograft: an experimental study. *Laryngoscope* 1996;106:334–337.
6. Treace H. Biomaterials in ossiculoplasty and history of development of prostheses for ossiculoplasty. *Otolaryngol Clin North Am* 1994;27:655–662.

7. Goldenberg RA, Emmet J. Current use of implants in middle ear surgery. *Otol Neurotol* 2001;22:145–152.

8. Austin D. Reporting results in tympanoplasty. *Am J Otol* 1985;6:85–88.

9. Bellucci R. Dual classification of tympanoplasty. *Laryngoscope* 1973;83:1754–1758.

10. Kartush J. Ossicular chain reconstruction: capitulum to malleus. *Otolaryngol Clin North Am* 1994;27:689–715.

11. Black B. Ossiculoplasty prognosis: the SPITE method of assessment. *Am J Otol* 1992;13:544–551.

12. Albu S, Babighian G, Trabalzini F. Prognostic factors in tympanoplasty. *Am J Otol* 1998;19:136–140.

13. Dornhoffer J, Gardner E. Prognostic factors in ossiculoplasty: a statistical staging system. *Otol Neurotol* 2001;22:299–304.

14. Moretz W Jr. Ossiculoplasty with an intact stapes: superstructure versus footplate prosthesis placement. *Laryngoscope* 1998;108(suppl 89):1–12.

15. Huttenbrink K. *Middle Ear Mechanics in Research and Otosurgery.* Dresden, Germany: Department of Oto-Rhino-Laryngology, University Hospital Carl Gustav Carus; 1997.

16. Goode R, Nishihara S. Experimental models of ossiculoplasty. *Otolaryngol Clin North Am* 1994;27:663–675.

17. Tonndorf J, Khanna S. *Mechanics of the Auditory System.* Chicago: Year Book Medical Publishers; 1976.

18. Fisch U. Reconstruction of the ossicular chain. *HNO* 1978;26:53–56.

19. Goldenberg R, Driver M. Long term results with hydroxylapatite middle ear implants. *Otolaryngol Head Neck Surg* 2000;122:635–642.

20. Pennington C. Incus interposition: a 15-year report. *Ann Otol Rhinol Laryngol* 1983;92:568–570.

21. House W, Sheehy J. Functional restoration in tympanoplasty. *Arch Otolaryngol Head Neck Surg* 1963;78:304–309.

22. Dornhoffer J, Colvin G, North P. Evidence of residual disease in ossicles of patients undergoing cholesteatoma removal. *Acta Otolaryngol* 1999;119:89–92.

23. Grote J. Tympanoplasty with calcium phosphate. *Arch Otolaryngol* 1983;110:197–199.

24. Macias J, Glasscock ME III, Widick M, Schall D, Haynes D, Josey A. Ossiculoplasty using the black hydroxylapatite hybrid ossicular replacement prosthesis. *Am J Otol* 1995;16:718–721.

25. Schwager K. Scanning electron microscopy findings in titanium middle ear prostheses. *Laryngol Rhinol Otol* 2000;79:762–766.

26. McGhee M, Dornhoffer J. The effect of Gelfilm in the prevention of fibrosis in the middle ear of the animal model. *Am J Otol* 1999;20:712–716.

27. Liening D, Lundy L, Silberberg B, Finstuen K. A comparison of the biocompatibility of three absorbable hemostatic agents in the rat middle ear. *Otolaryngol Head Neck Surg* 1997;116:454–457.

28. Hellstrom S, Salen B, Stenfors L. Absorbable gelatin sponge (Gelfoam) in otosurgery: one cause of undesirable postoperative results? *Acta Otolaryngol* 1983;96:269–275.

29. Li G, Feghali J, Dinces E, McElveen J, Van De Water T. Evaluation of esterified hyaluronic acid as middle ear-packing material. *Arch Otolaryngol Head Neck Surg* 2001;127:534–539.

Chapter 21

Endoscopic Middle Ear and Mastoid Surgery

Dennis S. Poe

Endoscopy has created new opportunities for minimally invasive techniques in middle ear and temporal bone surgery. Otologic surgery was revolutionized with the advent of the surgical microscope, but microscopes are limited to a direct line of sight visualization. Endoscopes bring the surgeon's eyes into the depths of the operating field, being designed with wide-angle lenses that produce panoramic views extending into recesses hidden from the microscope. Endoscopes offer the potential for reducing open surgical exposure, reducing operating time, improving cholesteatoma eradication, and minimizing surgically induced artifacts during middle ear exploration for perilymphatic fistulas.

EQUIPMENT

Rigid Hopkins rod and fiberoptic endoscopes can be used in otologic surgery, but generally rigid rod lenses are preferred because of their superior resolution. Fiberoptic endoscopes employ thousands of individual light fibers, with each one creating a single pixel of the resultant image. The cladding and cement between fibers creates a "chicken-wire fence" appearance when images are sharply focused.[1]

Endoscopic images have an inherent spherical distortion or "fish-eye view," and lack the three-dimensionality offered by the binocular operating microscope. Endoscopic magnification increases steeply as objects are brought into proximity with the lens and can approach the powers achieved with the operating microscope. Endoscopic surgeons learn to compensate for the variable magnification and two-dimensional images by watching how a structure and its surroundings are altered as the endoscope is moved in and out of proximity to it. The three-dimensionality of an image is re-created by its changes with endoscope motion.

Transtympanic endoscopy utilizes instruments of 1.9 mm in diameter or less. Operating room exposures permit the use of 2.7- to 4.0-mm diameters that yield larger images with improved lighting clarity. Endoscopes have 0-, 30-, 45-, and 70-degree view angles. Illumination is by a halogen or xenon fiberoptic light source generally providing between 150 and 300 W. Images may be viewed directly through an endoscope lens, or more commonly, a charge-coupled device (CCD) camera is attached to the endoscope lens to deliver the images onto a monitor.

ENDOSCOPY OF THE EXTERNAL AUDITORY CANAL AND TYMPANIC MEMBRANE

Endoscopes are useful in the office for inspecting areas of the ear that are inaccessible to the operating microscope and for photodocumentation. The panoramic views achieved with a 2.7- or 4-mm endoscope are excellent for otologic photography. Endoscopes are useful to inspect the tympanic membrane or medial external auditory canal when the microscopic view is limited by canal stenosis or other obstructions. Defects or recesses in the external canal and the depths of mastoid cavities may be easily visualized. Tympanic membrane retraction pockets may be inspected to determine their depths and the presence or absence of cholesteatoma debris.

OTOLOGIC MIDDLE EAR ENDOSCOPIC SURGERY

TRANSTYMPANIC ENDOSCOPY

Endoscopes may be passed through an existing perforation or myringotomy in the tympanic membrane to perform a limited middle ear exploration. The procedure may be done in the office or operating room. In the office, the patient is placed in the supine position in an exam chair. The ear is inspected through a speculum using an operating microscope. The tympanic membrane is anesthetized with topical phenol solution (United States Pharmacopeia) applied by dipping a 20-gauge (3-french) suction tip into the solution and dragging the bead of solution that adheres to the suction across the tympanic membrane over the incision site. An immediate blanching of the tympanic membrane is noted. Phenol is the preferred anesthetic because of its rapid onset of action and local cautery that produces a dry and bloodless field. A radially oriented myringotomy is made from the annulus to the malleus, overlying the site of anticipated pathology. An opening is created sufficiently large to atraumatically admit the endoscope and minimize the chance for inadvertent tearing of the tympanic membrane.

A drop of defogging solution is applied to the tip of the endoscope and the excess blotted away by touching a cotton sponge to the side of the lens. It is important to avoid direct contact with the lens as it often smears the solution and blurs the image.

A 0-degree endoscope is often used for the initial inspection of the middle ear because it yields a wide overall view of the middle ear. Close-up inspections in the area of suspected pathology are done with a 30-degree endoscope. It takes some practice to atraumatically maneuver an angled endoscope through a myringotomy because of its off-centered view.

Endoscopic images may be viewed directly through the lens or with use of a CCD camera delivering the image to a video monitor. Surgeons with little endoscopic experience find it easier to look directly into the endoscope eyepiece. Although the image appears very small to the eye, it yields an adequate examination and it is simpler to maintain control of the endoscope within the ear. The use of a CCD camera increases the difficulty of use by introducing potential disorientation from rotation of the camera on the eyepiece, operating while looking at a remote video monitor away from the surgical field, and maneuvering the increased weight of the endoscope system. Experienced en-

doscopists, however, usually prefer video monitor images that appear considerably larger to the eye and offer a better appreciation of detail in the surgical field.

A small ear speculum is placed deep into the external canal to help protect against inadvertent pain or bleeding from contact of the canal skin with the endoscope shaft. The speculum and endoscope shaft are held in the surgeon's nondominant hand, and the endoscope tip is guided atraumatically through the myringotomy using fine fingertip movements. The camera and eyepiece are held in the dominant hand, supporting the weight and assisting in guiding the endoscope. The endoscope may be rotated to a small degree in situ, but it is generally safer to make large rotations of the view angle into the appropriate direction prior to insertion into the middle ear to minimize the potential for tympanic membrane trauma. Once the endoscope lens has fully passed through the tympanic membrane, a wide view of the middle ear can be realized (Fig. 21–1). Close-up and angled views, especially around overhangs, are best done with a 30-degree endoscope (Figs. 21–2 and 21–3). It is important to repeatedly ensure that the camera is properly oriented to avoid inappropriate movements in the middle ear due to disorientation.

Patients may experience caloric-effect vertigo from the heat of a 300-W light source if it is in situ for more than 45 seconds. Withdrawal of the endoscope relieves the vertigo, so the examination may continue by removing the endoscope periodically or by reducing the intensity of the light source. Vertigo has not occurred using a 150-W light source. There have not been any reported cases of thermal injury,

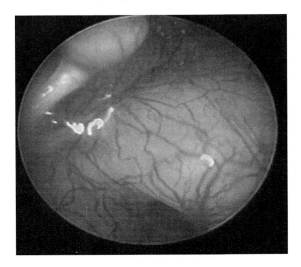

FIGURE 21–1 Transtympanic endoscopic view of middle ear with 1.9-mm, 0-degree angled Hopkins rod endoscope.

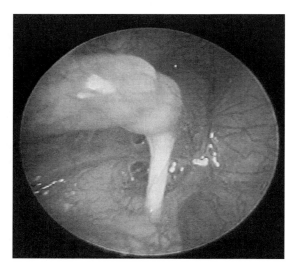

FIGURE 21–2 Transtympanic endoscopic view of superior mesotympanum with 1.9-mm, 30-degree angled Hopkins rod endoscope.

but elevations of temperatures to 50°C have been produced in dry temporal bones exposed for 2 minutes.[2]

At the conclusion of the exam, the myringotomy is inspected under the microscope to determine that the margins show no significant trauma and are nearly in approximation. Wide gaps or inadvertent tears may be repaired with adhesive Steri-Strips, Gelfilm, or cigarette paper. Tympanic membrane injuries are generally avoided by making the initial myringotomy sufficiently long to pass the endoscope easily. Water precautions and avoidance of nose-blowing are recommended for 2 weeks after the procedure.[1]

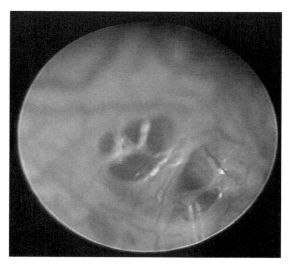

FIGURE 21–3 Transtympanic endoscopic view of round window niche with 1.9-mm, 30-degree angled Hopkins rod endoscope.

The author has performed 114 transtympanic endoscopic procedures in the office to date without any complications. There have been no cases of persistent hearing loss, vertigo, infection, or persistent perforation.

PERILYMPHATIC FISTULA EXPLORATION

Surgical exploration has previously been the "gold standard" for establishing the diagnosis of perilymphatic fistula. However, the criterion for determining the presence or absence of a fistula, the accumulation of fluid in either the round or oval window niches, has been demonstrated to be inaccurate because of the inability to distinguish between artifacts such as tissue transudates or injected anesthetics versus perilymph accumulating in the dependent window niches.[3] These artifacts can be reduced by a minimally invasive endoscopic exploration through a phenol cauterized myringotomy. The middle ear is visualized in as undisturbed a state as possible. A diagnostic endoscopic perilymphatic fistula exploration can be performed in the office. It may also be done in the operating room, especially if an open repair is anticipated after the diagnostic exam. A myringotomy is made radially halfway between the shadow of the round window niche and the distal end of the incus's long process, which are usually visible through the tympanic membrane.

It has been demonstrated that endoscopic and microscopic explorations have comparable resolution for the detection of a leaking fistula.[4] Endoscopic and microscopic observations of fistulas were compared in temporal bone specimens and in surgical cases. Seventeen patients suspected of perilymphatic fistula on the basis of clinical history or findings underwent both transtympanic endoscopy and microsurgical exploration under the same general anesthesia sitting. The endoscopic examinations were performed first and middle ear findings were noted. Subsequently, 1 mL of lidocaine 1% solution with 1:100,000 epinephrine was injected into the external auditory canal and a standard tympanomeatal flap was elevated. Eight of the 17 patients had no endoscopically visualized fistulas but were found to have repeated pooling of clear fluid in either the round or oval window on microsurgical exploration. The pooling would meet standard criteria for a fistula, but the previous endoscopic images had superior magnification, resolution, and visualization of the oval and round windows when compared to the microscopic views. It was concluded that the pooling of fluid seen on the microscopic views must be artifactual.[5]

Four cases of probable true perilymphatic fistulas were identified using both endoscopic and micro-

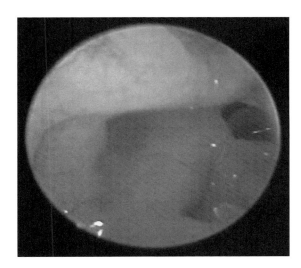

FIGURE 21–4 Transtympanic endoscopic view of round window perilymphatic fistula with 1.9-mm, 30-degree angled Hopkins rod endoscope.

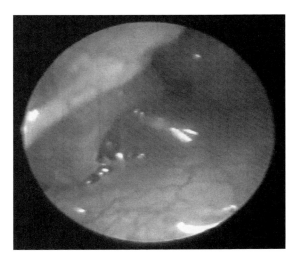

FIGURE 21–5 Transtympanic endoscopic view of persistent stapedial artery with 1.9-mm, 30-degree angled Hopkins rod endoscope.

surgical exams, and the fistulas were more readily identifiable with the endoscope (Fig. 21–4). Each case had involved significant trauma including barotrauma in three cases and perforating trauma in one case. Inadequate endoscopic examinations occurred in five cases, all of which had undergone previous surgery and had excessive bleeding after the lysis of middle ear adhesions.

The author has performed 75 transtympanic middle ear explorations for the identification of perilymphatic fistula and only five cases of true fistula have been identified. The low incidence of endoscopic fistula identification is in agreement with the findings of other authors, including Rosenberg et al,[6] who had 13 negative explorations, and Pyykkö et al,[7] who found only two fistulas out of 350 cases.

It may be concluded that the diagnostic specificity for identification of perilymphatic fistulas, that is, reducing the number of false positives, may be improved by middle ear endoscopy. The artifacts of surgically induced transudates and pooling of infiltrated anesthetic agents cannot be eliminated from open surgical explorations (Fig. 21–5).

Perilymphatic fistulas most likely occur in adults as the result of significant injuries such as barotrauma, head injury, penetrating trauma, and otologic surgery. Surgical exploration is indicated in patients with sensorineural hearing loss, persistent vertigo, or persistent disequilibrium due to the trauma. Every confirmed fistula case in the author's series had a positive subjective or objective fistula test. The diagnosis of perilymphatic fistula should be made only after the exclusion of other possible etiologies. Additional studies such as imaging stu-

dies and laboratory tests should be obtained on an individual basis.

ENDOSCOPY IN CHRONIC EAR SURGERY

Endoscopes may be employed in chronic ear surgery as an adjunct for the removal of cholesteatoma.[8–12] Residual disease most commonly occurs in the areas most difficult to expose under the operating microscope including the epitympanum, sinus tympani, and facial recess. Endoscopes are helpful to inspect these recesses and may be used to confirm the eradication of disease after microsurgical excision or to assist in the primary dissection of cholesteatoma. Tympanic membrane retraction pockets and shallow cholesteatomas that are limited to the attic, aditus ad antrum, facial recess, or sinus tympani are amenable to removal with endoscopic assistance, eliminating the need for mastoidectomy in many cases. The improved ability to remove cholesteatoma has reduced the incidence of residual disease and the number of planned second-stage operations. When a second-look procedure is necessary, it can often be performed through a transcanal approach with endoscopic assistance. Visualization into temporal bone recesses is far superior using endoscopes as opposed to surgical mirrors (Fig. 21–6).

Endoscopic techniques are not intended to replace microsurgical resection. There are several disadvantages with the use of endoscopes. There are no currently available satisfactory endoscope holders, so it is necessary to hold the endoscopes in the surgeon's nondominant hand, leaving only one hand free for surgical dissection. Bleeding usually neces-

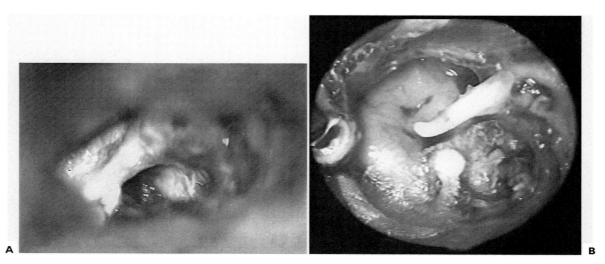

FIGURE 21–6 (A) Microscopic view of left ear with cholesteatoma in posterosuperior pars tensa retraction pocket. (B) Four-millimeter 0-degree Hopkins rod endoscopic view of the same ear.

sitates alternating between the use of a dissecting instrument and suction aspiration of blood, which markedly reduces the operating efficiency compared to two-handed techniques. It is recommended that dissection be performed with both hands using the operating microscope for dissection until reaching the limits of visualization and then switching to endoscopic techniques beyond the overhangs or into recesses. Endoscopes are usually reserved only for the limited times when dissection occurs in these difficult areas and are most typically used after most of the microscopic removal has been accomplished or for critical points when mobilization of disease out of a recess is needed. In many cases, micro-surgical resection of cholesteatoma matrix may become hindered by adhesions extending into deep recesses, especially the sinus tympani. "Blind" elevation may tear the matrix and leave residual disease but endoscopes may permit direct visualization of the adhesions, allowing for lysis, mobilization of the intact matrix, and resumption of microsurgical dissection. Alternating between the microscope and endoscope is often helpful for optimal eradication of cholesteatoma.

Cases of limited cholesteatoma or tympanic membrane atelectasis with deep retraction pockets are conventionally approached using an atticotomy or mastoidectomy for exposure. The removal of cholesteatoma matrix is frequently done in a piece-meal fashion, particularly when the disease is far anterior within the epitympanum, deep into the sinus tympani, or on the medial surface of the scutum. Second-stage operations are often recommended after microsurgical removal of cholesteatoma, as complete removal of disease is uncertain. Limited cholesteatoma cases are well suited for

endoscopic resection and can often be performed through a transcanal or postauricular-transmeatal approach without requiring atticotomy or mastoid-ectomy. Direct endoscopic visualization, allowing for complete removal of the intact matrix can obviate the need for second-look surgery.

TECHNIQUE

Surgery is usually performed using a CCD camera and video monitor, but if the endoscopy is expected to be a brief inspection, then viewing through the eyepiece is satisfactory and requires less setup time. Endoscopes with 30- and 70-degree view angles are most commonly used to inspect recesses. It is preferable to use the largest diameter suitable for introduction into the surgical field while allowing sufficient room to pass surgical instruments. Larger-diameter endoscopes yield superior image size and illumination. Endoscopes with 30-degree angulation and 2.7-mm outer diameter are useful for most shallow recesses. For visualizing deep into the facial recess, sinus tympani, or aditus, and looking far into the epitympanum and mastoid antrum, a 70-degree, 2.3-mm-diameter endoscope is used. The 70-degree endoscope lacks any forward view, so it is necessary to insert the endoscope nearly into the final position by looking along its shaft with the naked eye and noting its relationship to the ossicles or other important structures. The endoscope is tilted to bring the ossicles into view and, after noting their location, it is tilted to bring the area of pathology into view. The surgeon should periodically recheck the location of the ossicles, which may be out of the field of view, to avoid disorientation and inadvertent injury.

Large cholesteatomas and retraction pockets that extend deep into the epitympanum or mastoid antrum are beyond the reach of endoscopic resection and should be managed by conventional microsurgical techniques. Endoscopes may be appropriate to inspect for residual disease in the facial recess, sinus tympani, epitympanum, supratubal recess, and other recesses as needed. In the event that residual matrix is identified, excision may be accomplished using either endoscopic or microscopic dissection.

Small cholesteatomas and shallow retraction pockets may be removed in toto with endoscopic assistance. The atelectatic tympanic membrane or cholesteatoma matrix is initially elevated using conventional microsurgical techniques. The squamous epithelium is usually loosely adherent to the neck of the malleus and scutum, allowing for a good starting point for surgical dissection. Elevation of matrix continues until reaching firm adhesions typically encountered deeper in the aditus, facial recess, or sinus tympani. When it is determined that the matrix cannot be further mobilized without significant risk of tearing, the endoscope may be inserted to visualize the adhesions and facilitate their lysis with long angled dissectors.

Because endoscopic dissection is usually done one-handed, it is often helpful to obtain good hemostasis, placing Gelfoam soaked in 1:10,000 epinephrine solution into the middle ear for several minutes prior to the endoscopy. Hemostasis can be improved with frequent irrigation of the field, even with the endoscope remaining in situ. Persistent bleeding necessitates either alternating between suction and dissection or returning to the microscope to evacuate clots and improve hemostasis.

Two-handed dissection under the microscope is always more efficient and should be used whenever possible but discontinued again upon encountering difficult adhesions that disappear from the field of view. Careful elevation of retraction pockets usually results in the intact removal of even very thin squamous epithelium in the majority of cases, and when successfully accomplished a second-stage procedure is unnecessary (Fig. 21–7). Prototypical combined suction-dissectors can improve the efficiency of endoscopic dissection but are not yet commercially available.

After the removal of large epitympanic or antral cholesteatomas, it is often useful to smooth out the adjacent bony surfaces with a diamond drill to reduce the chance of residual disease. Exposure of the medial surface of the scutum, the epitympanic tegmen, and the supratubal recess can be improved with endoscopic assistance (Fig. 21–8).

Canal-wall-down (CWD) mastoidectomy has a significant advantage over intact-canal-wall exposure because of superior visualization into the sinus tympani, elimination of the facial recess, and exteriorization of the epitympanum, which results in significantly lower risk of residual disease. Thomassin et al[13] demonstrated that endoscopic-assisted canal-wall-up (CWU) surgery yielded a residual disease rate comparable with CWD surgery. Of 80 patients studied, 44 underwent intact-canal-wall mastoidectomy; 21 of these 44 patients (47.7%) were discovered to have residual disease at a planned second stage. The other 36 patients had endoscopic inspection for cholesteatoma during the

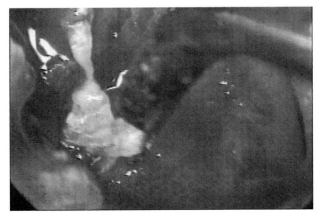

FIGURE 21–7 Endoscopic dissection of cholesteatoma using suction dissector.

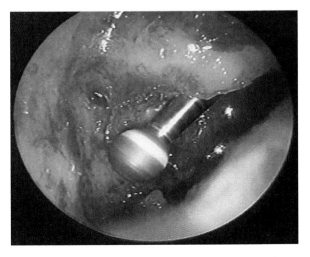

FIGURE 21–8 Endoscopic view of right mastoid cavity after intact canal mastoidectomy. Diamond drill is passed down bony canal to smooth tegmen bone and ensure cholesteatoma removal.

primary CWU operation and the rate of residual disease dropped to 5.5% as observed at the second-stage procedure. This rate is similar to published series of CWD operations and reflects the improved excision of disease made possible by endoscopic exposure.

SECOND-LOOK MASTOIDECTOMY

Endoscopic assistance in CWU mastoidectomy has significantly reduced the number of second-look procedures. When a second look is necessary, it can most often be done as a transcanal procedure because residual cholesteatoma most commonly occurs in the epitympanum, facial recess, or sinus tympani rather than in the mastoid cavity.[14]

McKennan[15] described performing an endoscopic approach to the mastoid through a small postauricular stab incision and doing a separate middle ear exploration when indicated. McKennan uses a transcanal approach with angled endoscopes to visualize the epitympanum and mastoid antrum. Initially, microsurgical elevation of a tympanomeatal flap is done followed by lysis of middle ear adhesions and hemostasis. A 70-degree, 2.3-mm-diameter endoscope is introduced into the middle ear and rotated 360 degrees to carefully inspect the epitympanum, supratubal recess, hypotympanum, sinus tympani, and facial recess. Lysis of some adhesions using long angled picks is usually needed to view beyond the scutum into the attic, aditus, and mastoid antrum. Satisfactory views well into the mastoid and superiorly up to the tegmen are usually obtained, and the postauricular incision is avoided in most cases (Figs. 21–9 and 21–10).

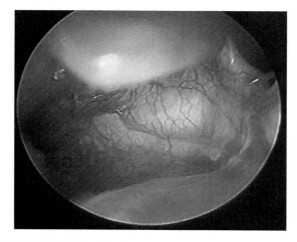

FIGURE 21–9 A 2.3-mm, 70-degree Hopkins rod endoscopic view of second-look case after primary cholesteatoma removal from cochleariform process and area medial to malleus head.

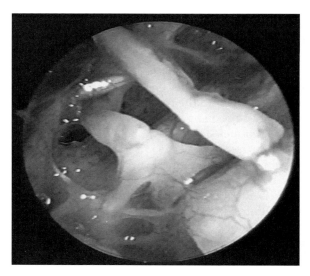

FIGURE 21–10 A 2.3-mm, 70-degree Hopkins rod endoscopic view of superior mesotympanum and epitympanum at primary surgery after removal of anterior epitympanic cholesteatoma.

When residual cholesteatoma is identified, it is possible to remove small lesions by endoscopic dissection.[15] Bulky residual disease usually requires microsurgical removal. Patients are counseled preoperatively about the possibility of reopening the postauricular incision if it is necessary for removal of cholesteatoma.

ENDOSCOPIC TYMPANOPLASTY

The repair of anterior marginal tympanic membrane perforations is commonly approached through a postauricular exposure, especially in the presence of a prominent anterior bony overhang that may obscure the anterior border. Anterior perforations can be managed through a transcanal approach with endoscopic assistance to visualize the anterior margin.[16] Marginal perforations are conveniently repaired with a laser "spot welding" technique[17] or with a cartilage "butterfly graft."[18] The laser technique uses an argon ion or other fiber-delivered laser to reach around the bony overhang and fuse the underlay graft to the perforation margins by coagulation. The cartilage graft technique uses a cartilage-perichondrial composite graft trimmed slightly wider than the perforation margin and filleted on its edge circumferentially. The graft is then inserted into the defect like a button and the margins settle into the graft's circumferential groove.

LASER STAPEDOTOMY

Laser stapedotomy minus prosthesis (STAMP) surgery can be accomplished without the insertion of a prosthesis.[19] An otosclerotic focus limited to the anterior third of the footplate may be managed by laser vaporization of the anterior crus and division of the stapes footplate between the anterior one third and posterior two thirds, making a transverse linear laser cut. These cuts release the posterior footplate and posterior crus, obviating the need for prosthesis. The procedure differs from previously described mobilization techniques that created a fracture through the otosclerotic focus and failed due to subsequent refixation. Division of the stapes footplate posterior to the otosclerotic focus can provide lasting air–bone gap closure.[19–21] The anterior crus and anterior footplate are rarely fully visualized using the operating microscope so the procedure may be facilitated with endoscopic assistance.

EUSTACHIAN TUBE ENDOSCOPIC SURGERY

Endoscopy of the eustachian tube has been performed through the middle ear and nasopharyngeal orifices and has given us new insights into tubal physiology and pathophysiology.[22,23] The cartilaginous tube is best studied by positioning an endoscope at the nasopharyngeal orifice and directing the view angle superiorly and laterally toward the lumen. Tubal movements are observed during swallows, yawns, and other maneuvers, captured on video, and studied in slow motion. Most tubal pathology involves mucosal edema that causes functional obstruction, but a number of patients have muscular or dynamic dysfunction. Endoluminal laser surgery is now being performed for the treatment of refractory tubal dysfunction when ventilating tubes have been inadequate.[21,22]

FUTURE PROGRESS

Minimally invasive endoscopic techniques are rapidly developing, but the gains in optics have outpaced progress in appropriate operative tools. Extralong angulated dissectors, angulated suctions, combined laser endoscopic probes, and specialized forceps are being designed and tested. Suction-dissectors improve on the one-handed techniques that are currently required when hand-holding an endoscope.

A practical endoscope holder may become available in the future but will always need to be used with caution to prevent injury to the middle ear or ossicles in the event of unexpected movement of the patient. Fixation of the endoscope holder to the patient's head minimizes the potential for movement-related injuries.

CCD cameras are becoming increasingly small and may ultimately be placed directly into the middle ear, eliminating the need for optical endoscopes. A tiny camera mounted on a thin cable would provide more flexibility and working space to better accommodate surgical dissection instruments.

Eustachian tube surgery is still in its infancy, but with experience there may be a significant role for laser treatment of refractory otitis media and tubal dysfunction in air travel and scuba diving. Surgery of the temporal bone and middle ear is expected to increasingly rely on minimally invasive techniques. It is anticipated that there will be improvements in patient outcomes, reductions in morbidity, and enhancements in our ability to maintain or restore function in the middle ear.

REFERENCES

1. Poe DS, Rebeiz EE, Pankratov MM, Shapshay SM. Transtympanic endoscopy of the middle ear. *Laryngoscope* 1992;102:993–996.
2. Bottrill ID, Perrault DF Jr, Poe DS. In vitro and in vivo determination of the thermal effect of middle ear endoscopy. *Laryngoscope* 1996;106:213–216.
3. Friedland DR, Wackym PA. A critical appraisal of spontaneous perilymphatic fistulas of the inner ear. *Am J Otol* 1999;20:261–279.
4. Poe DS, Rebeiz EE, Pankratov MM. Evaluation of perilymphatic fistulas by middle ear endoscopy. *Am J Otol* 1992;13:529–533.
5. Poe DS, Bottrill ID. Comparison of endoscopic and surgical exploration for perilymphatic fistulas. *Am J Otol* 1994;15:735–738.
6. Rosenberg SI, Silverstein H, Wilcox TO, Gordon MA. Endoscopy in otology and neurotology. *Am J Otol* 1994;15:168–172.
7. Pyykkö I, Selmani Z, Ramsay H. Middle ear imaging in neurotological work-up. *Acta Otolaryngol Suppl* 1995;520:273–276.
8. Rosenberg SI. Endoscopic otologic surgery. *Otolaryngol Clin North Am* 1996;29:291–300.
9. Bottrill ID, Poe DS. Endoscope-assisted ear surgery. *Am J Otol* 1995;16:158–163.
10. Yung MM. The use of rigid endoscopes in cholesteatoma surgery. *J Laryngol Otol* 1994;108:307–309.
11. Bowdler DA, Walsh RM. Comparison of the otoendoscopic and microscopic anatomy of the middle ear cleft in canal wall-up and canal wall-down temporal bone dissections. *Clin Otolarynol* 1995;20:418–422.

12. Karhuketo TS, Laippala PJ, Puhakka HJ, Sipila MM. Endoscopy and otomicroscopy in the estimation of middle ear structures. *Acta Otolaryngol* 1997; 117:585–589.

13. Thomassin JM, Korchia D, Doris JM. Endoscopic-guided otosurgery in the prevention of residual cholesteatomas. *Laryngoscope* 1993;103:939–943.

14. Youssef TF, Poe DS. Endoscopic-assisted second-stage tympanomastoidectomy. *Laryngoscope* 1997; 107:1341–1344.

15. McKennan KX. Endoscopic "second look" mastoidoscopy to rule out residual epitympanic/mastoid cholesteatoma. *Laryngoscope* 1993;103:810–814.

16. el-Guindy A. Endoscopic transcanal myringoplasty. *J Laryngol Otol* 1992;106:493–495.

17. Pyykkö I, Poe DS, Ishizaki H. Laser-assisted myringoplasty: technical aspects. *Acta Otolaryngol Suppl* 2000;543:1–4.

18. Eavey RD. Inlay tympanoplasty: cartilage butterfly technique. *Laryngoscope* 1998;108:657–661.

19. Silverstein H. Laser stapedotomy minus prosthesis (laser STAMP): a minimally invasive procedure. *Am J Otol* 1998;19:277–282.

20. Poe DS. Laser-assisted endoscopic stapedectomy: a prospective study. *Laryngoscope* 2000;110(suppl 95):1–37.

21. Silverstein H. Laser stapedotomy minus prosthesis (Laser STAMP): absence of refixation. Presented at the American Otological Society, Palm Desert, CA, May 13, 2001.

22. Fabinyi B, Klug C. A minimally invasive technique for endoscopic middle ear surgery. *Eur Arch Otorhinolaryngol Suppl* 1997;1:S53–S54.

23. Poe DS, Pyykkö I, Valtonen H, Silvolva J. Analysis of eustachian tube function by video endoscopy. *Am J Otol* 2000;21:602–607.

Chapter 22

CANALOPLASTY FOR ATRESIA

Larry K. Burton, Jr. and Colin L.W. Driscoll

Congenital aural atresia is thought to occur in 1 in 10,000 to 20,000 live births, with unilateral atresia being three times more common than bilateral atresia.[1-3] It occurs more often in males, and more often on the right side.[1] Although external ear and middle ear malformations often occur in combination, due to their similar embryologic origin from the first and second branchial structures, inner ear malformations are a less common association, owing to its derivation from the auditory placode and otic capsule. Surgery for canal atresia is one of the most complex surgeries performed by otologists, drawing on the techniques of canaloplasty, meatoplasty, tympanoplasty, and ossiculoplasty. A thorough understanding is required of the normal as well as variant surgical anatomy of the facial nerve, oval window, inner ear, temporomandibular joint, mastoid cavity, and tegmen tympani. This chapter discusses the history, embryology, classification, patient selection, surgical technique, postoperative care, risks, complications, and outcomes of surgery for canal atresia.

HISTORY

Kiesselbach[4] is credited with the first attempt at correction of congenital atresia in 1883. Unfortunately, that surgery resulted in facial nerve paralysis.[5] Although Dean and Gittens[6] described the first successful case with satisfactory hearing results in 1917, the high complication rates and the lack of middle ear microsurgical techniques limited surgery for atresia throughout the early twentieth century until 1947. In that year, both Ombredanne[7] in France and Pattee[8] in the United States separately reported a series of successful outcomes. Since that time, the development of tympanoplasty techniques and the

introduction of the operating microscope have made surgery for atresia both safer and more successful. Large case series have been reported by Gill,[2] Ombredanne,[9] Shih and Crabtree,[10] Jarhsdoerfer,[5,11] Marquet,[12] and De la Cruz.[13,14]

EMBRYOLOGY

The development of the inner ear, derived from the otic capsule, is greatly independent of the development of the middle ear and outer ear, which take their form from the first and second branchial structures.[15] The external ear develops around the primitive meatus by the fusing of the six primitive hillocks, derived from the first and second branchial arches (Table 22–1), the auricle assuming its primitive form by the end of the third month of development. The external auditory meatus develops from the first branchial groove as an ingrowth of epithelium from the primitive pinna that migrates inward toward the expanding first branchial pouch. During the sixth and seventh month of gestation, this solid core of tissue begins to hollow, creating the external meatus.

The middle ear cleft is created by an expansion of the first branchial pouch, its lateral wall fusing with the inward migrating tissue of the branchial groove to form the tympanic membrane. Along with the tympanic cavity, the first branchial pouch also expands to form the eustachian tube anteriorly as well as the mastoid cavity posteriorly. Within this expanding cavity, the ossicles develop from Meckel's cartilage (first branchial arch), which forms the malleus head and neck and incus body, as well as from Reichert's cartilage (second branchial arch), which forms the long processes of the incus and malleus as well as the stapes superstructure. The

TABLE 22–1 DEVELOPMENT OF THE AURICLE

First branchial arch	
1st hillock	Tragus
2nd hillock	Helical crus
3rd hillock	Helical rim
Second branchial arch	
4th hillock	Antihelix
5th hillock	Antitragus
6th hillock	Lobule

stapes footplate has a dual origin, forming from the second branchial arch as well as from the otic capsule. The ossicles assume their final shape by the fourth month of development, and by the end of the eighth month the middle ear cleft has expanded to include all of the ossicles.

The position of the facial nerve, the nerve of the second branchial arch, is dependent on the bony expansion of the middle ear as well as the expanding external auditory canal. The posterior and inferior expansion of the external canal accounts for the vertical course of the facial nerve through its mastoid segment. Failure of development of the external canal often results in an aberrant anterior displacement of the facial nerve through its descending portion, placing it at risk during drilling for canal atresia repair (Figs. 22–1 and 22–2).

The final form of the outer and middle ear structures, therefore, is dependent on the primitive structures involved as well as the time course of developmental arrest. Congenital aural atresia can range from a thin membranous canal thickening to complete absence of the tympanic bone, and from fused malleus–incus formations to near absence of the malleus, incus, and stapes superstructure. Nevertheless, only 4% of congenital malformations of the external and middle ear have associated inner ear deformities, owing to their separate embryologic origins.

CLASSIFICATION

Several classification schemes have been described to define the severity of canal atresia as well as to predict the likelihood of successful hearing restoration surgery. Classification systems can be helpful in choosing appropriate surgical candidates, in counseling patients, and in analyzing and comparing results. The first widely used classification system, descriptive in nature, was proposed in 1955 by Altmann[16] (Table 22–2). In 1985 De la Cruz[13] proposed a further classification of Altmann groups II and III into major and minor categories (Table 22–3), proposing that patients with only minor malformations stood a reasonable chance at hearing restorative surgery, whereas patients with major malformations had a low chance of success from

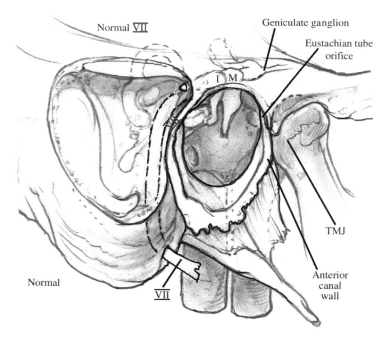

FIGURE 22–1 Normally developed ear, showing usual course of the facial nerve. I, incus; M, malleus; TMJ, temporal mandibular joint; VII, facial nerve.

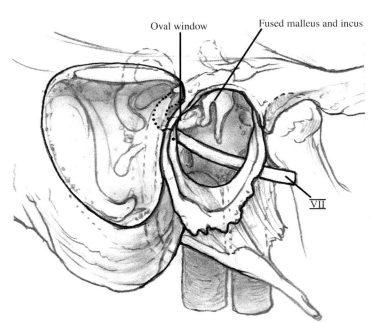

FIGURE 22–2 Aberrant anatomy in an atretic ear, with a fused malleus–incus complex as well as anterior and superior displacement of the facial nerve. VII, facial nerve.

TABLE 22–2 ALTMANN CLASSIFICATION OF CONGENITAL AURAL ATRESIA

Group I (mild)	External auditory canal (EAC) is present, although hypoplastic; tympanic bone is hypoplastic, and the tympanic membrane is small; tympanic cavity is normal or hypoplastic
Group II (moderate)	EAC is absent; tympanic cavity is small and its contents are malformed; an atretic plate is present and ossified
Group III (severe)	EAC is absent; the tympanic cavity is missing or severely hypoplastic

TABLE 22–3 DE LA CRUZ CLASSIFICATION OF CONGENITAL AURAL ATRESIA

Minor malformations (candidates for hearing restorative surgery)
  Normal mastoid pneumatization
  Normal oval window
  Reasonable oval window–facial nerve relationship
  Normal inner ear

Major malformations (candidates for bone-anchored hearing aids)
  Poor mastoid pneumatization
  Abnormal or absent oval window
  Abnormal facial nerve course
  Inner ear abnormalities

surgery, and were better managed by bone-anchored hearing aids to overcome their conductive hearing loss. Perhaps the most widely used classification system used to qualify patients for potential hearing restorative surgery is one proposed by Jahrsdoerfer et al[11] in 1992 (Table 22–4). A 10-point grading system evaluating a variety of middle and external

TABLE 22–4 JAHRSDOERFER GRADING SYSTEM OF CANDIDACY FOR SURGERY OF CONGENITAL AURAL ATRESIA

Parameter	Points
Stapes present	2
Oval window open	1
Middle ear space	1
Facial nerve normal	1
Malleus–incus complex present	1
Mastoid well pneumatized	1
Incus–stapes connection	1
Round window normal	1
Appearance of external ear	1
Total available points	10

Rating/Candidacy	
10	Excellent
9	Very good
8	Good
7	Fair
6	Marginal
≤5	Poor

ear structures as seen on high-resolution computed tomography (HRCT) scanning is used to predict the likelihood of success of hearing restoration surgery. Patients receiving total scores of 5 or below are not candidates for surgery, whereas patients scoring 6 or higher are considered for surgery.

PATIENT EVALUATION AND SELECTION

All children identified with a congenital ear deformity need a complete morphologic examination to uncover other potential malformations. Auditory brainstem response (ABR) audiometry of air (when possible) and bone conduction should ideally be performed within the first few days of life. In patients with bilateral hearing loss, a bone conduction aid should be fit within the first month of life, whereas in cases with unilateral hearing loss, a hearing aid is not necessary. The family history should be reviewed to identify other cases of atresia or hearing loss, and the details of the pregnancy are ascertained. All of the available information is used to determine whether the atresia is sporadic, non-syndromal, or syndromal.

Surgical and radiologic evaluations in the otherwise asymptomatic child can be delayed until shortly before surgical intervention is planned, typically at age 5 or 6. Because up to 14% of children with congenital aural atresia may present with a draining ear or acute facial palsy, these symptoms necessitate a radiologic evaluation to rule out congenital cholesteatoma. Computed tomography (CT) scan technology has evolved tremendously, and the very short scan times required for data acquisition now allow for very young children to be scanned without sedation in many cases. Therefore, once the child's mastoid has fully developed, a scan can be obtained that is useful for purposes of preoperative planning. Early scanning of affected children also has the benefit of identifying early the rare congenital cholesteatoma.

TIMING OF REPAIR

Traditionally, microtia repair has preceded atresia repair so that the reconstructive surgeon can operate in native tissue free from any altered blood supply or scarring, either of which could compromise a successful auricular reconstruction. Microtia repair is usually started at 6 years of age, when costal cartilage is of sufficient size for crafting an auricular frame. Because microtia repair is a multistage operation necessitating adequate healing time be-

tween surgeries, patients usually present to the otologist for atresia repair at 7 or 8 years of age. Because a completely reconstructed auricle with a rib cartilage graft remains a challenging endeavor, often with less than optimal results, some parents elect not to proceed with this type of reconstruction, choosing instead more limited reconstructive procedures or nothing at all.

Atresia repair can commence anytime after 2 months from the final stage of auricular reconstruction. The two absolute requirements for atresia repair for hearing restoration are radiographic evidence of an inner ear as seen on HRCT, and audiometric confirmation of cochlear function. The exception to this is surgery for congenital cholesteatoma, which is an absolute indication for surgery regardless of the age of presentation.

Atresia repair can be started earlier (age 5) under certain circumstances and with appropriate communication with the reconstructive surgeon. The requirements are that patients will not be undergoing a complete auricular reconstruction with a rib graft and that they will be cooperative with postoperative cleaning and care of the new ear canal. Often the existing deformed auricle can be reconstructed with more conservative otoplasty techniques to improve the cosmesis and functionality of the pinna. These reconstructions can be done after or even in conjunction with the canal atresia repair. Because the hearing results are not uniformly within the normal range, it is important to create an auricle and ear canal that is structurally accepting of a hearing aid.

SURGICAL PLANNING

As previously mentioned, HRCT scanning in the axial and coronal plane affords the best resolution and definition of the anatomy of the middle and inner ear. Specific attention is directed to evaluating the degree of temporal bone pneumatization, the course of the facial nerve (both its relationship to the oval window as well as its position in the mastoid segment), the existence of the oval window and stapes footplate, and the morphology of the inner ear. The thickness of the atretic plate, the existence of congenital cholesteatoma, and the size of the middle ear cavity are also determined.

SURGICAL TECHNIQUE

General anesthesia is used with an oral down-lead endotracheal tube. Muscle relaxation is avoided, and a facial nerve monitor is used in all cases. The use of nitrous oxide is usually avoided, but if used must be stopped at least 30 minutes prior to graft placement to prevent graft lateralization. The patient is placed supine, in a slight reverse Trendelenburg position, and the head is turned away from the surgeon as in most otologic procedures. A minimal amount of hair is shaved slightly behind and above the ear. Povidone iodine solution is used for skin preparation. As auricular reconstruction typically precedes atresia repair, a postauricular sulcus already exists. Local injection with 1% lidocaine with 1:100,000 epinephrine is injected subcutaneously in the area of the planned incision, taking care not to anesthetize the facial nerve.

The split-thickness skin graft (STSG) donor site, located on the ipsilateral upper lateral thigh or hip, is prepared with isopropyl alcohol, draped so as to allow harvest during the case, and covered with a sterile towel. We prefer to take the graft from an area that would be covered by underwear.

The location of the incision must take into account past and planned future incisions to prevent devascularization of tissue or limit future options. Most often a curvilinear incision 5 mm behind the postauricular crease is created. Ease of closure is facilitated by staying just posterior to the postauricular crease, a location that heals with excellent aesthetic results. It is important to understand that the facial nerve can be very superficial along the inferior part of the incision and is at risk of transection even with the skin opening. Temporalis fascia is harvested, crushed, and allowed to dry on the back of a Petrie

dish. The soft tissue over the mastoid is elevated from posterior to anterior until the root of the zygomatic process and the glenoid fossa are identified (Fig. 22–3). During this elevation the facial nerve is again at risk of being stretched. In normally developed ears, the 120-degree curve of the second genu directs the facial nerve in a mostly inferior direction throughout its mastoid segment. In atretic ears, the facial nerve can have a short vertical segment and a 60-degree angle at the second genu, directing the facial nerve in a more anterior direction and positioning it more superiorly in the mastoid segment. The nerve can exit the temporal bone and run right across the glenoid fossa and temporal mandibular joint.

An attempt is made to find a remnant of the tympanic bone, as this landmark points the way to the middle ear. In its absence, the drilling commences in an area defined by the glenoid fossa anteriorly, the root of the zygoma superiorly, and the cribriform area posteriorly (Fig. 22–4). By carefully hugging the tegmen tympani superiorly and the glenoid fossa anteriorly, one affords the best chance at avoiding the mastoid cavity posteriorly and an aberrant facial nerve inferiorly. The average depth of the atretic plate is 1.5 cm from the initial surface. As the drilling proceeds deeper, cutting burs are exchanged for diamond burs as an eggshell-thin piece of bone overlying the ossicles comes into view. The fused malleus–incus complex is encountered immediately deep to the thinned atretic plate, which is

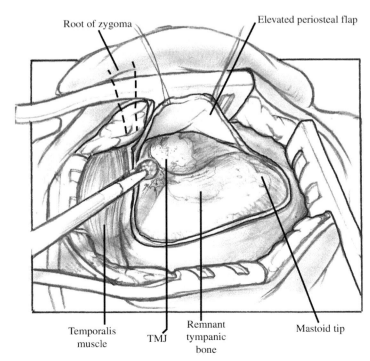

FIGURE 22–3 Initial exposure prior to drilling. The root of the zygoma, mastoid tip, linea temporalis, and temporal mandibular joint (TMJ) are all in view.

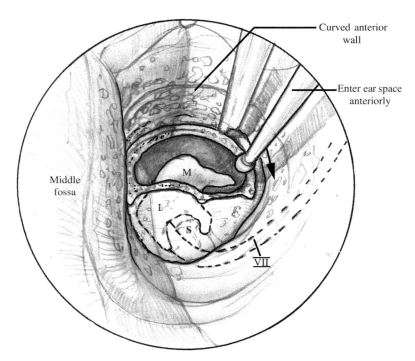

FIGURE 22–4 Drilling is commenced anteriorly and superiorly to avoid injury to an aberrant facial nerve. I, incus; M, malleus; S, stapes; VII, facial nerve.

unroofed with small right-angled picks, a laser, and/or diamond drills. The incus body or malleus handle is usually the first middle ear landmark to be seen, and its identity is confirmed by gentle palpation. The usual point of ossicular fixation to the bony atretic plate is anteriorly at the neck of the malleus, and no attempt is made early in the operation to free this attachment. The configuration of the ossicular mass can vary significantly as can the bony attachments. Regardless of the specific structure, it is important to maintain a bony bridge somewhere for stabilization of the ossicular chain to reduce the energy transferred to a mobile stapes.

Once the ossicular chain is encountered, special attention is required as the opening is enlarged posteriorly and inferiorly, because the facial nerve can be encountered in this position. Upon removal of the atretic plate, the ossicular chain is carefully assessed. In most cases the incus and malleus are fused, the handle of the malleus is malformed, the incus is attached to the stapes, and the neck of the malleus is fixed to the undersurface of the atretic plate (Fig. 22–5). Great care as well as sharp instrumentation is used while separating the malleus from its bony or periosteal attachments to the atretic plate. The transfer of vibrational energy to an intact ossicular chain can result in a postoperative sensory hearing loss, and avulsion of the stapes

footplate from the annular ligament can result in a traumatic perilymph fistula.

Crucial to a successful hearing result is confirming a mobile footplate as well as ossicular continuity of the malleus–incus complex to the stapes superstructure. In some cases, however, the stapes cannot be easily visualized and the surgeon must rely on gentle palpation. On the rare occasion that ossicular discontinuity is discovered, an ossiculoplasty is performed. In the uncommon instance of discovering a fixed footplate, a stapedotomy is not performed at this operation because both membranes at either end of the prosthesis (the oval window medially and the tympanic membrane laterally) are newly constructed and insecure, increasing the risk of hearing loss and postoperative vertigo. Indeed, if a fixed footplate is encountered, it is best to return at a second stage to perform a stapedotomy or to fit the patient with a hearing aid.

The final diameter of the canal is usually 1.5 cm at its medial extent, and it is positioned such that the center of the malleus–incus complex lies in the center of the canal. When enlarging the bony canal, it is important to appreciate the limits of dissection: the glenoid fossa anteriorly, the tegmen tympani superiorly, the mastoid cavity posteriorly, and the facial nerve inferiorly. Failure to create a large-enough canal predisposes to recurrent stenosis, and so an attempt is made to fashion a cone-shaped

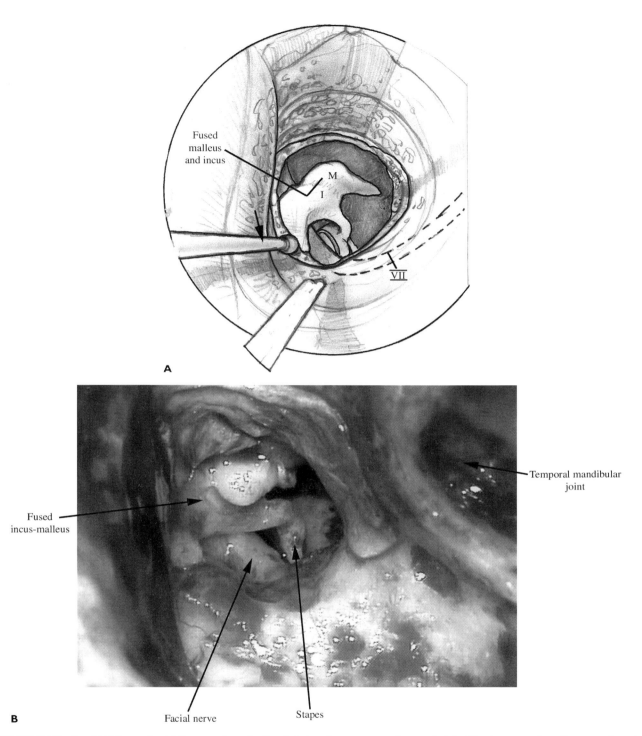

FIGURE 22–5   (A) View of middle ear after atretic plate has been removed completely. The incus and malleus are fused and yet in continuity to the stapes. The facial nerve rides high and anterior in its mastoid segment. VII, facial nerve. (B) Intraoperative photograph after removal of the atretic plate.

canal, wider at its lateral margin than at its medial margin.

A wide meatoplasty is created by debulking the posterior (deep) portion of the external ear in the area, which will overlie the ear canal. It is rarely a problem for a native or reconstructed external ear to be moved to a new position to align the canal with the external ear. An oval plug of skin is removed over the anterior (superficial) external ear, the external ear is positioned correctly over the canal, and subcutaneous sutures are used to stabilize the position of the external ear. The remainder of the procedure is performed through the meatoplasty.

The fascia graft is cut to size and placed lateral to the ossicles. The edges of the graft are reflected no more than 2 to 3 mm up the walls of the neocanal so that a minimal amount of fascia interposes between the skin graft and the underlying bone. If a substantial amount of graft is brought up the edges of the bony canal, capillary ingrowth from the underlying bone to the skin graft is prevented, predisposing to an avascular segment that requires serial debridement and may predispose to medial stenosis. Likewise the malleus–incus complex should protrude the graft slightly in its center portion to achieve the best chance at fibrous fixation, thus preventing graft lateralization. Small tabs can be made in the fascia graft to slip medial to the level of the neoannulus to further impede the tendency toward lateralization.

A split-thickness skin graft measuring 0.08 to 0.10 inch thick and 6 × 6 cm in size is harvested with a dermatome (Fig. 22–6). Thicker grafts have edges that tend to curl up, making precise positioning of the graft difficult and frustrating, and predisposing to future cholesteatoma formation. A graft that is too thin lacks the hardiness to withstand the environmental abuse. It is not uncommon for one edge of the graft to be thinner than the other. In this case the thinner edge is placed medially and the thicker edge is sutured to the new meatus. The final graft size is cut to 3 × 5 cm. The vertical slit of the graft is positioned anteriorly so that the skin edges do not grow into any exposed mastoid air cells. The bulk of the graft is placed deep into the canal, the medial edges overlapping the fascia tympanic membrane graft. Thereafter the graft is gently backed out of the canal until its medial edge is brought into proper position at the edge of the bony canal. This is technically easier than placing the skin graft in the canal only a shallow distance and thereafter trying to advance the leading edge deeper and deeper into the canal. The skin should overlap the fascia 1 to 2 mm. Key to a successful hearing result is a thin tympanic membrane; therefore, only a small portion of the skin graft is allowed to overlap the tympanic membrane fascia graft. Some surgeons prefer to cut small wedges out of the medial part of the graft to allow for complete coverage of the fascia without overlapping the skin. Others prefer to allow the epithelium to migrate across the fascia in the same

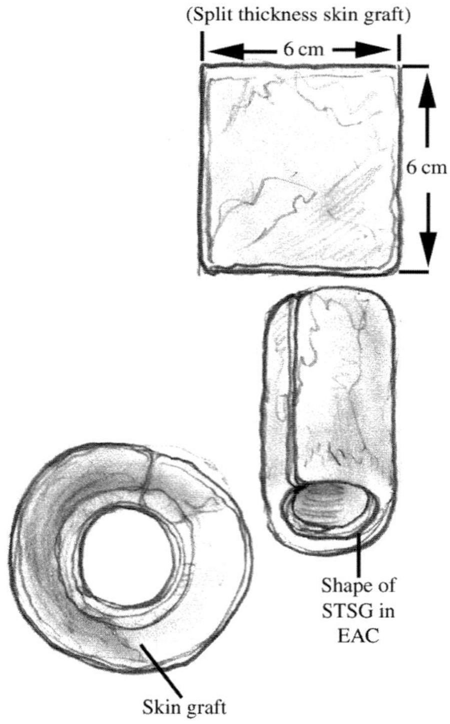

FIGURE 22–6 A 6 × 6 cm split-thickness skin graft (STSG) is harvested and trimmed to a final size of 3.5 cm. EAC, external auditory canal

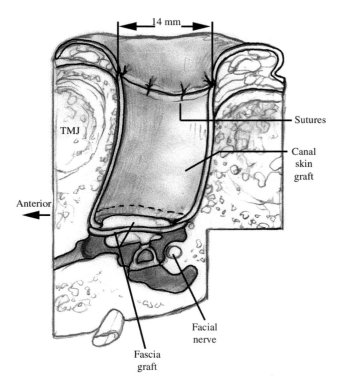

FIGURE 22–7 The neotympanic membrane of temporalis fascia lies under the split-thickness skin graft lining the canal. The skin graft is sutured laterally to the skin of the ear after creation of a large meatoplasty. TMJ, temporal mandibular joint.

fashion that occurs in a routine tympanic membrane repair. Excess skin is trimmed and the skin graft edges are sutured to the external ear skin with fast-absorbing chromic gut sutures. It is best to have some redundant skin remaining rather than to over-trim the graft, as the excess skin contracts over time (Fig. 22–7).

A 1-mm-thick reinforced Silastic button is cut and placed over the tympanic membrane graft, serving both to create and maintain a sharp anterior sulcus as well as serving as a buffer material between the tympanic membrane (TM) graft and the material used to pack the canal (Fig. 22–8). Were there no inert material between the TM graft and the canal packing, adhesions could form that could pull the graft laterally once the packing is removed in the postoperative period.

The ear canal is carefully packed with the surgeon's material of choice; we prefer to use Merocel soaked with Floxin Otic. Some surgeons use other materials such as a gauze fenestration pack, Gelfoam, or Pope Otowicks. Regardless of the material it is important to achieve good apposition of the skin graft to the canal wall.

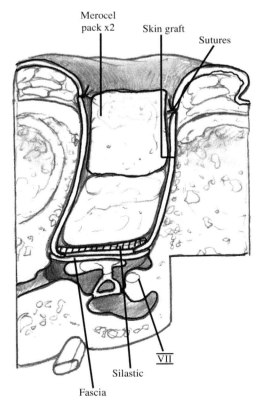

FIGURE 22–8 View upon completion of the procedure, with a Silastic button in place between the fascia graft and Merocel packing to stent the canal as it heals. VII; facial nerve.

The postauricular incision is closed with buried sutures, antibiotic ointment is applied, and a bulky mastoid dressing is placed. The patient is allowed to awaken from anesthesia and the facial nerve function is documented as soon as possible.

POSTOPERATIVE CARE

The patient is kept in the hospital overnight for observation, and the mastoid dressing is removed prior to the patient's discharge the morning after the surgery. Because the Merocel sponge canal packs must remain moist to maintain a pressure bolster against the skin graft, the patient is given a steroid-containing antibiotic otic preparation with instructions to place five drops in the ear three times a day until follow-up in 1 week. Water is kept out of the ear. At the first postoperative clinic visit, the canal packs are removed and the ear is cleaned. If there is any granulation tissue or healing areas (usually the case), the patient is continued on eardrops until the next visit. Patients are seen weekly for the first month for cleaning and debridement. The appointments are then gradually spread out based on the status of the ear. Healing is promoted and stenosis prevented by maintaining a clean ear canal. Lifelong follow-up at 6-month to 1-year intervals is often required, as the grafted canal skin is not self-cleaning and must be gently debrided of squamous epithelium to prevent chronic infection and subsequent stenosis.

After the ear has healed well, there are no activity restrictions. Patients are allowed to swim, but they may need to use drying or antibiotic drops afterward to prevent infections.

RISKS AND COMPLICATIONS

The major risks of the operation are injury to the facial nerve, a worsening of hearing, and canal re-stenosis. Although facial nerve monitoring is routinely used, it is no substitute for careful preoperative mapping of the facial nerve course on HRCT, attentive observation during surgery, and an appreciation for the possible anomalous course of the facial nerve as often encountered in congenital aural atresia surgery.

A high-frequency sensory hearing loss (6 to 8 kHz) can occur in up to 15% of cases, and in most cases is permanent. Although its etiology is not known with certainty, it is most often ascribed to vibrational energy transferred to the ossicles during drilling. It is, therefore, of paramount importance to switch to diamond burs as the atretic plate is thinned, to take special care to avoid drilling on the ossicles, and to use picks, sharp cutting instruments, and/or lasers when severing the final attachments of the ossicles to the bony atretic plate.

Re-stenosis is a frequent frustration to patients and surgeons alike, and patients with more severe forms of microtia have a higher incidence of re-stenosis. To prevent re-stenosis, a large canal (1.5 cm at the medial edge, tapering out more widely as one moves laterally) is created, as is a large meatoplasty (1.5 to 2 times larger than normal). Close follow-up is instituted, with intervals between visits lengthening as time progresses and debridement needs are lessened. Early (soft) stenosis can sometimes be reversed with triamcinolone injection, whereas late (firm) stenosis requires surgical revision.

OPERATIVE RESULTS

Postoperative audiologic results reported from various series are difficult to compare, as different classification systems are used in stratifying and selecting patients. Using the Altmann criteria, Federspil and Delb[1] reported correction of the air–bone gap to within 20 dB in 33 patients with grade I, II, or III stenosis as 50%, 63%, or 0%, respectively. Mean follow-up time was not reported, and complications included canal re-stenosis (43%) and postoperative infection (6%).

Chandrasekhar et al[14] reported outcomes on 92 patients undergoing canal atresia repair. Results were not subdivided by the degree of malformation encountered, but their patients achieved long-term closure of the air–bone gap to ≤30 dB in 60% of primary repairs and 54% of revision cases. They cautioned that short-term results do not predict long-term results, as 19% of their patients showed hearing deterioration over a 2-year period.

Shih and Crabtree[10] reported results of 39 cases of primary repair with a mean follow-up time of 5 years. As expected, better hearing results were obtained in patients with less severe deformities. Using the Altmann classification, 89% of patients with group I malformations obtained a postoperative pure-tone average (PTA) of ≤30 dB. Similar results were obtained in only 20% of patients with group II malformations and in 10% of patients with group III malformations. Complications included a 33% incidence of re-stenosis, a 31% risk of infection, and a 40% risk of hearing deterioration within 2 years after initial positive results, most often associated with re-stenosis.

De la Cruz and colleagues[13] reported their results of 56 primary atresia repairs, all ears having had Altmann group II or III abnormalities. Although no long-term hearing results were reported, 6-month postoperative closure of the air–bone gap to within 10, 20, or 30 dB was seen in 16%, 53%, or 73% of cases, respectively. Complications included delayed graft lateralization (25%), canal re-stenosis (9%), and the creation of one dead ear (2%). Cholesteatoma was found behind an atretic plate in 16% of cases.

Finally, using the 10-point grading system based on preoperative HRCT findings, Jarhsdoerfer and colleagues[11] reported results on 86 ears. Speech reception thresholds of 25 dB or better 4 weeks after surgery were obtained in 0%, 41%, 72%, 90%, and 88% in patients with scores of 5, 6, 7, 8, and 9, respectively. Neither long-term hearing results nor complication rates were reported.

SUMMARY

Surgery for congenital aural atresia has as its main goal the restoration of unaided, usable hearing. It is technically demanding, not without risk, and is purely elective except in cases of congenital cholesteatoma. Successful atresia surgery requires a variety of advanced otologic techniques in tympanoplasty, canaloplasty, meatoplasty, and ossiculoplasty, and successful hearing restoration surgery can be particularly gratifying to the patient and surgeon alike.

REFERENCES

1. Federspil P, Delb W. Treatment of congenital malformations of the external and middle ear. In: Ars B, ed. *Congenital External and Middle Ear Malformations: Management.* Amsterdam: Kugler; 1992:47–70.
2. Gill NW. Congenital atresia of the ear: a review of the surgical findings in 83 cases. *J Laryngol Otol* 1969;83:551–587.
3. Granstrom G, Bergstrom K, Tjellstrom A. The bone-anchored hearing aid and bone-anchored epithesis for congenital ear malformations. *Otolaryngol Head Neck Surg* 1993;109:46–53.
4. Kiesselbach W. Versuch zur Anlegung eines äusseren Gehöganges bei angeborener Missbildung beider Ohrmuscheln mit Fehlen der äusseren Gehörgänge. *Arch Ohrenheilk* 1882;19:127–131.
5. Jahrsdoerfer RA. Congenital atresia of the ear. *Laryngoscope* 1978;88(suppl 13):1–48.
6. Dean LW, Gittens TR. Report of a case of bilateral congenital osseus atresia of the external auditory canal with an exceptionally good functional result following operation. *Laryngoscope* 1917;27:461–473.
7. Ombredanne M. Chirurgie de la surdité: fenestration dans les aplasies de l'orielle avec imperforation du conduit: resultats. *Otorhinolaryngol Int* 1947; 31:229–236.

8. Pattee GL. An operation to improve hearing in cases of congenital atresia of the external auditory meatus. *Arch Otolaryngol Head Neck Surg* 1947;45:568–580.

9. Ombredanne M. Chirurgie des surdites congenitales par malformations ossiculaires. *Acta Otorhinolaryngol Belg* 1971;25:837–869.

10. Shih L, Crabtree JA. Long-term surgical results for congenital aural atresia. *Laryngoscope* 1993;103:1097–1102.

11. Jahrsdoerfer RA, Yeakley JW, Aguilar EA, Cole RR, Gray LC. Grading system for the selection of patients with congenital aural atresia. *Am J Otol* 1992;13:6–12.

12. Marquet JE, Declau F, De Cock M, De Paep K, Appel B, Moeneclaey L. Congenital middle ear malformations. *Acta Otorhinolaryngol Belg* 1988;42:117–302.

13. De la Cruz A, Linthicum FH Jr, Luxford WM. Congenital atresia of the external auditory canal. *Laryngoscope* 1985;95:421–427.

14. Chandrasekhar SS, De la Cruz A, Garrido E. Surgery of congenital aural atresia. *Am J Otol* 1995;16:713–717.

15. Van de Water TR, Maderson PF, Jaskoll TF. The morphogenesis of the middle and external ear. *Birth Defects: Original Article Series* 1980;16:147–180.

16. Altmann F. Congenital atresia of the ear in man and animals. *Ann Otol Rhinol Laryngol* 1955;64:824–858.

Chapter 23

CANALOPLASTY FOR CANAL STENOSIS

Robert A. Battista and Carlos Esquivel

The external auditory canal may be affected by numerous pathologic conditions. Over time, these conditions may result in narrowing of the canal with eventual stenosis. For the sake of discussion, the pathologies that cause stenosis can be broadly categorized as either bony or soft tissue. Both bony and soft external canal stenoses are unusual otologic conditions.

Modified mastoidectomy was considered the treatment of choice in early reports of acquired canal stenosis.[1-3] Currently, canaloplasty (also called canalplasty) is considered the most optimal treatment for both bony and soft tissue canal stenoses. Canaloplasty is a surgical means to restore the natural contours and patency of the ear canal.

This chapter discusses the anatomy of external auditory canal pertinent to the understanding of surgery of the ear canal, and the pathologies that may cause canal stenosis.

ANATOMY OF THE EXTERNAL EAR CANAL

The adult external ear canal is cartilaginous in its outer third and osseous in its inner two thirds. The average ear canal length is 6.5 cm, with an average diameter of 2.5 cm. At the junction of the cartilaginous and bony canal there is a slight angulation; the cartilaginous part is inclined slightly posterosuperiorly, and the bony part is inclined anteroinferiorly. As a result, the axis of the ear canal follows a lazy S shape. The anterior canal bone is very thick above and below the head of the mandible, but thin between these two points.[4] For this reason, the glenoid fossa is susceptible to injury during drilling in the anterior canal.

Skin over the cartilaginous canal is approximately 0.5 to 1 mm thick and consists of epidermis with papillae, a dermis, and a subcutaneous layer. The skin of the bony canal is approximately 0.2 mm thick, lacks a subcutaneous layer, and is continuous with the epithelial layer of the tympanic membrane. The thinness of the bony canal skin makes the periosteum prone to thermal irritation, which may lead to exostosis formation when a person swims in cold water.

The skin of the external canal contains hair follicles, sebaceous and ceruminous glands, which are a type of apocrine gland. The secretions of these glands combine with desquamated keratinocytes to form cerumen. Cerumen is relatively water-repellant and coats the surface of the canal skin to delay penetration of various substances through the skin. Some studies suggest cerumen has antibacterial qualities.[5]

The external auditory canal has a unique property in that is has a self-cleaning mechanism to keep the canal free of debris. In the normal ear canal, epithelial migration moves material laterally from the medial end of the canal. If such a mechanism did not exist, the lumen of the canal would gradually become occluded by keratin debris, and the transmission of sound would be impaired. Exostosis and chronic or recurrent external otitis are two of several conditions that may impair the self-cleansing mechanism of the ear canal.

Also of importance is the anatomic association of the chorda tympani and facial nerves with the bony external auditory canal. The chorda tympani passes just medial to the mid- to superior portion of the posterior fibrous annulus. The facial nerve may lie lateral to the posterior tympanic annulus in the lower part of the nerve's vertical segment.[6,7] To prevent damage to the chorda tympani and facial nerves, care must be taken when drilling in the region of the posterior bony canal in the region of the fibrous annulus.

CAUSES/PATHOPHYSIOLOGY

The most common bony diseases that may cause stenosis of the external auditory canal are exostosis, osteoma, and fibrous dysplasia. Exostoses of the external canal are rounded, multiple bony outgrowths that can occur because of chronic irritation of the external canal. The most common cause of exostoses is cold-water swimming. These lesions can continue to grow even after the ear canal is no longer exposed to a cold environment. Osteomas are singular, often pedunculated, benign bony tumors arising from the osseous meatus. There is no identifiable cause for external canal osteomas. Fibrous dysplasia is a benign disease of bone characterized by the abnormal proliferation of fibro-osseous tissue within cancellous bone.

Acquired soft tissue stenosis of the external canal is due to some insult to the canal that results in cicatrix formation. The insult may be the result of recurrent/chronic inflammation (infection, dermatologic disease), iatrogenic injuries (surgery, radiation), trauma (burns, chemical injury, repeated ear canal scratching, fracture), or neoplasm. In one large review, the leading cause of stenosis was chronic infection (54%) followed by prior ear surgery (20%).[8] When surgery or trauma is the inciting event, many years may elapse before the acquired soft tissue stenosis requires surgical treatment.[8]

Systemic diseases of the skin (e.g., psoriasis, lupus erythematosus, scleroderma) can affect the ear canal and eventually cause external canal obstruction. One important feature of psoriasis is that mild trauma to surrounding skin induces lesions localized to the area of injury.[9] Therefore, patients with psoriasis in or near the ear canal should be asked to avoid manipulation of the lesions, so as to prevent stenosis. Cutaneous (contact dermatitis) reactions to shampoos, medications, and foreign material in the ear canal can be severe and may require rapid medical attention to prevent scarring and stenosis of the soft tissue of the canal.

Acquired soft tissue stenosis of the external canal is uncommon. For postinflammatory acquired atresia, Becker and Tos[10] reported an annual incidence of 0.6 per 100,000. Many other large series of acquired soft tissue stenosis report, on average, treating one case of soft tissue stenosis per year.[4,11–13]

Many terms have been used to describe acquired soft tissue stenosis of the external canal including medial meatal fibrosis,[12–14] chronic stenosing exter-

nal otitis,[4] and postinflammatory acquired atresia.[10] The pathophysiology of acquired soft tissue canal stenosis is unknown because there are currently no experimental animal models. It is believed that the canal passes through several stages before developing the soft tissue stenosis. In the first stage of development, some type of insult (e.g., infectious, traumatic) produces granulation tissue of the ear canal, tympanic membrane, or combination of the two sites. The granulation tissue becomes infected and the tissue proliferates. This stage is considered the active or immature phase. Eventually, a mature stage ensues whereby the granulation tissue forms a well-developed fibrous plug lined by squamous epithelium. The disease process ceases to continue when the atresia reaches the lateral end of the bony canal.[15]

PATIENT PRESENTATION

Exostoses usually do not produce clinical symptoms. If the exostoses are large enough, patients may develop recurrent external otitis because the lesions may prevent the natural elimination of cerumen/desquamated epithelium from the external canal. Conductive hearing loss is possible when the exostoses tamponades cerumen against the tympanic membrane or when the external canal is occluded by the exostoses. For similar reasons, osteomas and fibrous dysplasia of the external canal can also present with recurrent external otitis or conductive hearing loss.

The ear canal must be narrowed considerably to develop clinically significant conductive hearing loss. Hearing loss does not become significant until there is an aperture of 3 mm or less. High-frequency conductive hearing loss is seen initially followed by lower-frequency loss as the aperture narrows below 3 mm.

The clinical presentation of patients with acquired soft tissue stenosis depends on the phase of the disease process at the time of presentation. When the disease is in the active phase, patients complain of chronic or recurrent discharge. During the mature phase, conductive hearing loss is the main complaint. Audiometric testing usually shows a 20- to 40-dB conductive hearing loss in the mature phase.[4,8,10–14] Volume measurements of the external auditory canal are also below normal.

As mentioned previously, there are many possible causes for acquired soft tissue stenosis of the ear canal. The clinical presentation may be the same whether the cause is benign or malignant. For this reason, the diagnosis of lesions of the external canal is made based on a careful history and cultures or biopsy.

RADIOGRAPHIC EVALUATION

A high-resolution computed tomography (CT) of the temporal bones is recommended for select cases of bony stenosis and for all cases of soft tissue stenosis (Fig. 23–1). CT is recommended for bony stenosis when the tympanic membrane cannot be visualized. For both bony and soft tissue stenosis, CT can help define disease medial to the stenosis. Becker and Tos[10] have reported a 9% incidence of cholesteatoma medial to soft tissue stenosis.

INDICATIONS FOR TREATMENT

Medical management may be employed initially in select cases of soft tissue stenosis. Surgery is an option for cases that fail medical management.

For both bony and soft tissue stenosis, surgical treatment is recommended when the patient develops chronic/recurrent external otitis or conductive hearing loss. Another indication for surgery is difficulty fitting a hearing aid.

Oncologic procedures are necessary when benign or malignant tumors cause canal obstruction. A description of these types of procedures is beyond the scope of this chapter.

MEDICAL MANAGEMENT

If identified early, soft tissue stenosis may be treated medically. Cases that may respond to medical therapy may include, but are not limited to, the early stages after surgery or radiation. Many options are available for medical management and would be based on each individual case. One option would include periodic dilatation of the external canal by placement of expandable ear wicks. Antibiotic-steroid otic drops are used and the ear is repacked every 4 to 10 days for 6 to 8 weeks. Local injections of Kenalog or Decadron should be used if there is little to no response to the dilatation technique within the first 4 weeks. For less severe cases, another option for treatment would include the use of steroid cream or drops on a daily basis for several weeks. If the ear canal opens with either of these techniques, periodic cleaning and frequent irrigations with acetic acid –alcohol solutions help to maintain patency. Patients who do not respond to these treatments are candidates for surgery.

SURGICAL MANAGEMENT

The main goal of surgery is to restore and maintain patency of the external auditory canal for normal sound transmission and maintenance of the canal's self-cleaning functions. If the ear is actively discharging, it is best to decrease the inflammatory process with cleansing and topical steroid-antibiotic therapy. Surgery can proceed when the ear is no longer draining.

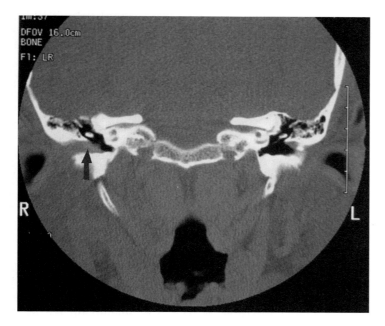

FIGURE 23–1 Coronal computed tomography (CT) of soft tissue stenosis with cholesteatoma (arrow) medial to stenosis and lateral to tympanic membrane. Stenosis due to psoriasis.

The authors prefer the postauricular approach for removal of both bony and soft tissue external auditory canal stenosis. The postauricular approach provides much better visualization and allows easier access for drilling compared to the endaural and transcanal approaches. In addition, the postauricular incision is more cosmetically appealing than the endaural incision. For exostosis removal, the postauricular incision allows for maximum preservation of canal skin and facilitates removal of the anterior exostosis, which is usually close to the tympanic membrane.

BONY STENOSIS

The procedure is begun by first injecting the ear canal skin with 1:100,000 epinephrine for hemostasis. A curvilinear postauricular incision is made approximately 1 cm behind the postauricular fold. The incision is carried directly down to bone inferiorly and down to the level of the temporalis fascia superiorly. A self-retaining retractor is placed, and the area of the spine of Henle is located by identifying the inferior border of the temporalis muscle. Dissection is carried anteriorly along the

mastoid bone in the region of the spine of Henle to identify the bony external meatus. Once the meatus is identified, the skin overlying the lateral surface of the posterior exostosis is elevated. The skin is elevated carefully with a Guilford or duckbill elevator as far medially as possible. Every attempt should be made to preserve as much canal skin as possible. Once elevated, the skin is retracted anteriorly with the blade of a House or Perkins bladed tympanoplasty retractor (Fig. 23–2). Placement of the tympanoplasty retractor allows further visualization of the medial skin dissection. Skin elevation is then completed as far medially as possible.

The posterior bony exostosis(es) is (are) removed using a medium-size diamond bur with suction-irrigation. The bony dissection is carried medially while keeping a protective shell of bone between the bur and the ear canal skin (Fig. 23–3). Bone removal is continued medially and posteriorly until the normal dimensions and contour of the ear canal are achieved.

The tympanic membrane and posterior annulus cannot be seen with this approach. Therefore, as drilling approaches the annulus, the surgeon may have to remove the tympanoplasty retractor and

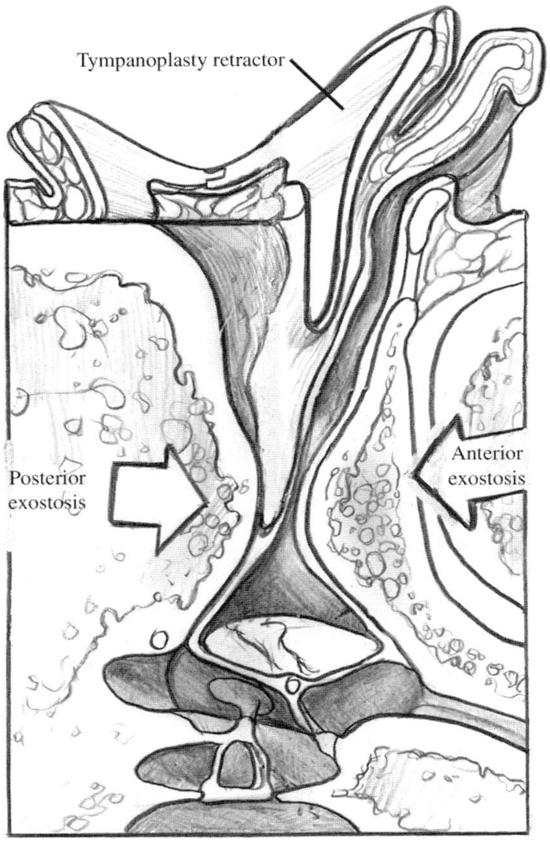

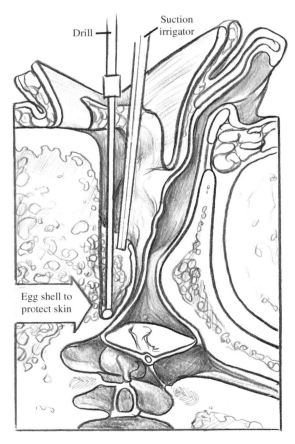

FIGURE 23–2 Retraction of posterior canal skin with tympanoplasty retractor.

FIGURE 23–3 Drilling of posterior canal wall for exostosis. Bony shell left to protect skin.

move the posterior canal skin posteriorly to judge the amount of remaining posterior bony stenosis. Care must be taken to avoid damage to the chorda tympani nerve, the posterior tympanic membrane, and the facial nerve. The facial nerve may lie lateral to the tympanic annulus in the lower part of its vertical segment.[6] Once the posterior bony removal is completed, the protective bony shell is fractured and removed. To facilitate removal, the ear canal skin must be thoroughly elevated off this shell prior to its removal.

If anterior exostosis(es) is (are) present, a laterally based posterior flap is created in the posterior canal skin. The laterally based flap is involuted into the meatus and held out of the way with the blade of the tympanoplasty retractor (Fig. 23–4A). The anterior exostosis is now exposed. To remove the anterior exostosis(es), an anterior, laterally based canal skin flap is created. The flap is formed by making a skin incision parallel to the tympanic membrane over the midportion of the anterior exostosis (Fig. 23–4B). Inferior and superior incisions made from the edge of this first incision are then extended laterally. The anterior, laterally based flap is elevated laterally and

held out of the way along with the posterior flap using a tympanoplasty retractor. The remaining skin over the anterior exostosis is elevated as far medially as possible. The exostosis is drilled in a fashion similar to that used to remove the posterior exostosis.

Anterior exostoses are often very close to the tympanic membrane. To protect the medial, anterior canal skin, a piece of tympanic membrane–size thin Silastic or the aluminum foil of a suture package is placed on the inside surface of the anterior canal skin to hold it down against the tympanic membrane during drilling. This material protects the anterior canal skin and tympanic membrane from the drill. At the completion of bony removal, the protective material is removed and all skin flaps are folded back into position over the new shape of the ear canal. The postauricular incision is closed in layers using 3-0 and 4-0 Vicryl suture, respectively, in a subcutaneous and subcuticular fashion.

The ear canal is then lined with a piece of thin (approximately 0.005 inch) Silastic. The Silastic helps to prevent blunting and stenosis of the ear canal during the postoperative period. The width of the

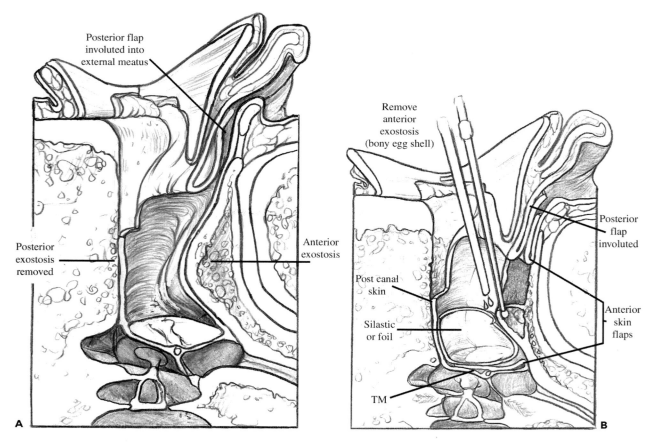

FIGURE 23–4 (A) Laterally based posterior flap involuted into external meatus. (B) Laterally based anterior flap created to expose anterior exostosis.

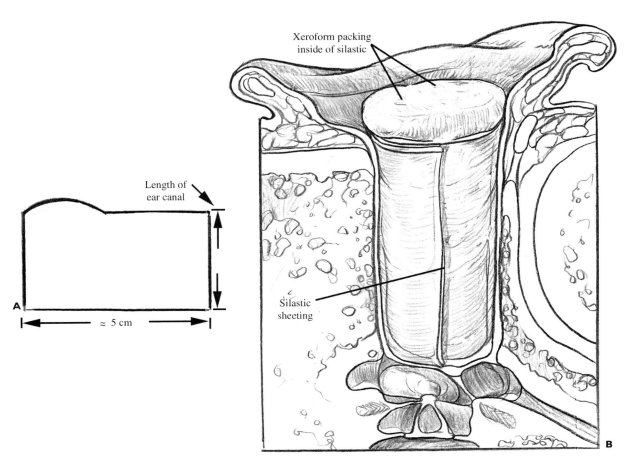

FIGURE 23–5 (A) Thin Silastic sheeting rounded in one end to accommodate additional length of anterior ear canal. (B) Silastic sheeting unrolled against canal skin with Xeroform packing used as a tamponade.

Silastic should be equal to the length of the ear canal from the posterior tympanic membrane to the external meatus. The length should be approximately 5 to 6 cm. One end of the Silastic should be rounded slightly wider than the other end to accommodate the additional length of the ear canal from the anterior drum to external meatus (Fig. 23–5A). To place the Silastic, it is rolled tightly along its width and positioned in the ear canal with the longer edge facing the anterior sulcus. It is allowed to unroll in the ear canal against the ear canal skin. This maneuver is facilitated by grasping the outside edge of the Silastic with bayonet forceps and the inside edge with cup forceps. The bayonet forceps stabilize the Silastic while the cup forceps are used to unroll it. Xeroform gauze is packed tightly inside the Silastic to keep the Silastic against the walls of the ear canal (Fig. 23–5B). A cotton ball impregnated with bacitracin ointment is placed in the meatus and a standard mastoid dressing is applied. Bacitracin ointment is applied to the cotton ball to prevent adherence to the Xeroform during removal of the cotton ball.

SOFT TISSUE STENOSIS

In addition to the ear, the volar forearm is prepped and draped in preparation for a possible skin graft. The procedure is then begun by injecting the ear canal skin with 1:100,000 epinephrine for hemostasis. If the soft tissue stenosis fills the entire external canal, a postauricular incision is made and the temporalis muscle identified in the same manner as that described for bony stenosis removal. If the soft tissue stenosis fills only a portion of the medial canal, a circumferential skin incision is made just lateral to the stenosis. This incision is connected to the external meatus through two canal incisions over the regions of the tympanomastoid and tympanosquamous suture lines. A postauricular incision is then made and the temporalis muscle found. The external meatus is identified and, if canal incisions have been made, the posterior, laterally based flap is involuted out of the way and held in place with a tympanoplasty retractor. The lateral edge of the stenosis is now in view.

The fibrosis is dissected circumferentially off bone using a Guilford or duckbill elevator. Dissection is

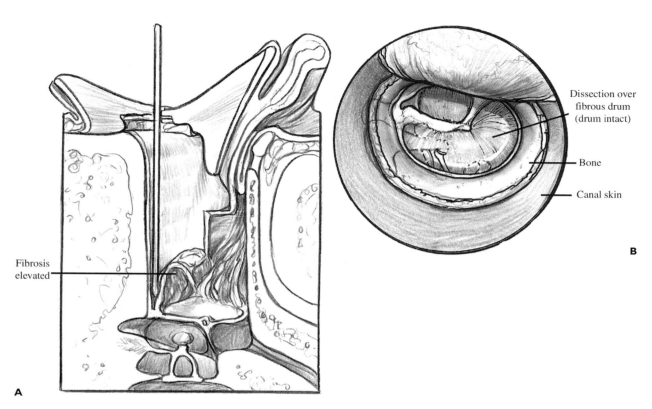

Dissection over
fibrous drum
(drum intact)

Bone

Canal skin

Fibrosis
elevated

A

B

FIGURE 23–6 (A,B) Dissection along posterior plane of soft tissue stenosis.

carried medially to the tympanic annulus (Fig. 23–6). When the stenosis is excessively thick, segmental removal of portions of the fibrosis may allow better visualization of the tympanic membrane. Care is taken when approaching the tympanic membrane to prevent a perforation. An avascular plane between the soft tissue stenosis and the fibrous drum should be developed. The plane can usually be established along the inferior annulus or over the short process of the malleus. Inadvertent elevation of the annulus may occur if dissection is begun posteriorly rather than inferiorly. Elevation of the annulus at this time will make dissection difficult. Every attempt should be made to preserve the fibrous layer of the tympanic membrane. After the fibrous plug is elevated from the tympanic membrane, the entire soft tissue stenosis is removed and sent for pathologic examination. To prevent recurrence, it is imperative that the entire cleaned fibrous annulus be visible, especially in the anterior sulcus.

Enlargement of the bony canal is necessary in all cases for three reasons. First, the bony anterior canal bulge often prevents complete visualization of the anterior sulcus. Fibrous tissue could be missed if the anterior bulge is left in place. The most common source of re-stenosis is in the anterior canal sulcus. Second, enlargement helps to maintain ear canal patency despite the tendency for soft tissue to

narrow the canal during the healing phase. Third, a large ear canal allows easier postoperative inspection and cleaning.

Bony canaloplasty is performed initially with a medium cutting bur and suction-irrigation. Grooves are drilled above and below the region of the glenoid fossa. The region between these two grooves is thinned using a diamond bur until an eggshell layer of bone is left over the glenoid fossa. Drilling must be performed carefully in the anterior canal because inadvertent entry into the glenoid fossa may result in herniation of fat into the ear canal. Herniation of fat may result in further stenosis. Additional drilling medial to the glenoid fossa is often necessary to completely expose the anterior fibrous annulus. A small diamond bur should be used in this area to minimize vibration to the ossicular chain. To prevent anterior canal blunting, the final angle between the tympanic membrane and anterior bony wall should be approximately 90 degrees. Any remaining fibrous tissue in the anterior sulcus should be removed at this time. The posterior canal wall is widened until mastoid air cells are visualized but not opened. A diamond bur should be used when working near the tympanic membrane. Once bony canaloplasty is completed, the surgeon should be able to view the entire annulus from one position of the microscope.

A posterior tympanotomy should be performed in cases with suspected middle ear disease. Up to 25% of cases of soft tissue stenosis may have middle ear pathology such as ossicular defects, cholesteatoma, or otosclerosis.[10] Sometimes a tympanic membrane perforation occurs during dissection over the drum. If it does, a standard underlay graft tympanoplasty should be performed.

Removal of the fibrous plug along with bony canaloplasty results in a wide ear canal. For this reason, a meatoplasty is often necessary. The meatoplasty should widen the external meatus sufficiently to allow easy visualization of all margins of the newly created external canal. Meatoplasty is performed through the postauricular approach by first removing a semilunar piece of conchal cartilage near the margin of the external meatus. The index finger of the nondominant hand is placed in the external meatus while the soft tissue overlying the conchal cartilage is carefully removed using cutting Bovie cautery. The nondominant hand is used to prevent inadvertent penetration of the cutting tool through the conchal skin. Once the cartilage is identified, a semilunar piece of conchal cartilage is removed using a No. 64 Beaver blade, which has a rounded tip scalpel that cuts at the tip as well as on one side. After conchal cartilage is removed, two incisions approximately 1 to 1.5 cm in length are made; the first is through the incisura and the second is made through conchal skin and cartilage at approximately the 4 o'clock position in a right ear and the 7 o'clock position in a left ear. Each of the two incisions must extend through all layers of subcutaneous tissue. A nonabsorbable suture is then used for permanent retraction of the posterior external meatus. After the meatoplasty is completed, the postauricular incision is closed in layers using 3-0 and 4-0 Vicryl suture in a subcutaneous and subcuticular fashion, respectively.

Finally, a thin split-thickness skin graft is obtained and used to cover all areas of exposed canal bone. The skin graft helps to prevent granulation tissue and re-stenosis, and speeds healing. For small defects, skin may be obtained from the non–hair-bearing region of the postauricular area. A No. 10 blade scalpel is used to shave an appropriate size graft. While obtaining the graft, the blade should be visible through the skin at all times to ensure a thin graft. Xeroform gauze is placed over the donor site. For large defects, the authors prefer to obtain the skin graft from the volar aspect of the ipsilateral upper arm. The skin of this area is ideal because it is thin and pliable and often lacks hair follicles. To obtain the graft, a rectangular area of skin of adequate dimensions (a 6 × 2-cm graft is necessary to cover the entire canal and drum) is infiltrated with lidocaine with 1:100,000 epinephrine. The harvest site is then lightly coated with mineral oil, and the arm is grasped firmly on the lateral aspect to provide tension on the volar surface. With a razor blade secured lengthwise in a curved clamp, a gentle back-and-forth slicing motion is used to harvest the graft. The proper thickness is obtained when the leading edge of the razor blade is barely visible beneath the skin graft. If performed properly, the graft thickness is approximately 0.010 to 0.012 inch in thickness.[16] The donor site is covered with Xeroform and wrapped with gauze. Both the postauricular and forearm donor sites heal with little or no cosmetic deformity.

The skin graft is then used to cover all areas of exposed bone in the external canal. The skin graft should also cover the tympanic membrane if the epithelial layer has been removed from the drum. When a graft is required to cover the drum, notches are cut on both sides of the graft. These notches correspond to the level of the anterior tympanomeatal angle. The anterior portion of the graft may be trimmed to a width slightly less than the posterior portion. In this way, the graft may fold around the posterior canal (Fig. 23–7A). The skin graft is placed in the ear canal with the short portion over the anterior canal wall. The notched area is folded at the anterior angle, whereas the larger area covers the drum and posterior canal (Fig. 23–7B). The graft should be sutured to the external meatus with a chromic suture if there is exposed bone near the external meatus. Suturing of the graft at the external meatus is necessary to maintain proper contact of the graft in this area. Compressed Gelfoam soaked in antibiotic-steroid otic solution is tightly packed into the anterior sulcus and around the tympanic annulus.

Regardless of the size of the skin graft, the ear canal is lined with Silastic as described previously for treatment of bony stenosis. The Silastic must extend up to the anterior sulcus to prevent blunting in this area. Xeroform gauze is packed tightly inside the Silastic to keep the Silastic against the skin graft and walls of the ear canal. A cotton ball impregnated with bacitracin ointment is placed in the meatus and a standard mastoid dressing is applied.

POSTOPERATIVE COURSE/PROGNOSIS

The mastoid dressing is removed by the patient on the first postoperative day. The patient is placed on prophylactic antibiotics for 5 days. Strict water precautions are observed using a cotton ball saturated with petroleum jelly or bacitracin ointment in

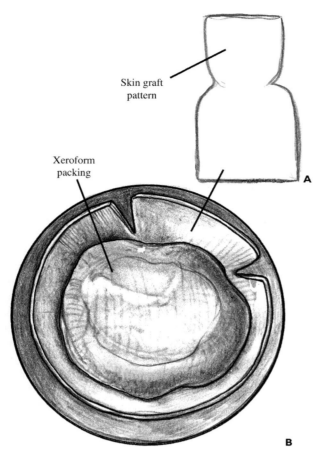

FIGURE 23-7 (A) Thin split-thickness skin graft with notch for bend at anterior sulcus. (B) Skin graft covering tympanic membrane and ear canal.

the meatus until the ear canal is healed sufficiently. The Xeroform and Silastic packing are removed at the first postoperative visit 3 weeks postoperatively. After packing removal, antibiotic-steroid otic drops are prescribed twice daily for 10 days. The second postoperative visit is at 5 weeks. If the canal is well healed and there is no evidence of infection, the drops are discontinued and the patient is seen several weeks later. If edema, granulation tissue, or infection is present, the drops are continued for an additional 7 days and the patient is seen in another 2 weeks. The patient is seen every 2 weeks until the ear canal is healed properly. Granulation tissue in the canal should be cauterized with silver nitrate or trichloroacetic acid. Cauterization shrinks the granulation tissue and promotes epithelialization.

Patients younger than 18 years old who have undergone canaloplasty for exostoses should limit cold-water exposure. Further exposure to cold water in this age group may increase the risk of exostosis recurrence.

Patients who require skin grafting are predisposed to infection and accumulation of debris. Skin grafts do not contain the normal apocrine and sebaceous glands, which normally cleanse and protect the ear canal from infection. In addition, patients with soft tissue stenosis may be prone to postoperative infection because of their previous history of chronic otitis externa. Therefore, patients undergoing canaloplasty for acquired stenosis should be examined at least every 6 months for the first 2 years after the ear canal is healed.

Hearing results after surgical treatment of bony stenosis are often excellent. Hearing results after repair of soft tissue stenosis are also good with air–bone gap closure to within 20 dB in 61 to 94% of cases.[10,11]

COMPLICATIONS

The following possible complications are associated with canaloplasty for acquired stenosis:

1. Temporomandibular (TMJ) dysfunction
2. Soft tissue re-stenosis
3. Tympanic membrane perforation
4. Taste disturbance
5. Hearing loss
   a. Conductive
   b. Sensorineural
6. Facial paralysis

TMJ dysfunction is caused by inadvertent entry into the glenoid fossa and may be helped with jaw mobility exercises. Soft tissue re-stenosis has been reported to occur in up to 18% of cases.[4,8,10–15] As mentioned earlier, medical management may be used to treat early cases of soft tissue re-stenosis. Revision surgery, with strict adherence to the principles mentioned in this chapter, is often helpful for more severe cases of re-stenosis. Taste disturbance is a potential risk due to the proximity of the chorda tympani nerve to the posterior fibrous annulus. When performing bony canaloplasty for exostosis, the medial extent of the posterior ear canal is approached without visualization of the tympanic membrane. This technique places the chorda tympani nerve at risk. An alternative technique to the one described is to remove the ear canal skin and perform a skin graft. Placement of a skin graft, however, results in the problems associated with skin grafting including delayed healing and the need for frequent ear cleaning. Conductive and sensorineural hearing loss may develop by unintentional contact of the ossicular chain with a drill or instruments. Facial paralysis may occur during drilling near the posterior fibrous annulus. A diamond bur should always be used when working near the tympanic membrane and the malleus. A diamond bur is less likely to run erratically than a cutting bur and cause damage to the tympanic membrane, ossicular chain, chorda tympani, and facial nerves.

REFERENCES

1. Anthony WP. Congenital and acquired atresia of the external auditory canal. *Arch Otolaryngol* 1957; 65:479–486.
2. Conley JJ. Atresial of the external auditory canal occurring in military service. *Arch Otolaryngol* 1946;43:613–622.
3. Work WP. Lesions of the external auditory canal. *Ann Otol Rhinol Laryngol* 1950;59:1062–1087.
4. Birman CS, Fagan PA. Medial canal stenosis: chronic stenosing external otitis. *Am J Otol* 1996;17:2–6.
5. Chai TJ, Chai TC. Bactericidal activity of cerumen. *Antimicrob Agents Chemother* 1980;18:638–641.
6. Williams B. The relationship of the facial nerve to the tympanic annulus and external auditory canal. *J Otolaryngol Soc Aust* 1988;6:95–96.
7. Adad B, Rasgon BM, Ackerson L. Relationship of the facial nerve to the tympanic annulus: a direct anatomic examination. *Laryngoscope* 1999;109:1189–1192.
8. Selesnick S, Nguyen TP, Eisenman DJ. Surgical treatment of acquired external auditory canal atresia. *Am J Otol* 1998;19:123–130.
9. Shea CR. Dermatologic diseases of the external auditory canal. *Otolaryngol Clin North Am* 1996;29:783–794.
10. Becker BC, Tos M. Postinflammatory acquired atresia of the external auditory canal: treatment and results of surgery over 27 years. *Laryngoscope* 1998; 108:903–907.
11. Cremers WR, Smeets JH. Acquired atresia of the external auditory canal: surgical treatment and results. *Arch Otolaryngol Head Neck Surg* 1993;119:162–164.
12. Keohane JD, Ruby RR, Janzen VD, MacRae DL, Parnes LS. Medial meatal fibrosis: the University of Western Ontario experience. *Am J Otol* 1993; 14:172–175.
13. Magliulo G, Ronzoni R, Cristofari P. Medial meatal fibrosis: current approach. *J Laryngol Otol* 1996;110: 417–420.
14. Katzke D, Pohl DV. Postinflammatory medial meatal fibrosis: a neglected entity? *Arch Otolaryngol* 1982; 108:779–780.
15. Bonding P, Tos M. Postinflammatory acquired atresia of the external auditory canal. *Acta Otolaryngol (Stockh)* 1975;79:115–123.
16. Harvey SA. Skin grafting in otology. *Laryngoscope* 1997;107:1199–1202.

Chapter 24

ENDOLYMPHATIC SAC SURGERY

Sarah L. Pertzborn and Patrick J. Antonelli

Meniere's disease can present in a variety of ways. The symptom constellation consists of episodic vertigo, fluctuating or progressive sensorineural hearing loss, aural fullness, and tinnitus. The vertigo is usually a hallucination of violent spinning that lasts 30 minutes to many hours, but not more than a day. In advanced cases, attacks of vertigo may be replaced by drop attacks (also known as crises of Tumarkin). The hearing loss is generally asymmetric, with the worse-hearing ear or ear with the most hearing fluctuation more often being responsible for the vestibular complaints. Changes in hearing, tinnitus, and aural fullness are often temporally associated with the onset of vertigo.

Clinical examination of patients with Meniere's disease is generally unremarkable, as most patients do not present during an acute flare. In such unusual situations, patients may manifest spontaneous nystagmus, diaphoresis, and pallor. Tuning fork testing reveals a sensorineural hearing loss in the affected ear. Between attacks, spontaneous or positional nystagmus is not commonly seen. The sensorineural hearing loss may also resolve completely during quiescent intervals.

Audiometry can be very helpful in the diagnosis of Meniere's disease. The classic audiometric presentation involves a low-frequency sensorineural loss, occasionally associated with a very mild "inner ear conductive" component. With time, all frequencies may be affected. The pattern of hearing loss is highly variable. Speech discrimination scores are in the expected range for a given sensorineural threshold.

Electrocochleography has been hailed as a means of detecting subclinical Meniere's disease (i.e., when audiometry is normal) by measuring an increased summating potential to action potential ratio (e.g., greater than 0.30). Electrocochleography has failed to gain widespread support because of its unclear sensitivity and specificity and the ability to diagnose Meniere's disease on the basis of history and audiometry alone.

Meniere's disease is widely believed to result from a buildup of pressure within the membranous labyrinth (also called endolymphatic hydrops). Inner ear fluid homeostasis remains poorly understood, so it is not clear whether Meniere's disease results from overproduction, underabsorption of endolymph, or both. Autoimmune and virally mediated etiologies have also found support. As the pathogenesis of Meniere's disease has been attributed to a variety of pathologies, it might be better considered a syndrome.

Most cases of Meniere's disease can be controlled nonsurgically, such as with a low-sodium diet and administration of thiazide diuretics. Intractable Meniere's disease may cause disability as a result of profound hearing loss or, more commonly, recurrent vertigo. Most of the surgery for intractable Meniere's disease is directed at controlling the episodic vertigo. Surgery for Meniere's disease should be considered only after maximal medical therapy, directed at the root cause and symptom control, has been exhausted (Table 24–1). The use of corticosteroids, either systemically or intratympanically, has yielded anecdotal benefits, but remains controversial. Corticosteroid administration should be more strongly considered in patients with possible bilateral Meniere's disease, as surgical intervention may render the vestibular and auditory systems nonfunctional.

TABLE 24–1   MEDICAL THERAPY FOR MENIERE'S DISEASE

Therapy

Low-sodium diet

Thiazide diuretic

Methazolamide

Corticosteroid administration (systemically or intratympanically)

Vestibular suppressants and antiemetics

SURGICAL TREATMENT OF MENIERE'S DISEASE

Surgery is indicated when medical treatment fails to relieve the acute attacks of vertigo and the frequency and severity of the vertigo is disabling. None of the surgical techniques for Meniere's disease has demonstrated any substantive benefit on hearing or tinnitus.

A variety of surgical therapies are used to treat the vertigo of intractable Meniere's disease. These include, in order of increasing invasiveness, aminoglycoside perfusion, endolymphatic sac shunt or decompression, and labyrinthectomy or vestibular neurectomy. The procedure selected depends on the individual's age, functional level, and degree of hearing impairment in both the affected ear and the opposite ear. Every effort should be made to preserve functional hearing.

Surgery is successful in relieving acute attacks of vertigo or drop attacks in most patients but varies according to the procedure used. Unsteadiness, however, may persist for a period of several weeks to months, until the central nervous system compensates for the loss of vestibular function in the operated ear. Compensation following surgery for Meniere's disease is dependent on other factors such as age, visual impairment, and other neurologic dysfunction.

AMINOGLYCOSIDE MIDDLE EAR PERFUSION

The ototoxic-vestibular more so than cochlear properties of gentamicin are used to chemically ablate the vestibular system. The drug is injected either through a needle or through a catheter that has been inserted through a myringotomy in the posterior aspect of the tympanic membrane. The drug is administered until the affected labyrinth is sufficiently suppressed or destroyed. Treatment may be stopped if the hearing is affected. Vertigo is con-

trolled in 80 to 90% of patients, and hearing is lost in up to 30%.[1] Some persistent imbalance, usually mild, is common after the treatment. Many patients choose this treatment option because it is the least invasive, it is done on an outpatient basis, it entails little risk, and it has a relatively high chance of successful control of vertigo.

ENDOLYMPHATIC SAC SURGERY

This procedure is thought to work by relieving endolymph pressure, that is, relief of hydrops. Most cases are done under general anesthesia on an outpatient basis. A more complete description of technique is given below. Endolymphatic sac decompression and sac shunting have been reported to be successful in 65 to 90% of patients.[2,3] Endolymphatic sac surgery is an attractive option when hearing is serviceable in the involved ear and when both ears are affected, or there is a significant chance of developing Meniere's in the contralateral ear (i.e., younger patients). Significant loss of hearing follows endolymphatic sac surgery in 1 to 2% of cases.[4,5] Patients may choose this option because it does not "burn any bridges" (i.e., all of the other surgical treatment options remain), though its chance of success is slightly lower than its alternatives.

Endolymphatic sac surgery has fallen into disfavor among some surgeons because of reports from a Danish "sham" endolymphatic sac surgery study that suggested that endolymphatic sac surgery yielded results no better than simple mastoidectomy.[6] Reanalysis of the Danish data and more rigorous evaluation in subsequent studies have since lent support to the benefits of endolymphatic sac surgery.

There are few contraindications to endolymphatic sac surgery. These include congenital inner ear dysplasias, such as enlarged vestibular aqueducts, which may be identified radiographically in patients that have had lifelong cochleovestibular dysfunction. Additionally, patients with tertiary syphilis and perilymph fistula may present similar to patients with Meniere's disease. These conditions must be ruled out before endolymphatic sac surgery is performed.

LABYRINTHECTOMY

This technique is covered in more detail in Chapter 25. Briefly, the vestibular labyrinth is surgically eviscerated through a standard mastoidectomy or a transcanal approach. Labyrinthectomy eliminates vertigo in 95% of cases.[7] This procedure causes total deafness in the operated ear (except in certain experimental procedures). Therefore, labyrinthectomy is generally recommended for patients with no usable hearing in the involved ear. As this procedure requires a surgery and the benefits are only slightly better than those observed with gentamicin perfusion therapy, this procedure has become much less common since the introduction of gentamicin therapy.

VESTIBULAR NEURECTOMY

This procedure requires a craniotomy and division of the vestibular nerve via either a middle fossa or suboccipital approach. Hearing is usually preserved, but up to 10% have profound hearing loss postoperatively.[8] Vertigo is eliminated in 85 to 90% of cases.[9,10] This treatment option has also become less common since the introduction of gentamicin therapy, as the results are similar and the latter does not require a craniotomy. This treatment option, however, should be considered by younger patients who are more critically dependent on their hearing for their daily activities (e.g., musicians).

ENDOLYMPHATIC SAC SURGICAL TECHNIQUE

The surgical suite is set up as it is for doing a mastoidectomy, with the bed turned either 90 or 180 degrees. The patient should be positioned with the nonoperative ear approximated to the contralateral shoulder. This improves visualization of the sac as it exits the labyrinth, toward the descending segment of the sigmoid sinus. As the endolymphatic sac may be in close proximity to the facial nerve, intraoperative monitoring should be considered.

An incision is made just outside the postauricular crease (Fig. 24–1). Lidocaine with epinephrine (1:100,000 or 1:200,000) may be infiltrated into the soft tissue prior to incision for vasoconstriction. The mastoid periosteum is divided in a cursive T (Fig. 24–2) and elevated to expose the entire mastoid cortex (Fig. 24–3). The cartilaginous ear canal is elevated off of the spine of Henle to allow full visualization of the posterior bony external auditory canal. A complete mastoidectomy is performed and the lateral semicircular canal is exposed (Fig. 24–4). Just posterior to the lateral canal, bone over the posterior semicircular canal is taken down until the latter canal can be appreciated. The endolymphatic sac will generally be apparent just caudal to the posterior canal. The mastoid segment of the facial nerve is identified, leaving a thin layer of bone overlying, as the sac may be medial to the nerve (Fig. 24–5). Failure to recognize the facial nerve may lead to injury on its posterior or medial surface. The sigmoid sinus is skeletonized and followed medially along the posterior fossa, up to the posterior semicircular canal (Fig. 24–6). The eggshell-thin bone over the sigmoid is fenestrated with a diamond bur, creating either an island of bone to remove in

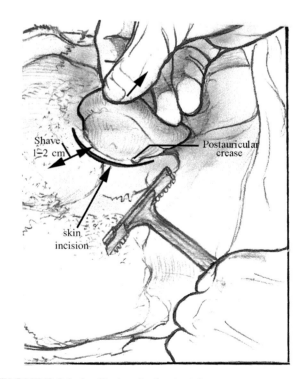

FIGURE 24–1 Postauricular incision.

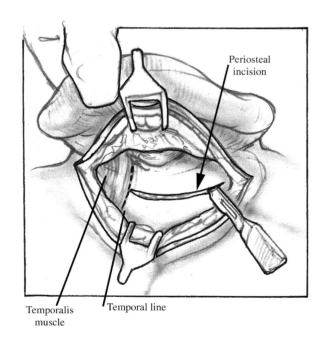

FIGURE 24–2 The mastoid periosteum is divided in a T fashion.

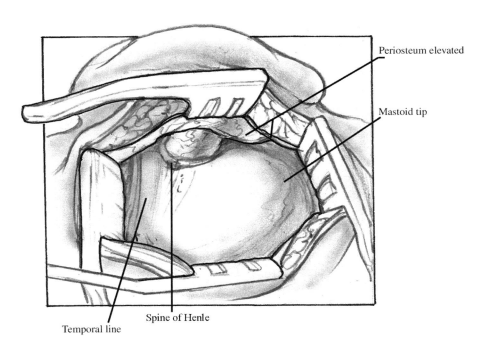

FIGURE 24–3   The mastoid periosteum is elevated until cortex is completely exposed, including the spine of Henle.

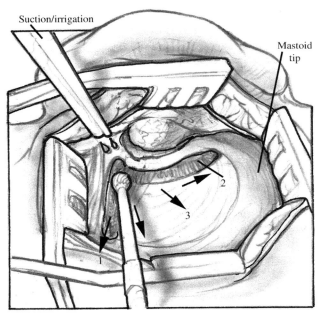

FIGURE 24–4   A mastoidectomy is performed with bone removed in a smooth plane and the deepest point of the dissection over the mastoid antrum.

toto or a slit from which to elevate the remaining bone. Bipolar cauterization of the sigmoid sinus improves visualization of the posterior fossa dura. Bone over the posterior fossa is then taken down, lateral to medial, up to the posterior semicircular

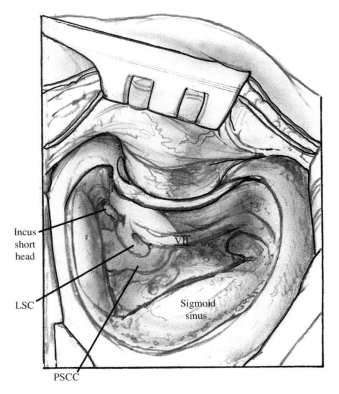

FIGURE 24–5   After completion of the simple mastoidectomy, the lateral and posterior semicircular canal (PSCC) and sigmoid sinus are exposed. The mastoid segment of the facial nerve is identified, but left covered with bone.

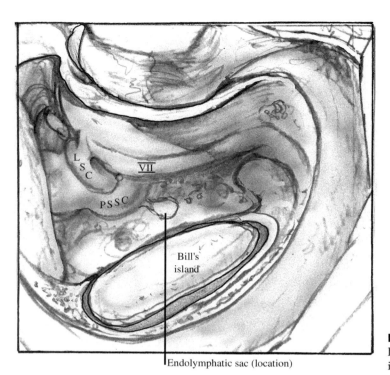

Endolymphatic sac (location)

FIGURE 24–6 The sigmoid sinus and vestibular labyrinth are skeletonized, with creation of an island of bone over the dome of the sinus.

canal and extending inferiorly as much as the sigmoid sinus will allow. The sac may be identified by elevating the dura and sac off the posterior face of the posterior semicircular canal and palpating the bony operculum more anteromedially (Fig. 24–7). The wound is thoroughly irrigated and closed in

layers with absorbable sutures. A mastoid pressure dressing is applied. This completes an endolymphatic sac decompression.

The endolymphatic sac may be opened and a shunt inserted (Fig. 24–8). The value of shunts has been questioned, relative to decompression, as

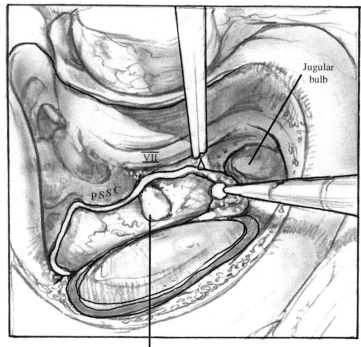

Endolymphatic sac exposed

FIGURE 24–7 Bone over the sigmoid sinus and posterior fossa cortex is removed up to the posterior semicircular canal. The endolymphatic sac and duct can be confirmed by palpating the operculum medial to the posterior canal.

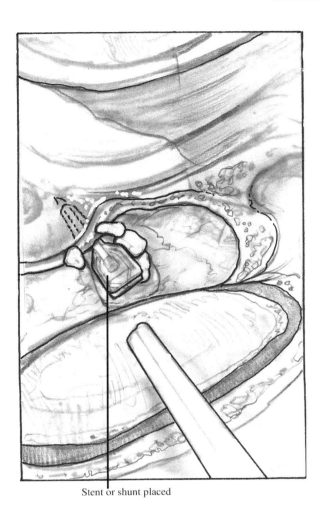

Stent or shunt placed

FIGURE 24–8   The endolymphatic sac may be incised and a shunt inserted into the sac lumen.

shunts typically become encased in fibrous tissue. Presumably this renders the shunt ineffective. The efficacy of endolymphatic sac decompression and shunt are equivalent.

POSTOPERATIVE CARE

Patients need not be admitted to the hospital. Patients traveling from long distances are encouraged to stay in a local hotel overnight to ensure that there are no significant postoperative difficulties in the immediate postoperative period.

The mastoid pressure dressing is removed on the first postoperative day. No special wound cares are necessary. Hair washing may be allowed on the third postoperative day. The first postoperative visit may take place as early as 1 week postoperatively or be delayed up to 6 weeks (e.g., for patients traveling long distances).

RISKS AND COMPLICATIONS OF ENDOLYMPHATIC SAC SURGERY

VERTIGO AND DYSEQUILIBRIUM

All surgery for vertigo is marked by a certain failure rate. Approximately 10 to 35% of patients have persistent vertigo with endolymphatic sac decompression or shunting.[2,6,11] Furthermore, control of hydrops exacerbations does not restore the vestibular system to normal. A certain degree of imbalance or dysequilibrium, usually mild, can be expected postoperatively. This is primarily a problem when relying on the vestibular system in the absence of visual cues (e.g., trying to balance in the dark while standing on soft carpet). Occasionally, such imbalance can be frustrating for patients, leading to dissatisfaction with the procedure if they are not properly counseled preoperatively. These symptoms are often improved with physical therapy.

HEARING LOSS

All surgery for vertigo also carries a certain risk for worsening hearing loss. Hearing loss in patients with Meniere's disease tends to fluctuate and progress, regardless of most treatments. Only 1 or 2% of patients experience a significant drop in hearing related to the surgical procedure.

TINNITUS

Tinnitus is usually not directly affected by surgery. Tinnitus often correlates well with hearing. As the hearing improves, so may the tinnitus. Tinnitus may in rare circumstances become much worse postoperatively.

FACIAL WEAKNESS

Temporary facial nerve weakness may occur after surgery secondary to edema of the nerve. This occurs in less than 1% of patients who have endolymphatic sac surgery. Facial function typically returns within several weeks. If the facial nerve is not identified and protected, nerve transection and prolonged palsy may result.

CEREBROSPINAL FLUID LEAK

Endolymphatic sac surgery carries a risk of dural fenestration, resulting in a cerebrospinal fluid leak. This may occur when arachnoid granulations are uncovered during drilling or through tears in congenital or age-related dural defects. Leaks through arachnoid granulations can be easily controlled by leaving cortical bone around the granulation and applying bone wax directly over the defect. Tears in dura may require packing with abdominal fat if they cannot be closed primarily.

INFECTION

Infection is extremely uncommon and usually responds to medical therapy. If infection occurs in the presence of a cerebrospinal fluid leak, meningitis may develop.

LONG-TERM PROGNOSIS

As with any surgery for vestibular disease, long-term outcomes wane slightly over time. Long-term studies are lacking. In many cases of recidivism, the ipsilateral ear is the cause, but in a significant percentage, the contralateral ear becomes problematic. When symptoms recur, patients should resume medical treatment (Table 24–1). Patients with persistent symptoms originating in the operated ear, despite ongoing medical therapy, may be considered for ablative therapy, ranging from aminoglycoside perfusion to vestibular nerve section.

REFERENCES

1. McFeely WJ, Singleton GT, Rodriguez FJ, Antonelli PJ. Intratympanic gentamicin treatment for Meniere's disease. *Otolaryngol Head Neck Surg* 1998;118:589–596.

2. Gianoli, GJ, Larouere MJ, Kartush JM, Wayman J. Sacvein decompression for intractable Meniere's disease: two-year treatment results. *Otolaryngol Head Neck Surg* 1998;118:22–29.

3. Paparella MM, Goycoolea M. Endolymphatic sac enhancement surgery for Meniere's disease: an extension of conservative therapy. *Ann Otol* 1981; 90:610–615.

4. Gibson WPR. The effect of surgical removal of the extraosseous portion of the endolymphatic sac in patients suffering from Meniere's disease. *J Laryngol Otol* 1996;110:1008–1011.

5. Welling DB, Pasha R, Roth LJ, Barin K. The effect of endolymphatic sac excision in Meniere's disease. *Am J Otol* 1996;17:278–282.

6. Bretlau P, Thomsen J, Tos M, Johnsen NJ. Placebo effect in surgery for Meniere's disease: nine-year follow-up. *Am J Otol* 1989;10:259–261.

7. Graham MD, Goldsmith MM. Labyrinthectomy: indications and surgical technique. *Otolaryngol Clin North Am* 1994;27:325–335.

8. De La Cruz A, McElveen JT. Hearing preservation in vestibular neurectomy. *Laryngoscope* 1984;94:874–877.

9. Brookes GB. The role of vestibular nerve section in Meniere's disease. *Ear Nose Throat J* 1997;76:652–656, 658–659, 663.

10. Thedinger BS, Thedinger BA. Analysis of patients with persistent dizziness after vestibular nerve section. *Ear Nose Throat J* 1998;77:290–292, 295–298.

11. Graham MD, Kemink JL. Surgical management of Meniere's disease with endolymphatic sac decompression by wide bony decompression of the posterior fossa dura: technique and results. *Laryngoscope* 1984;94:680–682.

Chapter 25

Transmastoid and Transcanal Labyrinthectomy

Tina C. Huang and Samuel C. Levine

Initial attempts to control vertigo are primarily medical; when those attempts fail, however, surgical approaches for control may be necessary. Multiple options exist including cochleosacculotomy, endolymphatic sac surgery, labyrinthectomy (transcanal and transmastoid) with or without vestibular nerve section, and vestibular nerve section (middle cranial fossa or retrosigmoid approach). Chemical labyrinthectomy has also become a commonly used option.

Surgical labyrinthectomy is a highly successful procedure for a patient with nonserviceable hearing in the affected ear. Jansen in 1895 was the first to describe ablation of the labyrinth during radical mastoidectomy for suppurative labyrinthitis. In 1904 Lake described the use of the transmastoid labyrinthectomy for control of vertigo in nonsuppurative vertigo. Cawthorn reported a wall-up mastoid approach for labyrinthine ablation in 1943.

Crockett in 1903 was the first to describe a transcanal procedure for control of vertigo by removing the stapes. Lempert in 1948 reported on the endaural approach with removal of the stapes and decompression of the labyrinth. The transcanal labyrinthectomy with removal of the vestibular end organs, however, was first described by Schuknecht in 1956. In addition to removal of the membranous labyrinth manually or with suctioning, various agents have also been injected into the labyrinth for further ablation, and the use of laser and ultrasound has also been described.[1–3]

PATIENT SELECTION

Labyrinthectomy is usually the option of last resort for patients with intractable vertigo. It has classically been described for Meniere's disease patients with-out useful hearing for whom medical management has failed. Vestibular suppressants, diuretics, and vestibular rehabilitation should be given an adequate trial before surgical procedures.

Labyrinthectomy is used in refractory cases and it is therefore important to confirm a unilateral peripheral vestibular deficit and rule out other central causes of vertigo. A careful history should be reviewed for any trauma, systemic diseases, and neurologic disorders. Patients with vertigo due to sequelae from head trauma, vestibular neuronitis, viral labyrinthitis, ischemic disease, neurologic disorders, and positional vertigo are less likely to benefit from labyrinthectomy. Careful counseling is needed for these situations. Therefore, it is recommended that all patients should have a full audiometric evaluation, electronystagmography including cold calorics, and imaging of the internal auditory canals, preferably using magnetic resonance imaging. Laboratory tests for syphilis, Lyme disease, autoimmune disorders, and thyroid function should also be obtained. High-resolution computed tomography of the temporal bones may also be obtained for surgical planning and to check for any anomalies of the facial nerve or labyrinthine structures.

Because surgical labyrinthectomy is expected to result in total sensorineural hearing loss in the operated ear, confirmation of severe hearing loss is needed. Candidates generally have greater than 50-dB speech reception thresholds (SRTs) and less than 50% speech discrimination scores (SDSs) in the affected ear. Those patients with less than 30 dB SRT and greater than 70% SDS are generally considered candidates for hearing preservation procedures.[4,5] These guidelines assume normal hearing in the contralateral ear. In cases where the contralateral hearing is poor, the decision for surgery must be done on a case-by-case basis. Assessment of the binaural hearing should be done in cases where the opposite ear is also affected. Some surgeons advocate even greater SRT and SDS thresholds in Meniere's patients because of the possibility of developing bilateral Meniere's.[5]

In addition, a unilateral peripheral vestibular deficit must be demonstrated. Although the absence of a caloric response on the affected side should be approached cautiously, patients have had relief of vertigo even with an absent cold caloric. Caloric testing tests only the horizontal canal. There should be some function on the contralateral side, however. Patients with bilateral vestibular deficits often do poorly after unilateral vestibular ablation secondary to inadequate compensation. They are unable to maneuver in the dark and have constant dysequilibrium and oscillopsia. Even patients with normal contralateral vestibular function may suffer persistent ataxia after ablation, although it is usually not disabling. The preoperative status of the patient must also be taken into account. Obesity, impaired vision, arthritis, peripheral neurologic deficits, and other conditions that may impair patients' maneuverability may negatively impact their postoperative recovery.

Finally, the decision of transcanal versus transmastoid labyrinthectomy must be made. Chemical labyrinthectomy is also an option and is discussed later in the chapter. Although a transcanal procedure is shorter, has lower morbility, and is a more direct route to the labyrinth, multiple studies have shown that the success rate of a transcanal labyrinthectomy is lower and the recurrence rate of vertigo higher. This is likely due to the incomplete removal of all of the vestibular end organs. In patients who are a substantial operative risk, however, it is a valid approach.

SURGICAL TECHNIQUE

TRANSCANAL LABYRINTHECTOMY

Patients must undergo general anesthesia for surgical labyrinthectomies because of the nausea and vomiting that accompany removal of the labyrinth. A facial nerve monitor may be used during the procedure due to the proximity of the horizontal segment of the facial nerve to the operative site. Preoperative antibiotics and steroids are not required. Anesthesiologists should be asked not to use paralytic agents if facial nerve monitoring is performed.

The patient is placed supine on the operating table with the affected ear up. The ear is prepped with antiseptic solution and draped accordingly. The operating microscope is also draped after checking for proper balance. A transcanal approach is sufficient for most patients; however, if the canal is narrow, an endaural or postauricular incision may be necessary for full exposure. Local anesthetic with 1:100,000 epinephrine is injected into the canal. Using the largest speculum possible in a speculum holder, a long tympanomeatal flap is raised. Part of the scutum is then removed either using a curette or a small bur to expose the horizontal segment of the facial nerve. Full exposure of the facial nerve and oval and round windows is required (Fig. 25–1A). A portion of the posterior bony canal may also need to be removed. The incus can be removed and the stapedial tendon sectioned (Fig. 25–1B). The stapes is carefully removed by rocking in an anteroposterior

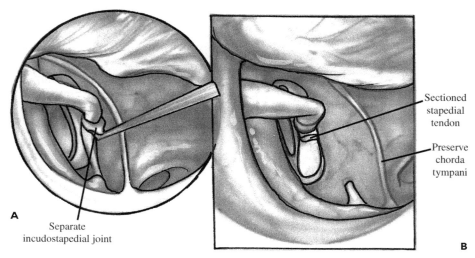

A — Separate incudostapedial joint

B — Sectioned stapedial tendon — Preserve chorda tympani

FIGURE 25–1 (A) Transcanal labyrinthectomy. A tympanomeatal flap has been raised and the incudostapedial joint separated. (B) Stapedial tendon is sectioned in preparation for removal of the stapes.

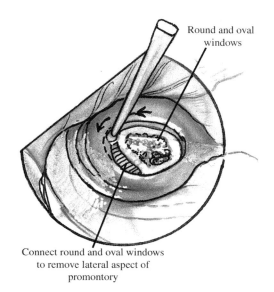

Round and oval
windows

Connect round and oval windows
to remove lateral aspect of
promontory

FIGURE 25–2 The oval and round windows are connected to remove the bony promontory.

motion to prevent fracture of the footplate. Avoid suctioning to prevent retraction of the utricle superiorly. The oval window is now enlarged using a microdrill, or the oval and round windows may be connected to remove the bony promontory (Fig. 25–2). The inferior portion of the round window niche is then removed to expose the posterior

ampullary nerve (singular nerve). Sectioning of the singular nerve facilitates a full labyrinthectomy, as the crista of the posterior semicircular canal is difficult to remove using the transcanal approach. The nerve is approximately 1 mm medial to the posterior edge of the round window niche at a 45-degree angle. Sectioning is done using a small pick (Fig. 25–3A). Any cerebrospinal fluid (CSF) leak that occurs can be controlled using bone wax.

Carefully examine the facial nerve for areas of dehiscence. The utricle is now removed using a 3- or 4-mm right-angle hook, whirlybird, or utricular hook. It lies in a recess that is deep and superior to the horizontal facial nerve (Fig. 25–3B). Irrigating with saline may be helpful at this point to free the utricle from the walls of the recess. Removal of the utricle usually also results in removal of the membranous horizontal and superior semicircular canals. The saccule is then removed by aspirating the medial portion of the vestibule. Fracture of the cribrose area, in the medial portion of the vestibule, results in a CSF leak from the internal auditory canal. The bony semicircular canals are then probed to destroy any residual neuroepithelium.

The vestibule can be packed either with Gelfoam or fat. This is not absolutely necessary, but leaving the windows open results in a pneumolabyrinth. Packing also helps contain any CSF leaks that may have occurred. The flap is then replaced and the

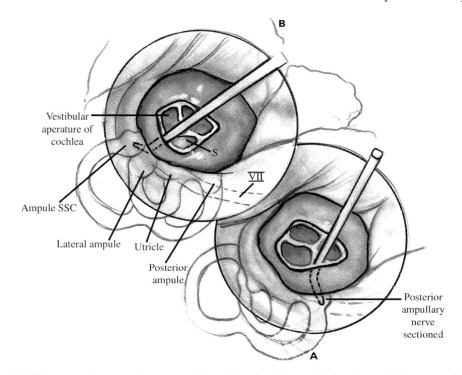

FIGURE 25–3 (A) The posterior ampullary nerve is sectioned with a pick. It is located 1 mm medial to the posterior edge of the round window at a 45-degree angle. (B) A hook is used to remove the utricle and semicircular canals, which are located deep and superior to the horizontal facial nerve. SCC superior semicircular canal; VII, facial nerve; S, saccule.

canal packed. If a postauricular incision was made, the incision is closed and a dressing placed.[6,7]

TRANSMASTOID LABYRINTHECTOMY

The patient is placed under general anesthesia and placed supine on the operating table. The table should be turned 90 or 180 degrees. The affected ear is up and the postauricular shave prep is extended several finger-breadths behind the ear. The exposure is usually a little more than that used in a standard mastoidectomy because of the need for greater exposure for the medial dissection. Place the facial nerve monitor leads and ensure that the monitor is working properly. A high-speed drill with multiple cutting and diamond burs should be available. Both monopolar and bipolar cautery should also be available. The postauricular area is then injected with epinephrine (1:100,000). If this is combined with local anesthesia, care must be taken not to inject at the mastoid tip and anesthetize the facial nerve. The anesthesiologist should be informed that nerve monitoring is taking place, and so paralytics should be avoided. If more than one anesthesiologist is giving agents during the procedure, it is important to communicate this instruction. In some operating room settings, this is instruction is posted in a prominent location. Preoperative antibiotics and steroids have not been shown to affect outcomes or postoperative infection rates.

The area is then prepped and draped in a sterile fashion. The surgeon should also check the operating microscope and ensure proper balance prior to draping. A postauricular incision is made and carried down to the temporalis muscle. Monopolar cautery is then used to make a T incision along the linea temporalis and down to the mastoid tip. A Lempert elevator is used to widely elevate the periosteum off the mastoid cortex, taking care to identify the spine of Henle anteriorly. The soft tissues are then held in place using self-retaining retractors. Any bleeding encountered during the dissection is controlled using electrocautery. A dry field is important for good visualization of the operative area.

A cortical mastoidectomy is then performed using a large cutting bur and continuous suction irrigation. The tegmen and sigmoid sinus are identified and the posterior bony canal thinned. The sinodural angle is opened widely for exposure of the vestibule. The antral air cell is entered and the horizontal canal, fossa incudis, and body of the incus should all be seen clearly (Fig. 25–4). The sigmoid sinus may also need to be decompressed for adequate exposure of the posterior semicircular canal. The bone over the sinus is carefully thinned and removed. Bipolar

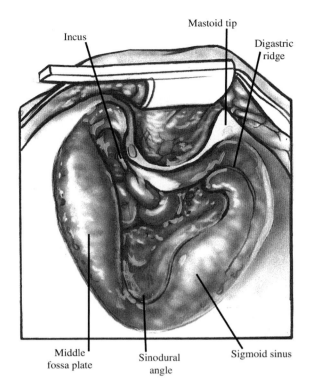

FIGURE 25–4 Transmastoid labyrinthectomy. A view of the horizontal canal, fossa incudis, body of the incus, tegmen, and sigmoid sinus after the cortical mastoidectomy.

cautery is then used to collapse the sinus. Leaving an island of bone covering the sinus requires the use of a retractor. No ill effects usually result from superficial coagulation and contraction of the sigmoid sinus. The vertical segment of the facial nerve is now carefully identified using a large diamond bur.

The lateral (horizontal) semicircular canal identified during the mastoidectomy is completely delineated. Many surgeons prefer to completely remove all air cells surrounding the labyrinth. The horizontal canal is "blue lined" and followed posteriorly to the posterior semicircular canal. This process is usually done with a diamond bur to also identify the relationship of the canals and the second genu of the facial nerve. The posterior canal is then delineated in a similar manner (Fig. 25–5). Removal of bone is carried medially on both canals, being careful to keep a flat plane of dissection without irregularities that might cause the bur to skip and injure the facial nerve. The posterior canal dissection requires much more bone removal and goes further medial. The area where the posterior and superior canals join is the common crus. The superior canal establishes the medial limit of the dissection (Fig.

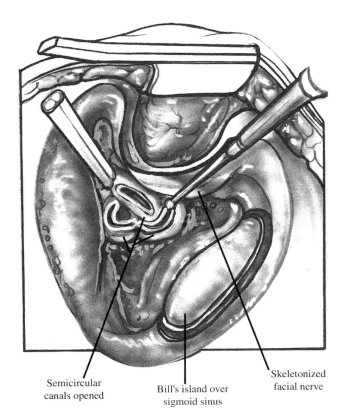

Semicircular
canals opened

Bill's island over
sigmoid sinus

Skeletonized
facial nerve

FIGURE 25–5   The decompressed sigmoid sinus and vertical segment of the facial nerve are identified prior to opening of the semicircular canals.

25–6A). The anterior ampullated end is immediately superior to the ampullae of the horizontal canal. The

superiormost point of dissection is the arcuate eminence. To see this point and the whole length of the canal, it may be necessary to angle the head of the microscope upward. The crus is then followed to the vestibule. The vestibule lies under (medial to) the facial nerve anteriorly. The bone covering the external genu of the facial nerve is thinned and the anterior and inferior portion of the posterior canal is opened to its ampulla. At the conclusion of drilling, it should be possible to see the open ampullae of all of the semicircular canals and the vestibule without any remaining bone dividing them. Once all the canals and vestibule have been opened, the neuroepithelium is removed with a right-angle hook (Fig. 25–6B).

The mastoid periosteum is now closed in layers. It is not necessary to pack the cavity with tissue unless a CSF leak has occurred. The area of the leak must be identified and repaired with tissue prior to packing of the cavity. A mastoid dressing is placed over the ear and the patient is brought out of anesthesia.[8–10]

POSTOPERATIVE CARE

The external dressing is removed the next day. Postoperative nausea, vomiting, and oscillopsia are to be expected. The degree of postoperative symptoms correlates with the degree of vestibular function preoperatively. A greater amount of vestibular function leads to greater symptoms once the labyrinth has been ablated. Symptoms can be controlled

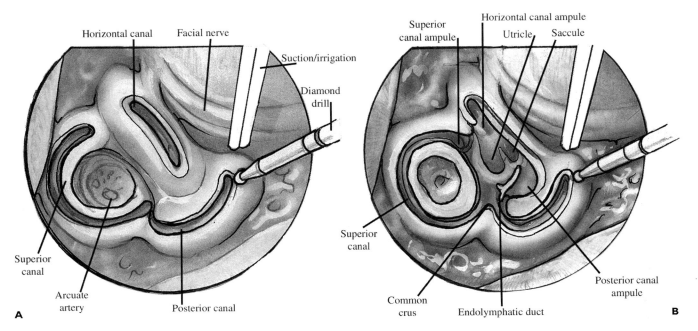

Horizontal canal   Facial nerve
Suction/irrigation
Diamond drill
Superior canal
Arcuate artery
Posterior canal
A

Horizontal canal ampule
Superior canal ampule   Utricle   Saccule
Superior canal
Common crus   Endolymphatic duct
Posterior canal ampule
B

FIGURE 25–6   (A) All three canals have been opened. The superior canal is the medial limit of the dissection and the arcuate artery is visible between the superior and horizontal canals. (B) The finished labyrinthectomy prior to removal of the neuroepithelium. All ampullae and the vestibule should be visible.

with vestibular suppressants; the use of suppressants should be conservative, however, as they may cause delayed or decreased compensation. Intravenous fluids should be given until the patient is able to ingest liquids without vomiting.

Patients are encouraged to sit up on the first postoperative day and begin ambulating as soon as possible. Vestibular rehabilitation is started while they are inpatients and continued after discharge. Follow-up in the clinic after 1 week to remove packing or sutures is common.

COMPLICATIONS

The complication rate for surgical labyrinthectomy is 1% or less. Complications include CSF leak, facial nerve injury, and failure to find the neuroepithelium. A CSF leak may occur in a transcanal labyrinthectomy when the cribrose bone is fractured. This is repaired using a tissue seal. In a transmastoid approach, the dura overlying the tegmen or the internal auditory canal may be damaged causing a CSF leak. These too are repaired with tissue. Facial nerve injury may be avoided in the transcanal approach by widely opening the scutum and posterior bony canal for adequate visualization of the horizontal portion of the facial nerve. Probing the portion for dehiscence will also indicate the areas to be avoided. Careful skeletonization of the vertical portion of the facial nerve and the external genu in the transmastoid approach prevents accidental injury to the nerve. Treatment of injury follows that of any iatrogenic facial nerve injury. Failure to find the neuroepithelium is more common in the transcanal labyrinthectomy. Again, care must be taken not to aspirate fluid from the vestibule prior to removing the utricle to prevent retraction of the utricle. The ampulla of the posterior semicircular canal is difficult to remove in a transcanal approach, and a singular neurectomy may be performed in conjunction with the labyrinthectomy to denervate the posterior canal. Wound infection rates for a transmastoid labyrinthectomy are also less than 1% and are treated with antibiotics. Meningitis is extremely rare and is treated with intravenous antibiotics. If meningitis occurs, it is almost always a result of a CSF leak.

Traumatic neuroma formation has been reported after both transcanal and transmastoid labyrinthectomies. A study by Ylikoski and Belal[11,12] on vestibular nerve morphology after labyrinthectomy found fibrosis and ossification and degeneration of the labyrinth in the majority of the temporal bones. The majority of the specimens, however, showed normal or only a slight decrease in the density of the vestibular neurons in the internal auditory canal. In addition, they found evidence of regeneration in nerve fibers and ganglion cells after labyrinthectomy with neuroma formation in several of the specimens. However, the significance of neuroma formation has yet to be shown. It has been postulated that there may be residual function in the neuroma leading to recurrent vertigo, but this has not been proven.[13] To prevent neuroma formation, complete excision of Scarpa's ganglion must be performed.[14]

RESULTS

Rates of control of vertigo after a transmastoid labyrinthectomy range from 90 to 98%; however, the recurrence of vertigo after a transcanal labyrinthectomy may be as high as 15%. This is likely secondary to the incomplete removal of neuroepithelium. Some debate exists over the success rate of surgical procedures to control non-Meniere's vertigo. Benecke[15] reported good success with labyrinthectomy for patients suffering from vertigo from a variety of reasons, and Hashimoto et al[16] reported on a small number of patients with ipsilateral delayed endolymphatic hydrops who were cured after transmastoid labyrinthectomy. Yazdi and Rutka[17] also had good results with their delayed endolymphatic hydrops patients.

Improvement in tinnitus is approximately 70%. Temporal bone specimens have shown that persistent cochlear hydrops may occur secondary to obstruction of the hook region of the cochlea and the ductus reunions.[18] This may result in persistent tinnitus and aural fullness.

Unfortunately, approximately one quarter to one third of patients develop permanent dysequilibrium of varying intensity. Eisenman et al[19] found a 55% incidence of balance dysfunction in patients undergoing a transmastoid labyrinthectomy. Pereira and Kerr[20] reported that even with an 89% cure rate, only 50% of their patients returned to work. Neither age nor relief of vertigo predicted a return to work. Although it has been assumed that elderly patients have poorer vestibular compensation, Gacek and Gacek[4] found that age was not a factor in developing unsteadiness. Levine et al[21] reported on long-term results of labyrinthectomy and found a decline in cure rates from 93 to 76% after 10 years. They proposed several different reasons for the decline, including increasing age with concomitant morbid conditions, vertebrobasilar insufficiency, and the development of bilateral Meniere's disease.

LABYRINTHECTOMY IN THE ELDERLY

Several articles have been published regarding the benefit of labyrinthectomy in patients over 65 years of age. The authors have not found that advanced age is a contraindication for vestibular ablation. Silverstein et al[5] and Dayal and Proctor[22] emphasize the importance of defining the cause of vertigo in this population. Dizziness and dysequilibrium rather than vertigo may be the primary complaint, and these conditions may be caused by conditions such as vertebrobasilar ischemia, poor vision, neuropathy with poor proprioception, and basal ganglia disease. Schwaber et al[23] found a 54% incidence of postoperative dysequilibrium with a 91% rate of vertigo control. Langman and Lindeman[24] report permanent dysequilibrium in 41% of patients who underwent a transmastoid labyrinthectomy and a 62.5% incidence in those who underwent a transcanal labyrinthectomy with an almost 100% cure rate for both procedures. A smaller group of patients treated by Dayal and Proctor had no permanent dysequilibrium and 100% control of vertigo. All the studies recommend a transmastoid approach if possible due to the better visualization and removal of neuroepithelium.[25]

COCHLEAR IMPLANTATION AFTER LABYRINTHECTOMY

A complete loss of hearing on the operated side is an expected outcome of surgical labyrinthectomy. This led to hesitation to perform this procedure in patients with poor hearing in the contralateral ear and for those patients with Meniere's disease due to the possibility of developing bilateral Meniere's disease. The incidence of bilateral Meniere's disease ranges from 2 to 73%.[5,17,26] Gacek[4] found that patients who had undergone surgical control of vertigo secondary to Meniere's had a less than 1% chance of developing bilateral disease. Regardless, the incidence of bilateral disease rises as follow-up increases. Not only is bilateral Meniere's disease disabling from a vestibular standpoint, but also there exists the risk for losing hearing in the only hearing ear.

Poor hearing in the contralateral ear may no longer be a contraindication for ablative procedures because cochlear implantation is possible for a previously labyrinthectomized ear. Multiple morphologic studies have been done on the cochlear nerve after labyrinthectomy that have found that although the organ of Corti showed severe degeneration, axons of the cochlear nerve remained intact.[11,12,18,27] Spiral ganglion cell densities were decreased, but they were not entirely absent and were present in numbers equal to those from successful cochlear implant users. Promontory electrical stimulation in postlabyrinthectomy patients generate auditory responses in multiple studies.[28–30] Because of these results, the authors of these studies now advocate surgical ablative approaches that do the least damage to the cochlea and cochlear nerve, that is, transmastoid labyrinthectomy as opposed to a transcanal approach.

Brackmann in 1975 was the first to implant a cochlear electrode array into a labyrinthectomized ear with positive auditory responses. Zwolan et al[31] implanted a prelingually deafened patient in the same procedure as a labyrinthectomy for intractable vertigo with good results. One of the technical challenges of postlabyrinthectomy cochlear implantation is obliteration of the vestibule with fibrosis and bony growth. Kemink et al[29] suggested placing an obturator in the scala tympani at the time of labyrinthectomy to maintain its patency. Facer et al[32] report on a patient who underwent implantation 18 months after a transmastoid labyrinthectomy with good results. Lastly, Morgan et al[33] implanted a patient who had undergone a chemical labyrinthectomy with gentamicin for Meniere's disease, again with good results.

CHEMICAL LABYRINTHECTOMY

Chemical ablation of the vestibular system is not a new technique. Streptomycin sulfate was developed in 1944 and was found to have ototoxic effects, primarily on the vestibular system. Fowler in 1948 was the first to use systemic streptomycin for the control of vertigo. Hanson reported not only cure of vertigo but improved hearing in several of his patients treated with systemic streptomycin. Since then, multiple studies have been conducted using systemic streptomycin with good control of vertigo and varying degrees of hearing loss.[34] Systemic administration of an ototoxic drug damages both ears, and the majority of patients with vertigo have disease in one ear. In addition, bilateral decreased vestibular function often led to permanent ataxia and oscillopsia.[35] In 1957 Schuknecht delivered streptomycin intratympanically with good relief of vertigo but complete loss of hearing in all of the patients. Shea was the first to use streptomycin in the inner ear via perfusion into the lateral semicircular canal with good results in 1988. Adair and Kerr[36] did a modification of the Shea procedure with a success rate of 94% but a hearing preservation rate of only 50%.

The first reported trial of intratympanic gentamicin therapy was by Beck and Schmidt in 1978.[37] Vertigo was controlled in more than 90% of the patients, but hearing preservation was achieved in only 42%. Gentamicin sulfate causes vestibular toxicity by damaging the hair cells of the vestibular epithelium. It also damages the dark cells, which in turn leads to a reduction in the volume of endolymph. The pathway of gentamicin entry into the inner ear through the middle ear may involve several routes. The most likely is via the round window membrane. The annular ligament of the oval window, blood or lymph vessels, and the small lacunae in the bony capsule are also possible routes of entry. Gentamicin sulfate, being an acidic solution, is generally buffered with sodium bicarbonate to a pH of 6.4 because acidic solutions also cause damage to both vestibular and cochlear hair cells.

No single protocol has yet been advanced for the administration of intratympanic gentamicin.[38] Initial studies were done on patients admitted to the hospital for close observation.[39,40] These often involved placing a tympanostomy tube. Some studies have attempted to deliver a specific drug quantity through a catheter or wick.[26,34,37,41] The tympanostomy tube should be placed in the posteroinferior quadrant of the tympanic membrane to ensure proximity to the round window niche. The courses of treatment consist of multiple injections a day for several days.[40] Newer studies aim at finding a course of outpatient treatment.[42–44] Often a tympanostomy tube is placed in the tympanic membrane and gentamicin is injected into the middle ear once a week until symptoms develop. The patient is placed supine with the treatment ear at a 30- to 45-degree angle and the patient is instructed to lie in that position for at least 30 minutes. The patient is also often instructed not to swallow during that time, as it has been shown that swallowing increases the rate of efflux from the eustachian tube.[45] Several researchers are using Gelfoam placed in the round window niche to try to prolong exposure of the round window membrane to the drug.[46] With the advent of otologic endoscopes, some physicians are advocating examination of the round window niche and clearing of adhesions overlying the round window membrane prior to tympanostomy tube insertion.[45]

Topical gentamicin results in rates of control similar to those of surgical labyrinthectomy. Complete control ranges from 78 to 90%, whereas 91 to 100% of patients exhibit substantial control. Hearing preservation ranges from 25 to 91%. A significant number of patients also develop permanent ataxia and dysequilibrium after treatment. The usual end points of treatment are the development of symptoms such as oscillopsia, deterioration of tandem gait, nystagmus using Frenzel's glasses, or deterioration in pure tone thresholds of 10 dB in three or more consecutive frequencies. The use of clinical end points may be one reason why such a high percentage of hearing deterioration is seen. Gentamicin exhibits a prolonged course of action and the delay in development of signs and symptoms may cause patients to receive excess amounts of the drug. Odvisk has found that more than 6 consecutive days of therapy increased the chance of hearing damage. Other studies have also found that increased duration of therapy increases the chance of hearing loss. Therefore, newer protocols have lengthened the time between treatments or give a short course of treatment, reevaluate, and continue treatment as needed.[47]

CONCLUSION

Surgical labyrinthectomy is an excellent procedure for control of disabling vertigo not relieved by medical therapy. Cure rates are in the 90% range. Surgical labyrinthectomy results in complete hearing loss in the operated ear, however, and a significant minority of patients experience permanent dysequilibrium following the procedure. Often the dysequilibrium is not disabling and the possibility of cochlear implantation after labyrinthectomy decreases the morbidity of hearing loss. In addition, chemical labyrinthectomy is now being widely used as an alternative to surgical procedures. With continued research into cochlea-sparing treatment protocols, chemical labyrinthectomy may become the procedure of choice for intractable vertigo.

REFERENCES

1. Nomura T, Okuno T, Mizuno M. Treatment of vertigo using laser labyrinthectomy. *Acta Otolaryngol (Stockh)* 1993;113:261–262.
2. Nomura Y, Okuno T, Young Y-H, Hara M. Laser labyrinthectomy in humans. *Acta Otolaryngol (Stockh)* 1991;111:319–326.
3. Snow JB, Kimmelman CP. Assessment of surgical procedures for Meniere's disease. *Laryngoscope* 1979;89:737–747.
4. Gacek RR, Gacek MR. Comparison of labyrinthectomy and vestibular neurectomy in the control of vertigo. *Laryngoscope* 1996;106:225–230.
5. Silverstein H, Arruda J, Rosenberg SI, Deems D, Hester TO. Direct round window membrane applica-

tion of gentamicin in the treatment of Meniere's disease. *Otolaryngol Head Neck Surg* 1999;120:649–655.

6. Goycoolea MV, Ruah CV, Lavinsky L, Morales-Garcia C. Overall view and rationale for surgical alternatives for incapacitating peripheral vertigo. *Otolaryngol Clin North Am* 1994;27:283–300.

7. Pulec J. Surgical treatment of vertigo. *Acta Otolaryngol Suppl (Stockh)* 1995;519:21–25.

8. Brackmann DE, Shelton C, Arriaga MA. *Otologic Surgery.* Philadelphia: WB Saunders; 1994.

9. Graham MD, Goldsmith MM. Labyrinthectomy: indications and surgical technique. *Otolaryngol Clin North Am* 1994;27:325–335.

10. Langman AW, Lindeman RC. Surgery for vertigo in the nonserviceable hearing ear: transmastoid labyrinthectomy or translabyrinthine vestibular nerve section. *Laryngoscope* 1993;103:1321–1325.

11. Ylikoski J, Belal A. Human vestibular nerve morphology after labyrinthectomy. *Am J Otolaryngol* 1981;2:81–93.

12. Ylikoski J, Belal A, House WF. Morphology of the human cochlear nerve after labyrinthectomy. *Acta Otolaryngol* 1981;91:161–171.

13. Linthicum FH, Alonso A, Denia A. Traumatic neuroma: a complication of transcanal labyrinthectomy. *Arch Otolaryngol* 1979;105:654–655.

14. Monsell EM, Brackmann DE, Linthicum FH. Why do vestibular destructive procedures sometimes fail? *Otolaryngol Head Neck Surg* 1988;99:472–479.

15. Benecke JE. Surgery for non-Meniere's vertigo. *Acta Otolaryngol Suppl (Stockh)* 1994;513:37–39.

16. Hashimoto S, Furukawa K, Sasaki T. Treatment of ipsilateral delayed endolymphatic hydrops. *Acta Otolaryngol Suppl (Stockh)* 1997;528:113–115.

17. Yazdi AK, Rutka J. Results of labyrinthectomy in the treatment of Meniere's disease and delayed endolymphatic hydrops. *J Otolaryngol* 1996;25:26–31.

18. Belal A. Pathology as it relates to ear surgery. IV: surgery of Meniere's disease. *J Laryngol Otol* 1984;98:127–138.

19. Eisenman DJ, Speers R, Telian SA. Labyrinthectomy versus vestibular neurectomy: long-term physiologic and clinical outcomes. *Otol Neurotol* 2001;22:539–548.

20. Pereira KD, Kerr AG. Disability after labyrinthectomy. *J Laryngol Otol* 1996;110:216–218.

21. Levine SC, Glasscock M, McKennan KX. Long-term results of labyrinthectomy. *Laryngoscope* 1990;100:125–127.

22. Dayal VS, Proctor T. Labyrinthectomy in the elderly. *Am J Otol* 1995;16:110–114.

23. Schwaber MK, Pensak ML, Reiber ME. Transmastoid labyrinthectomy in older patients. *Laryngoscope* 1995;105:1152–1154.

24. Langman AW, Lindeman RC. Surgical labyrinthectomy in the older patient. *Otolaryngol Head Neck Surg* 1998;118:739–742.

25. Rosenberg SI. Vestibular surgery for Meniere's disease in the elderly: a review of techniques and indications. *Ear Nose Throat J* 1999;78:443–446.

26. Corsten M, Marsan J, Schramm D, Robichaud J. Treatment of intractable Meniere's disease with in-

tratympanic gentamicin: review of the University of Ottawa experience. *J Otolaryngol* 1997;26:361–364.

27. Chen DA, Linthicum FH, Rizer FM. Cochlear histopathology in the labyrinthectomized ear: implications for cochlear implantation. *Laryngoscope* 1988;98:1170–1172.

28. Kartush JM, Linstrom CJ, Graham MD, Kulick KC, Bouchard KR. Promontory stimulation following labyrinthectomy: implications for cochlear implantation. *Laryngoscope* 1990;100:5–9.

29. Kemink JL, Kileny PR, Niparko JK, Telian SA. Electrical stimulation of the auditory system after labyrinthectomy. *Am J Otol* 1991;12:7–10.

30. Lambert PR, Ruth RA, Halpin CF. Promontory electrical stimulation in labyrinthectomized ears. *Arch Otolaryngol Head Neck Surg* 1990;116:197–201.

31. Zwolan TA, Shepard NT, Niparko JK. Labyrinthectomy with cochlear implantation. *Am J Otol* 1993;14:220–223.

32. Facer GW, Facer ML, Fowler CMF, Brey RH, Peterson AM. Cochlear implantation after labyrinthectomy. *Am J Otol* 2000;21:336–340.

33. Morgan M, Flood L, Hawthorne M. Chemical labyrinthectomy and cochlear implantation for Meniere's disease: an effective treatment or a last resort? *J Laryngol Otol* 1999;113:666–669.

34. Sataloff RT, McCarter A, Spiegel JR. Very high-dose streptomycin labyrinthectomy. *Ear Nose Throat J* 1996;75:239–243.

35. Hellstrom S, Odkvist L. Pharmacologic labyrinthectomy. *Otolaryngol Clin North Am* 1994;27:307–315.

36. Adair RA, Kerr AG. Streptomycin perfusion of the labyrinth in the treatment of Meniere's disease: a modified technique. *Clin Otolaryngol* 1999;24:55–57.

37. Pfleiderer AG. The current role of local intratympanic gentamicin therapy in the management of unilateral Meniere's disease. *Clin Otolaryngol* 1998;23:34–41.

38. Hirsch BE, Kamerer DB. Role of chemical labyrinthectomy in the treatment of Meniere's disease. *Otolaryngol Clin North Am* 1997;30:1039–1049.

39. Bagger-Sjoback D, Bergenius J, Lundberg A-M. Inner ear effects of topical gentamicin treatment in patients with Meniere's disease. *Am J Otol* 1990;11:406–410.

40. Murofushi T, Halmagyi GM, Yavor RA. Intratympanic gentamicin in Meniere's disease: results of therapy. *Am J Otol* 1997;18:52–57.

41. Nedzelski JM, Schessel DA, Bryce GE, Pfleiderer AG. Chemical labyrinthectomy: local application of gentamicin for the treatment of unilateral Meniere's disease. *Am J Otol* 1992;13:18–22.

42. Bath AP, Walsh RM, Bance ML. Presumed reduction of vestibular function in unilateral Meniere's disease with aminoglycoside eardrops. *J Laryngol Otol* 1999;113:916–918.

43. Harner SG, Kasperbauer JL, Facer GW, Beatty CW. Transtympanic gentamicin for Meniere's syndrome. *Laryngoscope* 1998;108:1446–1449.

44. Odkvist L. Gentamicin cures vertigo, but what happens to hearing? *Int Tinnitus J* 1997;3:133–136.

45. Silverstein H, Rosenberg S, Arruda J, Isaacson JE. Surgical ablation of the vestibular system in the treatment of Meniere's disease. *Otolaryngol Clin North Am* 1997;30:1075–1095.

46. Quaranta A, Aloisi A, De Benedeittis G, Scaringi A. Intratympanic therapy for Meniere's disease: high-concentration gentamicin with round-window protection. *Ann N Y Acad Sci* 1999;884:410–424.

47. Hone SW, Nedzelski J, Chen J. Does intratympanic gentamicin treatment for Meniere's disease cause complete vestibular ablation? *J Otolaryngol* 2000;29:83–87.

Chapter 26

Posterior Semicircular Canal Occlusion for Benign Paroxysmal Positional Vertigo

Pramit S. Malhotra and Rex S. Haberman II

Benign paroxysmal positional vertigo (BPPV) is an extremely common peripheral vestibular disorder. The origins of this pathology from free-floating particles in the posterior semicircular canal are well documented. Standard treatment is physical therapy utilizing particle-repositioning maneuvers. Physical therapeutic maneuvers successfully manage greater than 90% of patients with one or two attempts.[1] Patients who have failed particle-repositioning maneuvers and still have clear and persistent BPPV symptoms remain a clinical challenge. For a select group of patients, posterior semicircular canal (PSCC) occlusion is a therapeutic alternative.[2] This procedure involves the obliteration of the PSCC, and thus, prevents the canal from being motion sensitive. Success rates for this procedure for the symptoms of vertigo are reported near 100% in several studies.[3]

Diagnosis and Indications

BPPV manifests with a classic set of signs and symptoms. The classic symptoms are positional vertigo with the absence of hearing changes. Physical examination reveals the following:

1. Clockwise nystagmus with the left ear down during Dix-Hallpike maneuver
2. Counterclockwise nystagmus with the right ear down during Dix-Hallpike maneuver
3. Latency of 2 to 10 seconds
4. Fatigability
5. Vertigo
6. Reversal with sitting

It is essential that rotary nystagmus is observed during the Dix-Hallpike maneuver, confirming that the pathology is indeed from the PSCC.

Standard treatment with one or two Epley maneuvers successfully treats patients in the low 90% range.[1] Of the remaining patients, only a small subset will have symptoms troubling enough to warrant surgical intervention.

The two indications for PSCC occlusion after at least two particle-repositioning maneuvers have failed are as follows[4]:

1. Continuous symptoms for greater than 3 months
2. Recurrent symptomatic BPPV for 12 months or greater[5]

Contraindications

1. Only hearing or significantly better hearing ear
2. Active otomastoiditis

Preoperative Evaluation

The history should focus on confirming the diagnosis of BPPV as well as ruling out bilateral disease. Approximately 15% of patients may have bilateral BPPV.[3] Treatment should focus on the most symptomatic side first unless it is the significantly better hearing ear.

Physical exam should include a complete neuro-otologic exam with audiometry, electronystagmography (ENG) to confirm PSCC involvement, and magnetic resonance imaging (MRI) to rule out central pathology, and some clinicians request a variety of otologic-related metabolic labs.[6] A complete workup is essential before proceeding to the operative suite.

TABLE 26–1 SPECIAL INSTRUMENTS AND OTHER EQUIPMENT NEEDED FOR THE PROCEDURE

Fibrinogen glue (Tisseel, NHS Company, Hackensack, NJ)

Facial nerve monitor not routinely used

Mastoidectomy burs of choice

1- or 2-mm diamond bur

90-degree hook

Neurosurgical cottonoids

SURGICAL GOALS

The success of the surgery depends on two critical factors. The first is that the membranous labyrinth of the PSCC is not violated. Once the posterior semicircular canal is opened, no suctioning can be done in the proximity of the canal. The second critical factor is that the canal is packed tightly to avoid the possibility of a perilymph leak.

Special instruments are listed in Table 26–1.

ANESTHESIA

General endotracheal anesthesia is used.

OPERATIVE TECHNIQUE

After anesthesia induction and patient positioning, the postauricular incision is injected with 1% lidocaine with 1:100,000 epinephrine. The patient is prepped and draped as if for a tympanomastoidectomy. A No. 15 Bard-Parker blade is used to incise 0.5 cm posterior to the postauricular crease while palpating the mastoid tip to avoid excessive inferior dissection. The No. 15 blade is used to cut until the temporalis muscle superiorly and mastoid periosteum inferiorly is encountered. Blunt finger dissection is used over the top of the temporalis muscle to increase exposure. A No. 15 blade is used to incise the deep temporalis fascia, or true fascia, until muscle fibers are revealed beneath. Using a Brown-Adson and iris scissors, a 1.5-cm-square area of fascia is harvested. Two sets of fascia are trimmed into two different sizes in advance that are appropriately sized for packing the PSCC. A standard T incision is made in the mastoid periosteum, and it is elevated. Preparation of the fibrinogen glue should commence in anticipation of its use. A simple mastoidectomy is performed exposing the horizontal semicircular canal (HSCC) and PSCC. Thinning of the tegmen and development of the digastric ridge

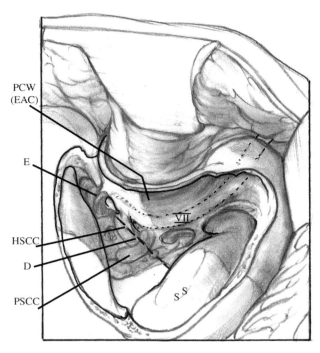

FIGURE 26–1 Donaldson's line along the plane of the horizontal semicircular canal (HSCC). D, Donaldson's line; E, epitympanum; EAC, external auditory canal; PCW, posterior canal wall; PSCC, posterior semicircular canal; SS, sigmoid sinus.

are unnecessary. Donaldson's line, which is a line drawn through the HSCC extending posteriorly, is identified (Fig. 26–1). This line bisects the PSCC in the middle of the area to be exposed.

The posterior half of the PSCC is identified and outlined with a diamond bur. A 1- or 2-mm diamond bur is then used to create a 5-mm bony island in the

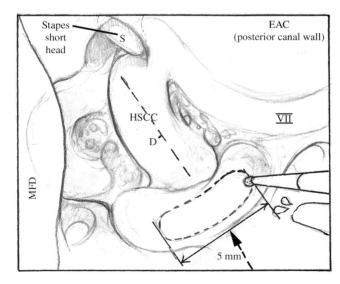

FIGURE 26–2 Creation of a 5-mm bony island.

middle of the exposed PSCC by blue-lining the canal around the bony island. It is critical that the membranous labyrinth be kept intact (Fig. 26–2). Set the suction aside and switch to neurosurgical cottonoids for blotting. Gently remove the bony island with a 90-degree hook while not violating the membranous labyrinth (Fig. 26–3). Often, the membranous labyrinth partially collapses with wicking. Select the appropriate-sized temporalis fascia piece and mix with one to two drops of fibrinogen glue. It will begin to get sticky and malleable, and then is ready for packing. Now pack the exposed ends of the PSCC with temporalis fascia atraumatically (Fig. 26–4). The intervening PSCC between the packed ends should be drilled away (Fig. 26–5). The remaining pieces of temporalis fascia are draped over the exposed packed ends of the PSCC. Several drops of fibrinogen glue are placed on the draped temporalis fascia. The soft tissues are closed and dressing applied per surgeon preference.

TIPS AND PITFALLS

It is critical that once the PSCC is opened, or even blue-lined, all suctioning cease in this area. This is the single most important factor in avoiding a dead ear. The PSCC can be packed with a variety of materials with temporalis fascia and/or muscle as the most common choices. Some authors have had good success with bone dust, and moderate success with bone wax. The majority of surgeons advocate the use of fibrinogen glue to aid with a watertight closure. The preparation of the fibrinogen glue should begin in advance of its need by 20 minutes. Packing the canal tightly is of utmost importance.

COMPLICATIONS

All patient should be counseled on the following possible complications:

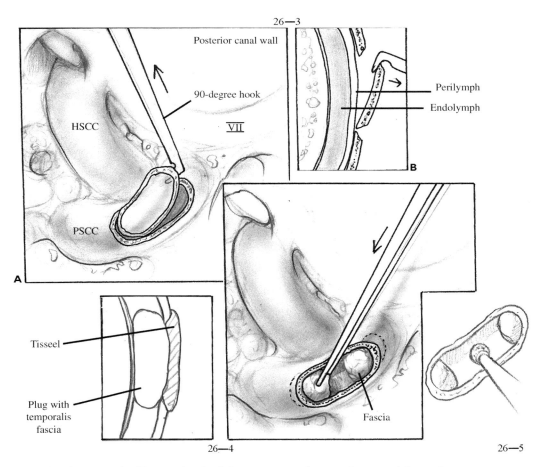

FIGURE 26–3 (A,B) Removal of bony island while preserving the membranous labyrinth.
FIGURE 26–4 Plugging the posterior semicircular canal (PSCC) with temporalis fascia and fibrinogen glue.
FIGURE 26–5 Removal of the intervening PSCC remnant.

1. Two percent risk of complete hearing loss[3]
2. Chance of persistent or worse symptoms
3. All patients have dysequilibrium for 6 to 8 weeks postoperatively, and a hospital stay of 2 to 4 days until they get accustomed to the dysequilibrium.

POSTOPERATIVE CARE

Some physicians perform this procedure as outpatient surgery, whereas others do it as an inpatient procedure that entails on average a 3-day hospital stay. Patient recovery is much faster with the addition of vestibular rehabilitation. Vestibular suppressants slow recovery by delaying compensation. Patients are given the following instructions and cautions:

1. No strenuous activity for 3 weeks.
2. They may have hearing loss for 3 to 4 weeks.
3. Dysequilibrium lasts for 6 to 8 weeks.
4. Motion sensitivity lasts for 2 to 3 weeks.

REFERENCES

1. Ruckenstein MJ. Therapeutic efficacy of the Epley canalith repositioning maneuver. *Laryngoscope* 2001; 111:940–945.
2. Parnes LS, Mcclure JA. Posterior semicircular canal occlusion for intractable benign paroxysmal positional vertigo. *Ann Otol Rhinol* 1990;99:330–334.
3. Zappia JJ. Posterior semicircular canal occlusion for the benign paroxysmal positional vertigo. *Am J Otol* 1996;17:749–754.
4. Walsh RM, Bath AP, Cullen JR, et al. Long term results of posterior semicircular canal occlusion for intractable benign paroxysmal positional vertigo. *Clin Otolaryngol* 1999;24:316–323.
5. Pace-Balzan A, Rutka JA. Non-ampullary plugging of the posterior semicircular canal for benign paroxysmal positional vertigo. *J Laryngol* 1991;105:901–906.
6. Pulec JL. Ablation of posterior semicircular canal for benign paroxysmal positional vertigo. *Ear Nose Throat J* 1997;76:17–22, 24.

Chapter 27

Basic Neurotologic Procedures

G. Mark Pyle

This chapter provides a brief overview of approaches to the internal auditory canal, posterior fossa, and petrous apex. This discussion is not intended as a detailed reference for the neurotologic subspecialist. There are a number of approaches to the posterior and middle cranial base, which are not addressed here. The reader is referred to other extensive discussions of these procedures in the literature.[1,2]

TRANSLABYRINTHINE (TL) APPROACH

The most common indication for TL surgery is a vestibular schwannoma of any size in an ear with nonserviceable hearing. Existing classification schemes for hearing include those described by Gardner and Robertson[3] and Samii and Matthies.[4] Controversy persists in approach selection for patients with larger tumors (greater than 2 cm of cerebellopontine angle tumor component) who have good hearing. Some institutions may favor a TL approach for these tumors because the rate of hearing preservation is low. At my institution, I offer a hearing preservation approach even in patients with larger (up to 3 cm in diameter) tumors who have Gardner class 1 hearing preoperatively. A number of variables including patient characteristics, tumor size and location, patient preference, and the results of preoperative studies determine the feasibility of hearing preservation. All of these factors must be taken into consideration when deciding on a TL approach.

The TL route is frequently combined with other bone flap craniotomies performed in conjunction with neurosurgery. Retrolabyrinthine and TL bone work is frequently performed as part of the transpetrosal approach for other lesions of the middle and posterior cranial base. The TL approach is also used in total facial nerve decompression for trauma when the patient has lost hearing.

There are several advantages to the TL approach when compared to other routes to the posterior cranial base. In comparison to the retrosigmoid approach, it offers direct complete exposure of the internal auditory canal (IAC). The TL approach also offers better anterior and superior exposure than the classical retrosigmoid approach. Facial nerve decompression or mobilization is facilitated through this approach. The TL route offers excellent exposure for placement of an auditory brainstem implant if required.[5] There is less cerebellar retraction, and all bone work is performed extracranially, which may limit postoperative headache. Cerebrospinal fluid (CSF) leak is almost nonexistent in the TL approach.[6]

The primary disadvantage of this approach is the obvious loss of hearing. In larger tumors, with a wide inferior brainstem attachment, a high jugular bulb can limit the approach. This route is contraindicated in patients with active chronic otitis media and mastoiditis.

A thorough otologic and neurotologic history and physical examination should be performed on all patients. The patient's subjective assessment of dysequilibrium, imbalance, and tinnitus intensity are reviewed. A comprehensive neurologic review of systems should be included, with particular attention to any cranial nerve symptoms. A past medical history of chronic ear disease or prior otologic surgery should be elicited. A family history of intracranial neoplasm or neurofibromatosis is of obvious importance. In addition to the standard otologic and head and neck examination, cranial nerve function and vestibular function should be assessed. Subtle physical findings may include a diminished corneal reflex, and drift and past pointing to the ipsilateral side.

All patients undergo complete audiometric testing including pure tone and speech audiometry. Electrocochleography (ECoG) and auditory brainstem response (ABR) testing are performed as a preoperative baseline if hearing preservation is being considered. Preoperative vestibular testing, including electronystagmography (ENG), is also useful. Preoperative evaluation by the balance physical therapy team, including platform posturography, may prove useful in selected patients who require vestibular retraining postoperatively. All patients have undergone magnetic resonance imaging (MRI) with contrast enhancement. High-resolution computed tomography (HRCT) of the temporal bone is not required but may delineate anatomic abnormalities including a high jugular bulb, sclerotic mastoid, or anteriorly placed sigmoid sinus. Widening of the IAC also correlates negatively with hearing preservation. All options, including observation and radiosurgery, must be thoroughly discussed with the patient. All elements of informed consent are included in a surgery-specific consent form for TL surgery, and the external canal is painted with gentian violet preoperatively.

The TL procedure should be performed in a larger operating suite. This provides ample room for equipment including the operating microscope, intraoperative monitoring systems, dissection tools including pneumatic drills, and cavitating ultrasonic aspirators. Increased room size is also needed for added personnel including neuroanesthesia, nursing staff, the multidisciplinary surgical team, intraoperative monitoring personnel, and observers.

For the routine TL approach, the head is rotated 30 to 45 degrees to the contralateral side with the chin gently flexed toward the shoulder. The surgeon is seated on the same side as the anesthesia service, which is located toward the feet. The operating room nurse is positioned directly across from the surgeon. The first assistant and microscope base are positioned at the head of the table. Arterial line placement and facial nerve monitoring are always performed. Intravenous mannitol (0.5 g/kg) and dexamethasone are given for larger tumors.

A limited hair shave is done, and adhesive drapes are applied. A previous abdominal incision or the left lower quadrant is also prepared for harvesting an abdominal fat graft. The head is secured with tape and an incision is outlined (Fig. 27–1). The incision is infiltrated with 1% Xylocaine with 1:100,000 epinephrine prior to the skin prep.

The incision is made with a knife or an electrocautery device. The incision is normally beveled

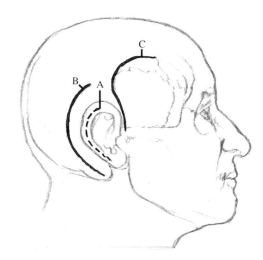

FIGURE 27–1 Outline of incisions for the translabyrinthine (A), retrosigmoid/transmeatal (B), and middle cranial fossa (C) approaches.

anteriorly to provide increased surface area for closure. Muscle and periosteum are incised and elevated using the cautery or periosteal elevators. All soft tissue is removed from the lateral cranial base to completely expose the mastoid process, digastric ridge, external auditory canal, and retrosigmoid region. The anteriorly based flap is retracted and held in position with fishhook retractors.

Bone work is begun with an extended mastoidectomy. Initial drilling may be done without microscopic control. The sigmoid sinus and a limited amount of retrosigmoid dura are completely skeletonized. The mastoid tip is removed and the facial nerve, jugular bulb, and superior petrosal sinus are identified. All bone is removed from the middle cranial fossa dura. The inferior limit of the dissection is the jugular bulb, which is completely exposed or down-fractured. Usually the upper limit is the superior petrosal sinus and middle fossa dura, but the TL approach can be extended superiorly if needed.

A modified labyrinthectomy is performed. The posterior cranial fossa dura and the superior petrosal sinus are traced medially, followed by removal of the posterior canal, common crus, and superior canal. In this way the facial nerve is protected and the lateral semicircular canal is removed in the final portion of the labyrinthectomy. The vestibule is widely opened and the ampullated ends of the lateral and superior semicircular canals are removed. During anterior dissection, care must be taken to avoid injury to the tympanic segment of the facial nerve. Skeletonization of the facial nerve significantly improves exposure, and the shoulder of a large diamond bur and continuous suction irrigation are used.

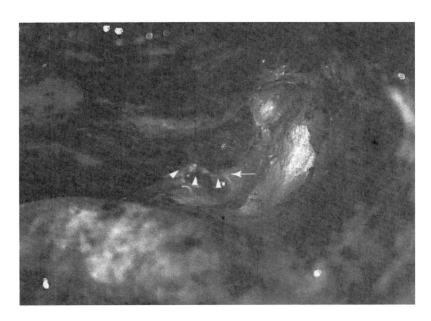

FIGURE 27–2 Photograph of left translabyrinthine approach demonstrating remaining superior meatal bone (arrow). The asterisk indicates internal auditory canal (IAC) with tumor, and arrowheads show posterior fossa dura (PFD).

The next step in the bone work is the identification of the porus acusticus. A large trough is created between the jugular bulb inferiorly and the IAC superiorly. The cochlear aqueduct is located in this region and is widely opened to allow egress of cerebrospinal fluid. Once the inferior aspect of the IAC is identified, dissection is continued superiorly with identification of the superior portion of the porus acusticus. There is a dense wedge of bone located between the superior aspect of the internal canal and the posterior fossa dura (Fig. 27–2). Bone removal in this area is important to provide adequate exposure and facilitate dissection of the facial nerve. The lateral dissection of the IAC is carried out last. This includes identification of the vertical and horizontal crest as well as the labyrinthine segment of the facial nerve. The egg-shelled bone is removed from the dura. An island of bone may be left over the sigmoid sinus. Once all of the bone work is completed, the dura of the internal auditory meatus is opened. This incision can be extended posteriorly toward the sigmoid sinus. Superior and inferior extensions of this incision can then be made toward the jugular bulb and petrosal sinus. Wide reflection of the posterior fossa dura provides complete exposure of the cerebellopontine angle.

Dissection within the IAC is begun laterally. The superior and inferior vestibular nerves are sectioned sharply. The facial and cochlear nerves are identified. Facial nerve dissection is facilitated with the use of stimulus dissecting instruments. I leave the cochlear nerve intact as the tumor is dissected from lateral to medial (Fig. 27–3). This results in less traction on the facial nerve. Hemostasis is controlled with bipolar cautery and small pledgets of absorbable gelatin and thrombin. Care must be taken to dissect any vascular

loops located within the IAC. Small tumors can usually be removed in an en-bloc fashion. Larger tumors require debulking using microinstruments or a cavitating ultrasonic aspirator. The role of the neurosurgeon varies based on tumor size, but at my institution all cases of vestibular schwannoma are done in a multidisciplinary manner.

Once tumor removal is complete and hemostasis has been assured, the abdominal fat graft is harvested. I also perform closure of the eustachian tube via the facial recess during the fat graft harvest. The middle ear and attic are closed with a muscle graft followed by bone wax, closing the facial recess. The abdominal fat graft is cut into bilobed strips. These strips are layered together to serially close the defect in the posterior fossa dura. A compressive mastoid dressing is placed for 48 hours.

Bleeding during temporal bone dissection is usually easily controlled with bone wax, bipolar cautery, or a diamond drill. Hemorrhage from the sigmoid sinus and jugular bulb or superior petrosal sinus can be troublesome, however. Bleeding from the sinus can often be controlled with a large pledget of absorbable gelatin sponge moistened with topical thrombin and placement of a cottonoid followed by gentle pressure. The complex can be left in place and held with the arm of a self-retaining retractor while dissection is allowed to continue. Bleeding from the jugular bulb may require a firm oxidized cellulose pack. Care must be taken to avoid embolization of the packing material. Ligation of the internal jugular vein or complete occlusion of the sigmoid sinus has not been required in my experience. Bleeding from the petrosal sinus may be controlled with small clips posteriorly and with packing anteriorly. Bleeding from the subarcuate artery is easily controlled with

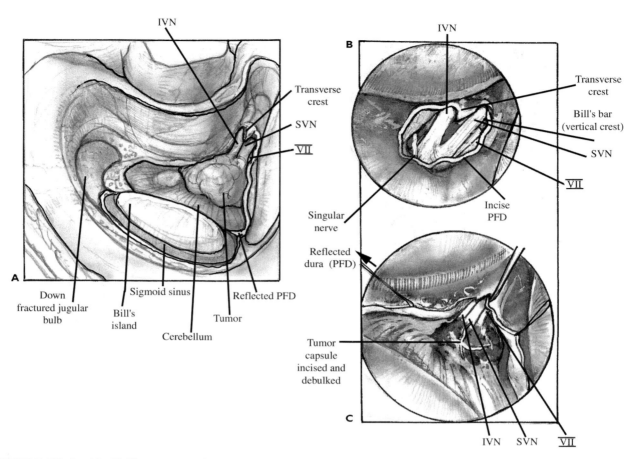

FIGURE 27–3 (A–C) Illustrations of tumor dissection from internal auditory canal. PFD, Posterior fossa dura; IVN, inferior vestibular nerve; SVN, superior vestibular nerve.

the diamond drill. During tumor work, I have found that a suction bipolar is very effective for controlling bleeding and facilitating tumor dissection.

In my experience, the TL approach to the IAC has the lowest rate of CSF leak. In the last 200 consecutive operative cases of vestibular schwannoma from 1995 to 2001, only one of the 57 TL cases leaked. This is most likely due to the fact that my colleagues and I now close the eustachian tube through the facial recess approach in all cases. If it occurs, initial treatment of CSF leak consists of bed rest and lumbar drainage. The overall incidence of facial paresis has been dramatically reduced over the past decade. New techniques in tumor debulking, sharp dissection, and intraoperative facial nerve monitoring have led to excellent rates of facial nerve preservation. Despite these results, iatrogenic injury to the facial nerve does occur. Complete facial nerve decompression of the labyrinthine segment and perigeniculate region is facilitated with the TL approach. Transtemporal rerouting of the facial nerve with direct anastomosis is rarely needed in schwannoma surgery. Intraoperative facial nerve

monitoring may be useful as a predictor of postoperative facial nerve outcome.[7]

Patients are monitored for the first 24 hours in the neurosurgical intensive care unit. Antibiotics are discontinued after the third postoperative dose. Steroids are not given unless cerebellar edema or transient facial paresis develops. Standard neurologic checks are performed for the first 24 hours. The Foley catheter and sequential compression stockings are discontinued when the patient is ambulatory, which usually occurs on the first or second postoperative day. Antihypertensives, narcotics, antivertiginous drugs, antiemetics, and muscle relaxants are used as needed for symptom control. Medication is titrated to allow for accurate mental status examination. All of my patients receive balance retraining on the second or third postoperative day. Any patient with facial weakness is instructed in lateral taping and lubrication of the eye until facial nerve recovery. Patients are normally discharged on the third or fourth postoperative day. The first postoperative visit occurs 1 week later when sutures are removed and the patient is examined. Patients normally return to work, depending on occupation, in the next 4 to 6 weeks. At 1 month the patient is counseled regarding the possible use of a transcranial contralateral routing of signal (CROS) hearing aid. Patients with delayed vestibular compensation are offered a more formal platform-based vestibular program.

RETROSIGMOID-TRANSMEATAL (RS) APPROACH

The most common indication for this approach is the removal of vestibular schwannoma or cerebellopontine angle tumors with hearing preservation. The approach is also useful for selective vestibular neurectomy in unilateral Meniere's syndrome. Another indication is for microvascular decompression of the seventh and eighth nerve complex in those patients with hemifacial spasm or severe vertigo. Presenting symptoms are similar to those mentioned in the previous section.

Studies determining a patient's candidacy for hearing preservation have already been described. ABR and ECoG are always performed as a baseline for intraoperative monitoring. It should be noted that MRI with gadolinium enhancement may not predict actual tumor extent into the IAC.[8] The position of the vestibular labyrinth in relation to the posterior aspect of the porus acusticus is important in calculating the lateral extent of meatal bone removal. In those patients with more than 1 cm of tumor extension into the cerebellopontine angle and good hearing, I perform the retrosigmoid transmeatal approach. With larger tumors, patients

are informed of the lower success rate with hearing preservation so that they do not have unrealistic expectations.

The patient is positioned supine with a large roll under the ipsilateral shoulder to facilitate rotation of the head and neck. In this approach I always use pin fixation of the head. The head is turned laterally at 45 degrees, the neck is flexed, and the vertex is tilted slightly down. In obese patients, or those with limited mobility of the cervical spine, a modified park bench or lateral position may be planned. All auditory and facial nerve monitoring electrodes are placed. The active electrode for ECoG can be placed on the tympanic membrane or middle ear promontory. The scope of this chapter does not allow a detailed description of intraoperative monitoring techniques. Usually direct eighth nerve monitoring, ECoG, and ABR are used together.

There are some differences in surgical equipment between the TL and RS approaches. The pneumatic dissection tool should have a craniotome attachment in addition to the standard burs. The working distance for bone and tumor dissection is longer in the RS approach. I use a longer set of drill attachments and longer microinstruments for dissection.

The curved hockey-stick incision is made and an anteriorly based flap is secured with fishhooks. Initial bone work is performed with complete identification of the sigmoid sinus and transverse sinus. The posterior emissary vein is identified, bipolared, and sectioned. The mastoidectomy is limited and as few air cells as possible are opened to lessen the possibility of CSF leak. Skeletonizing the venous structures facilitates turning the bone

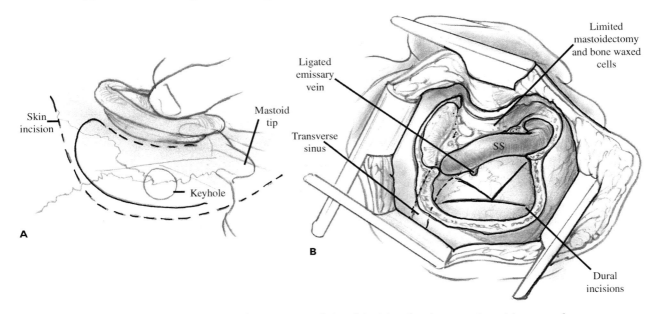

FIGURE 27–4 (A,B) Illustrations of initial exposure and dural incision for the retrosigmoid approach.

flap, which is removed with the craniotome and preserved for later replacement (Fig. 27–4).

Neurosurgical colleagues open the dura, release CSF from the cistern, and gain tumor exposure (Fig. 27–5). They may also perform additional debulking in large neoplasms to provide better exposure of the posterior aspect of the temporal bone.

The neurotologist returns to the operating room for the temporal bone dissection. A U-shaped incision is made in the dura extending from the jugular fold to below the level of the tentorium. Small pledgets of absorbable sponge are placed in the subarachnoid space to limit bone dust exposure. Labyrinthine landmarks including the vestibular aqueduct and singular canal are useful indicators during dissection.[9] Once established, IAC dissection is continued from the porus laterally to the level of the vestibule. The vestibular labyrinth must be avoided. The common crus and posterior canal are at greatest risk. The endolymphatic sac is also left undisturbed. Normally, several millimeters of the IAC can be carefully exposed (Fig. 27–6). It is very important to completely skeletonize the IAC circumferentially, at least 180 degrees, rather than simply unroofing the internal auditory meatus.

After the bone work is completed, an inferior incision is made along the meatal dura. If distal tumor extent is present, lateral dissection may require the use of endoscopes and angled internal canal dissectors. Sharp dissection is required to identify the appropriate cleavage plane. Sharp technique is also important to limit traction on the cochlear nerve in hearing preservation. If the tumor

is small, it should be removed en bloc if possible. Identification of the normal proximal eighth nerve allows placement of an active electrode for direct eighth nerve monitoring. Frequent communication between the audiologist and surgeon is important during the tumor work. In larger tumors, additional debulking is frequently required once the tumor has been removed from the IAC and the course of the distal facial and cochlear nerves has been determined. The scope of this chapter does not allow for detailed description of the vasculature of the posterior cranial fossa, which is well described elsewhere.[10] This is a crucial part of the procedure, and all significant vessels should be carefully dissected from the tumor in the proper plane and preserved.

Closure is initiated with a careful search and occlusion of exposed air cells in the region of the meatus. Endoscopic control may reveal distal tumor or previously undiscovered air cells.[11] The internal auditory meatus is sealed with a large piece of prepared free temporalis muscle. The dura is normally closed primarily, but may require augmentation with autogenous grafts or manufactured dura substitutes. The bone flap is returned over a large pad of absorbable gelatin sponge and secured with miniplates. Routine closure is then performed. Primary cranioplasty is not usually required.

As previously mentioned, the incidence of complete facial paresis is now uncommon, although patients with larger tumors may have a significant delay in neural recovery. Cerebrospinal fluid leak is somewhat more common in this approach than in

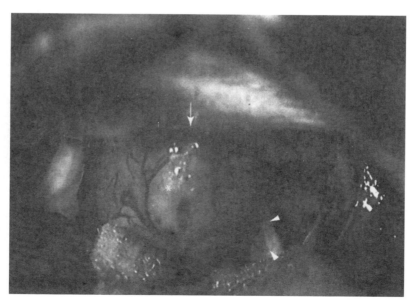

FIGURE 27–5 Photograph of small tumor in cerebellopontine angle prior to transmeatal bone work. Arrow indicates porus acusticus. Arrowheads indicate eighth nerve.

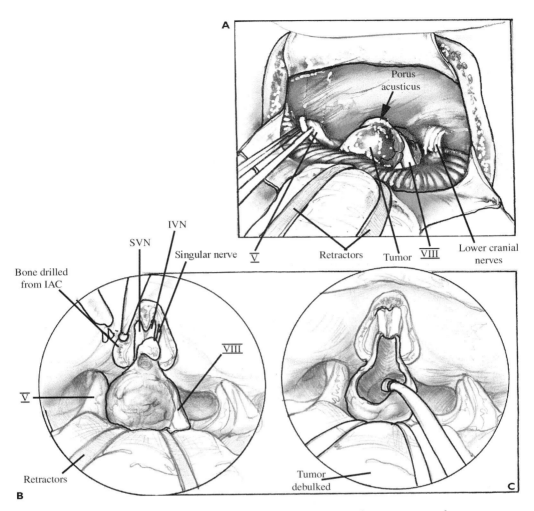

FIGURE 27–6   (A–C) Illustrations of completed bone work prior to meatal tumor removal.

the TL approach. If initial measures including bed rest and short-term lumbar drainage are ineffective in closing the leak, then reoperation can be performed. If hearing has been maintained, a transmastoid approach without closure of the eustachian tube can be used.

Hearing loss may occur due to direct mechanical injury to the cochlear nerve or more likely due to interruption of the blood supply of the cochlea. Sharp dissection, preservation of microvasculature, intraoperative monitoring, one-piece tumor removal, and limiting cautery are all important in lowering the potential for hearing loss. It is also possible that early bone work with decompression of the IAC may improve perfusion pressure during extended tumor dissection for larger schwannomas.[12] Other serious complications including stroke or hemorrhage are rare. These may occur early in the postoperative period, and the surgeon must be vigilant and immediately evaluate any questionable change in mental status or the neurologic examination. Addi-

tional postoperative procedures are similar to those described in the previous section. If sutures or staples are used for the skin closure, they are normally removed between 10 and 14 postoperative days. Facial function is assessed and eye care is initiated.

Audiometric testing and vestibular evaluation are performed at 1 month. Patients having difficulty with vestibular compensation are referred for postoperative platform-based balance retraining therapy. Patients who have lost hearing may be candidates for transcranial amplification. All patients undergoing a retrosigmoid approach are followed with imaging. I recommend a 1-year postoperative MRI study and a final study done 4 years postprocedure. In the uncommon case of residual or recurrent schwannoma, radiosurgical treatment is the primary mode of therapy. This may not be required unless significant growth is demonstrated. Translabyrinthine removal of residual growing neoplasm can also be entertained if there is a nonhearing ear.

MIDDLE CRANIAL FOSSA (MCF) APPROACH TO THE IAC AND PETROUS APEX

The MCF approach is commonly used for patients with small vestibular schwannomas, good hearing, and limited extension into the cerebellopontine angle.[13] The approach is also useful for lesions of the anterior petrous pyramid, including cholesterol cysts and epidermoids of the petrous apex. The MCF approach can be extended anteriorly and posteriorly for other lesions of the cranial base. The exposure is frequently performed for complete facial nerve decompression secondary to trauma or in cases of Bell's palsy with a poor prognosis. Finally, patients who exhibit symptoms and imaging evidence of superior semicircular canal dehiscence syndrome are candidates for middle fossa exposure to repair the dehiscent canal.[14]

A complete history and physical examination should be performed. A careful evaluation of fifth cranial nerve function including testing of facial sensation and corneal reflex should be included. Schirmer's test can be performed in those patients with a history of a dry eye. In facial nerve decompression candidates, detailing the time course of facial paralysis and associated symptoms is very important. Assessment should include electroneuronography and standard needle electromyography. Otoscopy may reveal pathology in the middle ear cleft related to a petrous apex lesion. All patients undergo complete audiometric testing, baseline ABR, ECoG, and vestibular testing.

Imaging analysis normally includes both MRI and CT techniques. Both modalities have the capability to be loaded simultaneously on the intraoperative navigation workstation. One can use the CT image during bone work and the neurosurgeon may refer to the MR images for his intracranial work. When more extensive lesions of the middle cranial base are present, carotid artery status may need to be evaluated with preoperative test occlusion.

The patient is supine on the operating room table with the head turned 45 degrees. The final head position depends on tumor characteristics and individual patient mobility. Navigation may be useful to plan the surgical trajectory. Patient registration for the navigation system can be performed at this time. Accuracy may be improved through the use of pin fixation as well as bone-anchored anatomic markers. Intraoperative auditory electrodes and facial nerve electrodes are placed for monitoring. The surgeon and first assistant are positioned at the head, with the microscope base near the side of the anesthesia team. Images for navigation can be observed at the workstation or as a heads-up display in the microscopic field.

The incision is made (Fig. 27–1) and carried down to the temporalis fascia. The frontotemporal branch of the facial nerve and the blood supply to the temporalis muscle are always preserved. There are a number of ways to divide the temporalis, but in general the technique should preserve the integrity of the muscle for later use as a rotation flap if required.

Classically, a 4 × 5-cm rectangular flap extending two-thirds anterior and one-third posterior to the

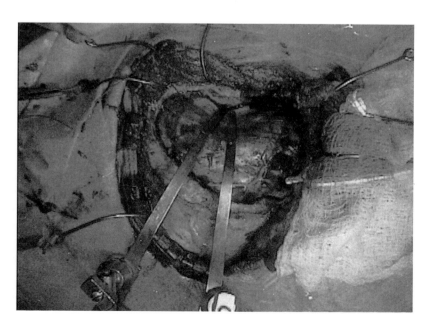

FIGURE 27–7 Photograph of self-retaining retractor system in place.

zygomatic root is removed. The creation of a rectangular flap with straight edges allows use of the traditional self-retaining MCF retractor systems. I perform a wider, more anterior, craniotomy and utilize a lower profile retractor system with the dura retractors secured to a system applied to the head holder as described by Greenberg.[15] This allows for a flexible approach and additional dural elevation if required (Fig. 27–7). Dura is elevated from the middle fossa floor in a posterior to anterior direction. The petrous ridge, superior petrosal sinus, arcuate eminence, greater superficial petrosal nerve, and middle meningeal artery are all useful landmarks. Identification of the petrous carotid artery and dissection of the trigeminal ganglion are required for more anterior lesions of the petrous apex (Fig. 27–8). Several techniques for identification of the internal auditory meatus have been described.[13] Drilling is begun on the meatal plane as medially as possible with initial identification of the porus. A large quantity of bone can be removed posteriorly and medially between the superior semicircular canal and the IAC. Extensive bone removal can also be done anteriorly along the petrous ridge. The canal can be skeletonized medially, but laterally, approaching the fundus, the IAC dissection is limited by the cochlea anteriorly and the superior canal posteriorly.

The vertical crest and labyrinthine segment of the facial nerve are identified. The bone is thinned and finally removed with small curettes (Fig. 27–9). The facial nerve may be displaced superiorly over the tumor, so care must be taken when the dura is incised prior to tumor removal. Tumor removal begins laterally with sharp sectioning of the superior and inferior vestibular nerves. Tumor involving the inferior compartment must be carefully dissected from the overlying facial nerve. As in the retrosigmoid approach, hemostasis should be accomplished with limited use of electrocautery. A dural incision may be extended into the posterior fossa for dissection of the cerebellopontine angle component of the tumor. Dissection must free any vascular loops extending into the meatus or adherent to tumor in this region. An extension of the MCF approach can be accomplished with ligation of the superior petrosal sinus and incision of the tentorium.[16] This allows for a more panoramic view of the posterior fossa and can be employed for larger tumors.

Anterior extension of the MCF approach is my favored route for complete excision of cholesterol granuloma or nonexteriorized epidermoid tumors of the anterior petrous pyramid. Simple drainage of cysts can also be performed via a transmastoid route.[17] An anterior MCF approach is also useful to

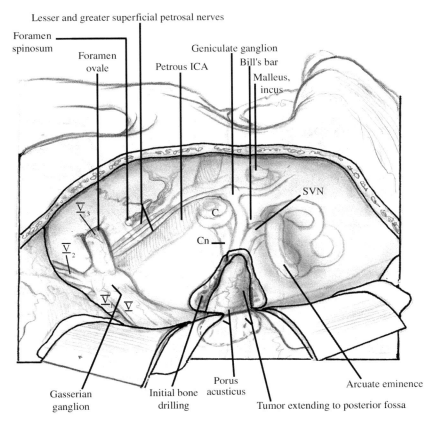

FIGURE 27–8 Illustration of middle fossa landmarks prior to bone removal.

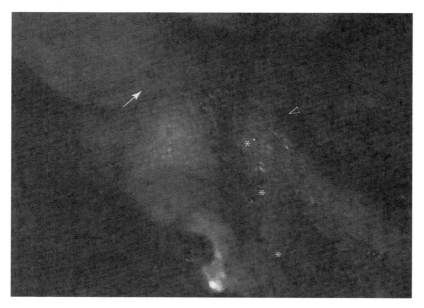

FIGURE 27–9 Photograph following exposure of the IAC (*) in those patients with left vestibular schwannoma. Arrow, arcuate eminence; arrowhead, geniculate ganglion.

assist in the removal of meningioma and other lesions of the anterosuperior cerebellopontine angle. This exposure requires extension of the previous incision. In addition, zygomatic osteotomies can be performed, with inferior reflection of the zygomatic arch, to allow for more basal exposure. The neurotologist frequently performs the bone work along the anterior middle fossa floor to facilitate exposure for neurosurgical tumor extirpation. This approach is begun similar to the MCF approach mentioned previously. Anterior exposure necessitates sectioning the middle meningeal artery. A key component of this dissection is identification of the horizontal petrous segment of the internal carotid artery. Larger lesions may also require sacrifice of the greater superficial petrosal nerve. Once the IAC, carotid artery, and cochlea are identified, drilling can proceed from posterior to anterior along the course of the superior and inferior petrosal sinus. For most lesions the trigeminal ganglion is identified and preserved. Large cholesterol cysts can be completely excised after they are unroofed (Fig. 27–10).

The middle cranial fossa approach is often combined with the transmastoid approach for complete facial nerve decompression in cases of traumatic or viral paralysis. Some indications dictate more limited MCF exposure and less bone work. These include the repair of tegmen cerebrospinal fluid fistulas, meningoceles, and dehiscent superior canals.

Bleeding can be a troublesome complication during middle fossa surgery. Methods for hemostasis have already been described. The middle menin-

geal artery can usually be controlled with bipolar cautery or firm packing of the lumen. In most other instances a combination of saline irrigation, careful cautery, gentle packing, and patience results in adequate hemostasis. Extensive lesions with possible involvement of the petrous carotid artery obviously require proximal and distal vascular control. Temporal lobe infarction or injury may occur as a

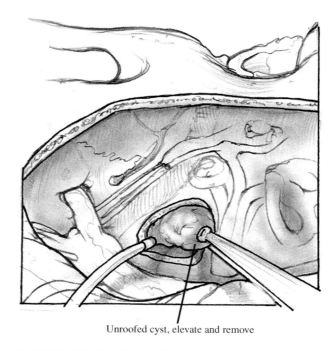

Unroofed cyst, elevate and remove

FIGURE 27–10 Illustration demonstrating removal of left petrous apex cholesterol cyst via middle fossa exposure.

complication during extended middle fossa surgery due to traction or damage to the vein of Labbé. The use of specialized retractor systems with extensive removal of bone along the floor of the middle fossa has limited the need for temporal lobe retraction. Lumbar drainage can be utilized to allow for addition relaxation if required.

Facial paralysis is an uncommon complication of middle cranial fossa surgery. If an injury does occur, complete decompression, rerouting, or grafting are facilitated through the available exposure. Resection of facial nerve neuromas frequently requires end-to-end anastomosis with or without a cable graft.[18] Cerebrospinal fluid leak can occur following the middle cranial fossa approach. Any exposed mastoid air cells must be thoroughly sealed with bone wax. Large tegmen defects may require bone grafts. I normally use a large sheet of autologous temporalis fascia supplemented with free or pedicled temporalis muscle held in place with fibrin glue. Persistent postoperative leak that does not respond to bed rest and lumbar drainage may require reexploration through the middle fossa. Finally, injury to the labyrinth may cause sensorineural hearing loss and postoperative vertigo or dysequilibrium. The structures most at risk are the cochlea and the superior semicircular canal.

Postoperative care for MCF approach is similar to the previous protocols. The patient is typically discharged on the third or fourth postoperative day after adequate pain control, oral intake, and initial vestibular compensation have been established. Suture removal is carried out approximately 10 days after surgery. I frequently use glue on the incision, which eliminates this requirement. In cases where extensive work has been done in the region of the temporomandibular joint, physical therapy may improve mandibular range of motion and limit spasm. In those cases where facial nerve decompression has been performed, facial nerve retraining is initiated in a neuromuscular retraining clinic at the onset of recovery.

REFERENCES

1. Jackler RK, Driscoll C. *Tumors of the Ear and Temporal Bone.* Philadelphia: Lippincott Williams & Wilkins; 2000.
2. Sekhar LN, Janecka IP. *Surgery of Cranial Base Tumors.* New York: Raven Press; 1993.
3. Gardner G, Robertson JH. Hearing preservation in unilateral acoustic neuroma surgery. *Ann Otol Rhinol Laryngol* 1988;97:55–66.
4. Samii M, Matthies C. Management of 1000 vestibular schwannomas (acoustic neuromas): hearing function in 1000 tumor resections. *Neurosurgery* 1997;40:248–260.
5. Otto SR, Shannon RV, Brackmann DE, et al. The multichannel auditory brainstem implant: performance in 20 patients. *Otolaryngol Head Neck Surg* 1998;18:291–303.
6. Falcioni M, Mulder J, Sanna M. No cerebrospinal fluid leaks in translabyrinthine vestibular schwannoma removal. *Am J Otol* 1999;20:660–666.
7. Beck DL, Atkins JS Jr, Benecke JE Jr, et al. Intraoperative facial nerve monitoring: prognostic aspects during acoustic tumor removal. *Otolaryngol Head Neck Surg* 1991;104:780–782.
8. Selsnick SH, Rebol J, Heier LA, et al. Internal auditory canal involvement of acoustic neuromas: surgical correlates to magnetic resonance findings. *Otol Neurotol* 2001;22:912–916.
9. Kartush JM, Telian SA, Graham MD, et al. Anatomic basis for labyrinthine preservation during posterior fossa acoustic tumor surgery. *Laryngoscope* 1986;96:1024–1028.
10. Lang J. *Clinical Anatomy of the Posterior Cranial Fossa and Its Foramina.* New York: Thieme; 1991.
11. Valtonen HJ, Poe DS, Heilman CB, et al. Endoscopically assisted prevention of cerebrospinal fluid leak in suboccipital acoustic neuroma surgery. *Am J Otol* 1997;18:381–385.
12. Lapsiwala SB, Pyle GM, Badie B. Correlation between auditory function and internal auditory canal pressure in patients with vestibular schwannomas. *J Neurosurg* 2002;96:872–876.
13. Slattery WH, Brackman DE, Hitselberger W. Middle fossa approach for hearing preservation with acoustic neuroma. *Am J Otol* 1997;18:596–601.
14. Minor LB, Solomon D, Zinreich JS, et al. Sound and/or pressure induced vertigo due to bone dehiscence of the superior semicircular canal. *Arch Otolaryngol Head Neck Surg* 1998;124:249–258.
15. Greenberg IM. Self-retaining retractors and handrests. In: Wilkins RH, Rengachary SS, eds. *Neurosurgery.* New York: McGraw-Hill; 1996: 346–360.
16. Wigand ME, Haid T, Berg M. The enlarged middle cranial fossa approach for surgery of the temporal bone and of the cerebellopontine angle. *Arch Otorhinolaryngol* 1989;264:299–302.
17. Wilson DF, Hodgson RS. Transmastoid infralabyrinthine approach to petrous temporal bone. *Skull Base Surg* 1991;1:188–190.
18. Wiet RJ, Pyle GM, Schramm DR. Middle fossa and intratemporal facial nerve neuromas. *Otolaryngol Head Neck Surg* 1991;104:141–142.

Chapter 28

Cochlear Implant Surgery

Phillip A. Wackym and Jill B. Firszt

Although cochlear implantation began in earnest in the early 1970s, it was not until December 1984 that the Food and Drug Administration (FDA) approved a single-channel device for implantation in postlingual adults. Since then, dramatic improvements in speech processor design and sound quality have led to significant improvements in quality of life for many implanted patients. This chapter presents specific details relating to cochlear implantation surgery.

Patient Positioning and Preparation

For both children and adult patients, the standard otologic position is used: supine with the head placed on a foam doughnut and turned away from the operated ear. Surgical preparation should always include review of the computed tomography (CT) scans or magnetic resonance imaging (MRI) to determine the cochlear anatomy and whether the cochlea is filled with fluid, fibrous tissue, or neo-ossification. With the wide array of available cochlear implant electrode designs, it is particularly important to be certain that the appropriate electrode array has been ordered and is available in the operating room.

Soft Tissue Incisions and Approach

Over the years, several variations of scalp and skin incisions have been utilized in cochlear implant surgery. Although several flaps have been utilized with consistently good results, two fundamental principles must be adhered to: first, the blood supply of the flap must be ample for survival of the flaps; and second, the skin incisions must not overlie the cochlear implant itself. With this evolution in flap design has also come changes in philosophy regarding the amount of hair that must be shaved. Fig. 28–1 shows a commonly utilized skin and scalp incision design that is used by most cochlear implant surgeons. The only hair shaved is that necessary to allow draping of the field around the incisions. The postauricular incision is designed to be at the hairline and is thereby camouflaged. The posterior scalp extension length can be varied depending on the implant design, and because the internal magnet and receiving coil can be placed lateral to the skull for the Nucleus Contour device (Cochlear Corp., Melbourne, Australia) and the HiRes 90K Bionic Ear device (Advanced Bionics Corp., Sylmar, CA), shorter scalp incisions are required for these devices, thereby permitting a minimally invasive approach. A pocket can be developed beneath the existing scalp flap to receive these portions of the device. For the CII Bionic Ear and Med-El C40+ (Medical Electronics AB, Innsbrück, Austria) devices, the entire ceramic receiver portion of the device must be inset into the skull, and therefore the scalp incision must be somewhat longer. This issue is of no functional consequence and does not produce additional morbidity in patients. Moreover, this scalp incision is placed within the patient's hair and is not seen once the incision is healed and the hair has regrown.

There are differences in the soft tissue approach used for adults and that used for children. For young children the incisions are carried through the skin, pericranium (periosteum), and temporalis muscle, directly down to the bone. The soft tissue flaps are elevated en bloc, and subperiosteal elevation is completed to expose the sites of bone work neces-

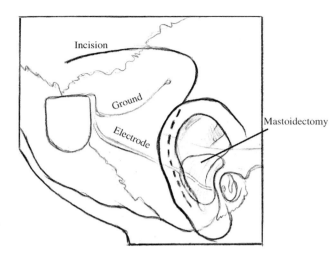

FIGURE 28–1 Common design for skin incision used during cochlear implantation.

sary to accomplish cochlear implantation. Important points to consider and accomplish during this aspect of the surgery are adequate exposure of the external auditory canal and zygomatic root, and ample elevation of the soft tissue necessary to protect the soft tissue from the surgical drill.

With adults and older children, it is possible and desirable to develop two tissue planes. The first is in an avascular subgaleal plane lateral to the pericranium, and temporalis fascia and mastoid periosteum superiorly and anteroinferiorly, respectively. Once these flaps are elevated, incisions through the periosteum are made, first along the temporal line superiorly with a perpendicular extension down to the mastoid tip. The superior limb of this incision is carried posteriorly over the skull, and a periosteal flap is then elevated. These flaps are used to close the wound in two layers, which further helps in protecting the receiver portion of the cochlear implant and thereby minimizes the risk of extrusion.

Several pieces of temporalis fascia or pericranium are then harvested and kept sterile in the moist gauze sponge on the back table and are used for sealing the cochleostomy, placing fascia between the facial nerve and electrode array, and in helping to retain the electrode array at the juncture of the trough housing the electrode array and the mastoid cavity. Once hemostasis has been achieved either with the bipolar electrocautery or with the monopolar cautery, it is at this point that the monopolar cautery is taken off of the operative field and turned off within the operating room. Once the cochlear implant has been opened and placed on the operative field, it is necessary to remove the monopolar cautery to prevent current-induced damage to the internal device.

For both adults and children, the elevated soft tissue flaps are protected with 1 × 3-inch cottonoids or moistened gauze sponges (Kendall Vistec sponges, TYCO Healthcare Group LP, Mansfield, MA) and retracted from the bone with dural fish hooks (DermaHooks, Weck Closure Systems, Research Triangle Park, NC) and rubber bands. Alternatively, after placement of the cottonoids and/or moist Vistec sponges, self-retaining retractors can be used.

RECEIVER BED AND ELECTRODE ARRAY TROUGH

Preparation of the receiver bed begins by selection and design of the placement. It is important to place the receiver bed posterior enough to accommodate the ear level hook or behind-the-ear speech processor. Placement of the receiver bed in a position that is too far anterior is a common mistake made by inexperienced cochlear implant surgeons. The consequence of this misplacement is extrusion of the receiver following skin erosion due to the ear hook or behind-the-ear speech processor placing pressure on the skin overlying the receiver. Another consideration in designing the position of the receiver bed is the anticipated position of a hat band, should the patient frequently wear hats or wish to wear hats. Each device manufacturer provides templates that are used in designing the shape of the receiver bed and these accurately represent the size of the receiver. The CII Bionic Ear device also utilizes a plastic template that is of the size and shape of the internal device.

There are specific differences in how the receiver bed is designed and these will be described in separate subsections of this portion of the chapter; however, general techniques are described first. Although it is possible to inset the receiver in some adult patients, virtually all young children and the majority of older children and adults require a craniotomy that extends down to the dura and allows the insetting of the receiver. The technique for accomplishing this includes completing a craniectomy of the dimensions necessary for accommodating the receiver. The outer cortex and diploic layers are removed and the inner cortex of the skull is thinned until the dura is visible through the bone. Next, the craniotomy is performed using a 2-mm coarse diamond bur and is carried down to the dura without violating this layer. The surrounding bony edges are then smoothed to remove any rough edges, and conformation of the template to the craniotomy is completed to be certain that the receiver fits in the created space. It is estimated that 6 months are required for the bone to regrow across this gap and provide stable bone beneath the cochlear implant receiver; however, this important issue has not been systematically studied using CT imaging.[1] This is an important consideration when making a decision for a patient with a cochlear implant in place to undergo an MRI, and consequently should be performed prior to MRI scanning. For young children a small (usually 2.5 or 3 mm in diameter) cutting bur is used to remove the outer cortex and diploic layer, whereas for older children and adults a 5-mm cylinder burr is helpful because it allows perpendicular walls to be created around the receiver site while simultaneously dissecting bone with the cutting flukes located on the tip of this cylinder bur.

Figure 28–2 shows the two methods available to create the tie-down suture holes through the bone. Four sites for suture tie-downs are created so that two separate 3-0 nylon sutures can be used to secure the cochlear implant receiver.

Bone wax is useful in controlling hemostasis, and if there is epidermal bleeding, placement of strips of Surgicel (Ethicon Inc., Somerville, NJ) are placed into the epidural space to achieve hemostasis and prevent postoperative epidural hematoma formation. Specific details necessary to create the receiver beds for the Nucleus Contour device, the Clarion CII and HiRes 90K devices, and the Med-El C40+ device are described below.

NUCLEUS CONTOUR

The Nucleus Contour device has two options regarding creation of the receiver bed. The first is to create the cylindrical well to receive the deepest portion of this cochlear implant. It is common in very young children to require a craniotomy down to the dura and creation of the bony island as described above. For the majority of adults and older children, this is not necessary and a craniectomy is all that is required. The remaining portion of the internal

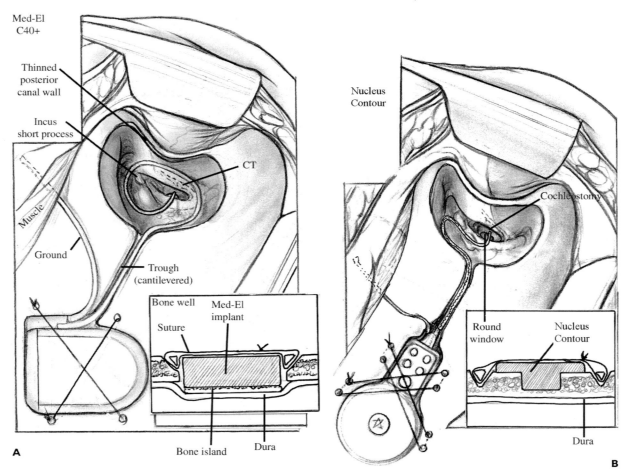

FIGURE 28–2 Securing the internal receiver-stimulator to the skull requires (A) four holes drilled through the skull into the bone bed (Med-El C40+ or CII Bionic Ear), or (B) eight channels drilled in pairs (Nucleus Contour or HiRes 90K Bionic Ear).

device is placed lateral to the skull, and, in parti-cular, the magnet and loop antenna have a very low profile and are barely palpable beneath the scalp flap. The remaining rectangular portion of the internal device/receiver is palpable, and for this reason it is especially important for this device to be placed well posterior to the position that will be occupied by the behind-the-ear speech processor. Another option for this device is to create a receiver bed that will accommodate most of the volume of the Nucleus Contour receiver. This is done in the same manner as described above and the advantage of this is that it allows a more integrated placement of the internal device, but it does require creation of a complex bony island and craniotomy, which re-quires additional surgical time.

The Nucleus Contour device has a separate ground electrode, which is placed beneath the temporalis muscle that is located lateral to the principal electrode array. A trough is created be-tween the internal receiver device and the area of the mastoidectomy. A 2-mm cutting bur is used to create this trough, and an important point is to complete the dissection such that one of the bony margins is cantilevered over the tract created in the bone. This further helps in securing and protecting the elec-trode array.

CLARION CII AND HIRES 90K BIONIC EAR

The internal device for the CII Bionic Ear is the largest of the internal devices made by the three companies presently in the United States market-place. The depth of this device is 6 mm; conse-quently, virtually all patients receiving this device require a craniotomy to inset it. The special con-sideration in preparing the receiver bed for this device is principally related to the fan-tail that allows the electrode array to leave the internal receiver device. Accommodation for this structure is critical to avoid excessive pressure or bending of the electrode array. It is important to dissect the bone underlying the fan-tail down to the same level that the floor of the receiver bed will be placed into. A 2-mm cutting bur is used to create the trough that accommodates the electrode array. The Clarion devices have the ground electrode built into the primary electrode array, and therefore a second electrode carrier containing the ground electrode is not used with these devices. The trough utilizes a cantilevered segment of the bone on either the superior or inferior aspect of this trough, and is helpful in keeping the electrode array from becom-ing exteriorized on the lateral aspect of the skull (Fig. 28–3).

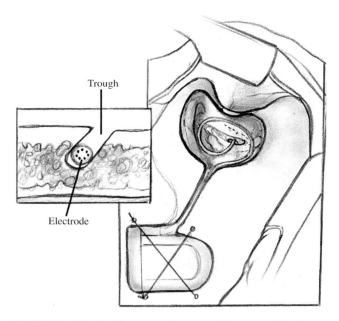

FIGURE 28–3 The trough created between the bone bed and the mastoidectomy site is cantilevered to facilitate retention of the electrode array beneath the surface of the skull.

The HiRes 90K Bionic Ear has a Silastic carrier surrounding the components and has a position for a replaceable internal magnet within the center of the loop antenna. The issues specific to the HiRes 90K Bionic Ear receiver bed are similar to those described in the Nucleus Contour device. The design of the HiRes 90K Bionic Ear differs from the Nucleus Contour device principally in the midportion of the internal device between the magnet and loop antenna and the electrode array. The design allows for a more tapered device, which theoretically results in fewer problems with extrusion and skin erosion than are experienced with the Nucleus Contour device. Thus, it is possible to create the smaller internal well, relative to the CII Bionic Ear device, to accommodate the most medial aspects of this device while allowing the remainder of the device to be positioned lateral to the skull. It is also possible to create a larger complex receiver bed that would accommodate this entire component, as has been described in the Nucleus Contour device subsection. The trough to accommodate the electrode array is the same as is necessary to accommodate the CII Bionic Ear electrode array.

MED-EL C40+

The biggest difference in the receiver bed for the Med-El C40+ is that the electrode array and ground electrode emanate from the side of the cochlear implant instead of from the proximal end of the cochlear implant, as is the case with the Nucleus Contour, CII Bionic Ear, and HiRes 90K Bionic Ear devices. Accommodation for this design feature requires that the bony trough begins at the side of the implant internal device and must be positioned so that one of the holes necessary to secure the implant can be placed.

Because the depth of the Med-El C40+ is 3.9 mm, some of the adult patients do not require a craniotomy down to the level of the dura, and creation of a bone island. This is necessary, however, in virtually all children and in many adults. The same principles described in earlier sections apply with this device, both in terms of creation of the bony island and the trough necessary to accommodate the electrode array. The ground electrode is separate and is placed beneath the temporalis muscle, as is the case with the Nucleus Contour device.

During the creation of the craniotomy and bone island necessary to accommodate the receiver-stimulator, inadvertent dural injury may occur. If this violation is small, placement of fascia is done through the opening, so that tissue remains both medial to and lateral to the dura in a dumbbell-shaped manner, and the hole is easily sealed. It is also important to determine that no parenchymal injury has occurred in this clinical setting.

MASTOIDECTOMY, FACIAL RECESS APPROACH, AND COCHLEOSTOMY TECHNIQUES

MASTOIDECTOMY

The important point in considering the mastoidectomy for placement of a cochlear implant is that this is much smaller than that utilized for chronic ear disease. In contrast to the standard method of saucerizing the mastoid cavity, this is not performed in cochlear implant surgery. There are two areas that need to be skeletonized, and the single most important one of these is the bony external auditory canal. If the bony external auditory canal is not thinned appropriately, then the angle through the facial recess and the size of the posterior aspect of the mastoidectomy become much more difficult and much larger, respectively. It is important to skeletonize the bony external auditory canal, but not to violate the integrity of this structure. Should this occur, the greatest postoperative risk is that of the electrode array extruding through the skin of the external auditory canal. Consequently, it is necessary to reinforce this area with either a graft composed of thick AlloDerm (LifeCell Corp., Branchburg, NJ) or a bone graft harvested from the cortex of the skull. The

second area that needs to be skeletonized is that of the tegmen mastoideum. This allows greater ease in completing the facial recess and developing the cochleostomy. An additional advantage is that of providing better exposure and consequently better light delivery, which results in better visualization within the facial recess and middle ear. It is also important to continue this action forward into the zygomatic root for the same reasons (Fig. 28–4). In contrast, the posterior as well as inferior aspects of the mastoidectomy are not saucerized. It is also important to create bony overhangs in these inferior and posterior aspects of the mastoidectomy cavity that are helpful in retaining the electrode array, which is ultimately coiled into the mastoid. These differences in the mastoidectomy technique also facilitate performance of cochlear implantation in very young children (6 to 12 months of age).

For those individuals who have undergone a canal-wall-down mastoidectomy procedure in the past and require cochlear implantation to rehabilitate their hearing loss, a two-stage procedure is required. First, mastoid obliteration with removal of all epithelium, oversewing the external auditory canal, and filling the resulting dead space with abdominal fat is performed. Three to 6 months later, cochlear implantation can be undertaken. If no active disease is present, a one-stage procedure may be considered; however, this is not recommended due to the risk of bacterial contamination.

FACIAL RECESS APPROACH

Once the mastoidectomy has been completed, the facial recess dissection is performed. The size of the facial recess is the same for individuals of any age, and based on the anatomic measurements of human temporal bones, the facial recess is of adult size at by at least 2 weeks of age.[2] Facial nerve electromyography is appropriate during this portion of the operation, and this cochlear implant surgeon (P.A.W.) always uses facial nerve electromyography during the dissection of the facial recess and during creation of the cochleostomy as well as insertion of the electrode array (NIM-2, Medtronic Xomed Inc.). A general guideline for determining the position of the facial recess is a direct inferior extension of the short process of the incus. Because there is no mechanical function of the incus in an ear receiving a cochlear implant, there is no adverse consequence for removing the incus buttress, which normally is preserved to maintain the suspensory ligament attached to the incus in this position. This has the advantage of delivering additional light into the middle ear and allows direct extension in an inferior direction below the short process of the incus. The

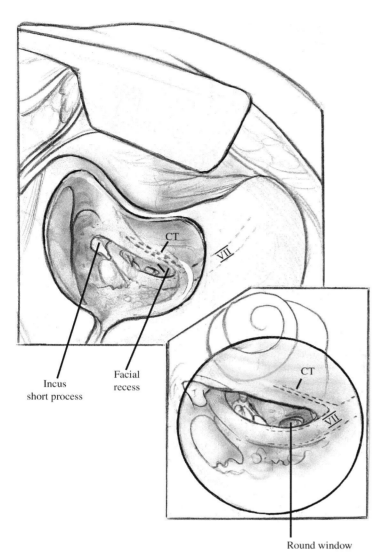

Incus
short process

Facial
recess

CT

VII

Round window

FIGURE 28-4   The mastoidectomy necessary for placement of a cochlear implant is limited, relative to that required to treat chronic ear disease. Skeletonization of the external auditory canal is important to facilitate access via the facial recess approach (posterior tympanotomy). Overhanging bone is created posteriorly and inferiorly to facilitate retention of the coiled electrode placed within the mastoid at the conclusion of the procedure. Skeletonization of the tegmen mastoideum and dissection into the zygomatic root facilitates light delivery into the mastoid and subsequently into the middle ear via the facial recess. CT, chordae tympani nerve.

vertical segment of the facial nerve is skeletonized, and a 1.5-mm diamond bur with a long shaft is helpful during this portion of the dissection. The dissection is carried inferiorly to the level of the chorda tympani nerve, and in some of the patients undergoing cochlear implantation surgery the chorda tympani nerve is divided to provide adequate access and visualization of the round window niche. Preoperative counseling of the patient or the parents is necessary so that they understand the consequences of dividing the chorda tympani nerve. The lateral limit of the facial recess is the tympanic annulus, and for the majority of patients this should be partially skeletonized to maximize the size of the facial recess.

Although it is possible to create a small facial recess, most experienced cochlear implant surgeons do not do this and prefer widely opening the facial recess. This provides much better visualization of the

round window niche and delivers additional light via the microscope into the middle ear. These factors facilitate completion of the cochleostomy and insertion of the electrode array. The tympanic annulus can be well visualized, with exposure of the promontory and epithelium of the middle ear also readily apparent.

During the facial recess dissection, violation of the tympanic annulus and tympanic membrane results in contamination and direct communication with the external auditory canal. This raises the possibility of postoperative infection and cholesteatoma formation. There are two options if this occurs, and one is to repair this area and stage the cochlear implantation. The other is to repair this area with a medial graft, which could be composed of temporalis fascia or thin AlloDerm. This is then supported with Gelfoam and/or muscle grafts. Should this be necessary, an important point is that the incus should be disarticulated and removed. This provides better access to the annulus and tympanic membrane for adequate apposition of the reconstructed material to the native tissue from the tympanic cavity side, and obviates the need for external auditory canal skin incisions and development of a tympano-meatal flap.

Cochleostomy

Placement of the electrode array within the scala tympani is accomplished via a cochleostomy. This cochleostomy is positioned relative to the round window membrane, and the single most important aspect in being able to appropriately place the electrode array within the scala tympani is visualization of the round window niche. The electrode

inserted within the scala tympani is shown in Figs. 28–5 and 28–6, and the specific electrode insertion techniques are described later. This landmark is critical to determine the relative position of the basal portion of the scala tympani. When completing the facial recess a temptation that often impacts the inexperienced cochlear implant surgeon is to begin preparing the cochleostomy when only the promontory is visualized. This leads, however, to the most common reason for failure to place the electrode array: the inadvertent opening into the hypotympanic air cell tract and extracochlear insertion of the electrode array.[3] If the drilling begins too inferiorly, dissection in this area can resemble an ossified basal turn of the cochlea. Often the hypotympanic air cell tract appears like the open scala tympani following successful completion of a cochleostomy. The ob-

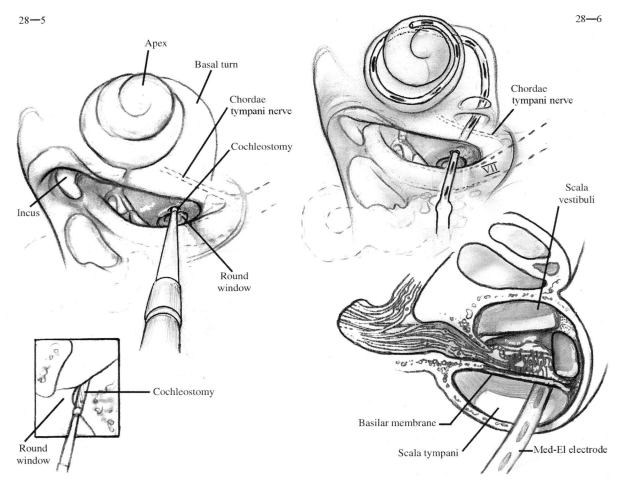

28—5

28—6

FIGURE 28–5 Cochleostomy position relative to the round window niche. It is important to visualize the bony overhang of the round window niche before beginning the cochleostomy. Removal of this overhang and subsequent exposure and visualization of round window membrane ensures that the cochleostomy is positioned with the midpoint centered on the lower margin of the round window, and located anterior in position to the round window membrane.

FIGURE 28–6 Electrode insertion through the cochleostomy follows the scala tympani.

vious result is an incomplete electrode insertion and ultimately no activation of the primary afferent neurons in the spiral ganglion. Another important anatomic landmark to keep in mind when experiencing difficulty in identifying the scala tympani is the position of the intratemporal internal carotid artery. With anterior dissection, when the scala tympani has not been adequately identified, the posterior aspect of the intratemporal carotid artery can be exposed, and this is an especially important consideration when performing cochlear implant surgery in children between the ages of 6 and 12 months. A high index of suspicion must be maintained during the surgical dissection, if the round window membrane and round window niche are not visualized at the beginning of the creation of the cochleostomy. This also underscores the importance of identifying this key landmark before beginning the cochleostomy. Those factors that help in the visualization of the round window niche include a wide facial recess and skeletonization of the bony external auditory canal.

Once the round window niche has been visualized, the use of a 0.6-mm diamond bur with a long shaft allows dissection of the niche until the round window membrane is directly seen. It is important to position the cochleostomy anterior to the round window membrane, as utilizing this position facilitates the angle of insertion of the electrode array. Should the round window be opened and the electrode array inserted through the round window, the angle of insertion is too acute and results in excessive pressure on the electrode array against the lateral wall of the cochlea during the attempted advancement of the electrode array. This excessive force applied to the electrode array can result in damage.

The design of the cochleostomy varies depending on the electrode array used. The smallest cochleostomy is associated with the Med-El C40+ electrode array, and the diameter of the cochleostomy only needs to be 1.3 mm in diameter. For the Med-El C40+, the diameter of the electrode array increases from $\approx$ 0.5 $\times$ 0.6 mm at the apex (distal tip) to $\approx$ 1.3 mm at the proximal, thicker part of the array just before the marker ring. The marker ring is $\approx$ 1.5 mm in diameter. Thus, the cochleostomy can be as small as 1.3 mm, and should be no larger than 1.5 mm to allow proper sealing of the cochleostomy with the marker ring. Small strips of fascia should be placed around the cochleostomy to further seal the perilymphatic space from the middle ear. The cochleostomy required for placement of the Nucleus Contour electrode is typically 1.5 to 2 mm. The electrode array itself has a diameter at the tip of $\approx$ 0.5 $\times$ 0.6

mm, and the diameter at the basal portion of the array is 0.8 mm.

In the past, the largest cochleostomy size was associated with the Clarion devices. For the old HiFocus I electrode array, a round cochleostomy was prepared and this measured 2.5 mm in diameter. In contrast, the present HiFocus electrode utilizes a round cochleostomy, 1.5 mm in diameter, when the metal insertion tube is used; however, a 2-mm cochleostomy is necessary when the Teflon insertion tube is used. The electrode array itself has a diameter at the tip of 0.6 mm and the diameter at the basal contact is 0.8 mm.

With all three devices, once the cochleostomy has been created it is important to irrigate the scala tympani via the cochleostomy to remove air bubbles and to wash bone debris from the scala tympani. This bone debris, if left in place, will induce ossification at this site, and it is important to minimize this because of the potential need for reimplantation in the future should a device fail. This is particularly important in young children being implanted between the ages of 6 and 12 months, as there is a higher likelihood that they will encounter a device failure at some point during their entire life span than an adult patient receiving a cochlea implant. Lactated Ringer's solution with a 5-cc syringe and a 24-gauge suction tip is ideal for the irrigation and refilling of the scala tympani.

SECURING THE RECEIVER

Once the bone work has been completed and the cochleostomy opened, the internal device is then secured in position with the retaining sutures. Two separate nylon sutures are used for this purpose. It is important during this process to be cognizant of the position of the electrode array so that excessive force or kinking is not encountered during the tightening of these sutures. It is also important that hemostats or other instruments not be used along any portion of the suture that will remain in the patient, as this weakens the material. Using a single throw in the first portion of the knot allows the second throw of the suture to slide along the monofilament nylon to achieve the appropriate level of tension and position of the internal device relative to the lateral aspect of the skull. It is also important that the knots be placed overlying the bone and not overlying the internal device. A total of eight knots are placed into each suture, and a medium-length tail to the suture is created when cutting the suture. After both of these retaining sutures are placed, then the ground electrode is placed beneath the temporalis muscle for both the Med-El C40+ and Nucleus Contour devices. To accomplish this, a Freer elevator is used to elevate the periosteum and temporalis muscle, and while maintaining this in position the ground electrode is placed medial to this and then the elevator is retracted out of the surgical field. The Nucleus Contour device has a second extracochlear electrode that is attached to the receiver-stimulator device.

ELECTRODE INSERTION

The electrode insertion is specific for each device, and the following subsections describe the technique used for each electrode insertion. The standard electrodes are described below, and descriptions of special electrode designs are provided in the section dealing with ossification of the cochlea.

NUCLEUS CONTOUR ELECTRODE

The Nucleus Contour electrode is a perimodiolar design and is preformed to conform to the modiolus. There is a stylet that is positioned within this electrode array that maintains the electrode in a straight configuration. The electrode array is curved, consisting of 22 half-banded platinum electrodes, variably spaced over 15 mm. The diameter of the intracochlear portion ranges from 0.5 to 0.8 mm. Overall, the length of the electrode array distal to the first of three silicon marker rings is 24 mm; the electrode is designed to be inserted 22 mm, however, and a platinum band is present at this position to use as a guide for depth of insertion. The half-banded electrodes face the modiolus with a width of 0.3 mm, and a geometric area ranging from 0.28 to 0.31 mm^2. In addition to the electrodes, there are 10 support bands that together with the stylet stiffen the electrode array. Of all available electrodes, this is the stiffest electrode, and consequently it is relatively easy to insert. The greatest disadvantage of this current electrode design is that once the stylet has been removed, it cannot be replaced. This is problematic should the electrode insertion be difficult because of anatomic variations. Manual positioning of the electrode tip within the opening of the cochleostomy is performed, and guiding the tip into this position is facilitated by the use of a claw-shaped instrument held in the dominant hand. Once the electrode tip is retained within the opening of the cochleostomy, bimanual advancement of the electrode array using two claw-shaped instruments held opposing each other, as close to the cochleostomy as possible, facilitates advancement of the electrode array within the scala tympani. The Nucleus Contour electrode array has three Silastic bands outside

of the electrode array that represent the proximal limit, and these should remain outside of the cochleostomy. Once this level is reached, the stylet is withdrawn by holding the electrode array in place with a single claw-shaped instrument or the specially designed alligator forceps, whose jaws do not close completely, and either instrument is held with the nondominant hand. A small right-angle hook is placed into the loop of the stylet and this is withdrawn. Fascia grafts are then placed around the cochleostomy site to seal it, and fascia grafts are also placed between the electrode array and the facial nerve within the facial recess. In addition, I place fascia between the electrode array and the tympanic annulus.

CII BIONIC EAR AND HiRes 90K BIONIC EAR

There is one electrode array system available for the two devices manufactured by the Advanced Bionics Corporation (CII Bionic Ear and HiRes 90K Bionic Ear): the HiFocus electrode system. This electrode is banana-shaped and curved toward the modiolus, consisting of 16 contacts, spaced every 1.1 mm over 17 mm. The diameter of the intracochlear portion ranges from 0.6 to 0.8 mm. Overall, the length of the electrode array designed to be inserted into the cochlea is 23 mm. The electrodes face the modiolus with a width of 0.4 mm and length of 0.5 mm. The HiFocus electrode system utilizes an insertion tube through which the insertion tool allows advancement of the electrode array. Both a metal (outer diameter of 1.5 mm) and a Teflon (outer diameter of 2 mm) insertion tube are included, and selection is based on surgeon preference. Gentle pressure along a thumb-driven advancement mechanism is required to insert the electrode. Should errors occur in electrode insertion, the electrode is easily reloaded into the insertion tube/insertion instrument, and additional attempts at electrode insertion can be made. The major advantage of this method is that uniform pressure during insertion can be made. Subsequent to insertion, fascia grafts are placed around the cochleostomy site to seal this area. Fascia grafts are also placed between the electrode array and the facial nerve within the facial recess as well as between the electrode array and the tympanic annulus.

MED-EL C40+

The Med-El C40+ system has three separate electrode designs. The standard electrode is the longest electrode available in the marketplace and is tapered in design. Twelve pairs of electrode bands are distributed over the ≈ 31.5 mm electrode array length. The contacts are spaced over ≈ 26.4 mm with ≈ 2.4 mm between each contact. As described in a later section, for cochleas that are partially ossified, a compressed electrode is also available, and for severely ossified cochleas, a split electrode array is available. Once the cochleostomy is complete and the internal receiver secured, the electrode array is then held in the nondominant hand. A claw-shaped instrument is then used to help guide the tip of the electrode into the cochleostomy, and once this is retained at the edge of the cochleostomy, two separate claw-shaped instruments are used to advance the electrode array. The advancement is facilitated if small segments of the electrode array are inserted with each subsequent movement. Unfortunately, the design of the Med-El claw is too narrow to accommodate the electrode array. Thus the electrode is incompletely engaged, and damage to the Silastic carrier material is possible with the use of this claw. Most experienced cochlear implant surgeons in the United States do not prefer the claw provided by the Med-El Corporation. The use of the Cochlear Corporation's claw-shaped instruments is adequate for this purpose, and this is the way that this author inserts the Med-El electrode array. There is a circumferential ring that represents the limit of the electrode array to be inserted, and this is located 31.5 mm from the distal tip. Once this is sealed at the cochleostomy, the manufacturer states that an adequate seal will be obtained if the cochleostomy is created at the optimal size. In addition, I place strips of fascia around the cochleostomy site around the electrode array, and free fascia grafts are placed between the facial nerve and the electrode array as well as between the electrode array and the tympanic annulus.

OSSIFICATION OF THE COCHLEA

During the opening of the cochleostomy if some ossification of the cochlea is encountered, but once drilling past 1 to 4 mm of the basal cochlea a normal scala tympani is encountered, then the compressed electrode array may be the appropriate array for insertion. The C40 + compressed electrode (C40 + S) is designed with the same number of electrode contacts ($n = 12$ pairs), but the total length of the electrode array is 18 mm as compared to 31.5 mm. The C40 + S electrode contacts are arranged closer together on the apical end of the array. These 12 pairs of electrodes are spaced over ≈ 12.1 mm. There is an insertion test device designed to replicate the electrode array, which can be used to determine whether a standard array or a compressed array is

the appropriate electrode to be inserted. With this, the insertion test device is advanced through the cochleostomy and the depth of insertion is determined. If it is apparent that the standard electrode array if inserted would result in electrodes being extracochlear in location, then the compressed electrode array should be used and fully inserted.

For more severely ossified cochleas, both the Med-El Corporation and the Cochlear Corporation manufacture split electrode arrays. The Med-El split electrode design (C40 + GB) has two compressed electrode arrays with five and seven pairs of electrode contacts, respectively (Figs. 28–7 and 28–8). These electrode arrays are inserted via two cochleostomies. They have a constant ≈ 0.5 × 0.6-mm diameter up to the fixation rings that are located ≈ 8.3 mm (on the longer array) and ≈ 6.1 mm (on the shorter array) from the apex. The Nucleus system also has a second electrode design, which is a split electrode array to be used for implantation of severely ossified cochleas.

SPECIAL CONSIDERATIONS REGARDING SECURING THE ELECTRODE ARRAY

For all three devices manufactured for the U.S. marketplace, securing of the electrode array at the cochleostomy site and at the facial recess is important. The cochlea and facial recess are the same size at birth as they are throughout adulthood and therefore, it is important to secure the electrode array at the cochleostomy with the fascia graft, which will scar in place and bridge the surrounding promontory to the electrode array. A second site of stabilization at the facial recess, with fascia grafts between the facial nerve and the electrode array as well as between the electrode array and the tympanic annulus, will further stabilize this relationship with the electrode array to the cochlea and facial recess (Fig. 28–9). This is important in children because of the relationship between head growth and the cochlear implant. The distal sites of stabilization at the cochleostomy and facial recess will secure the electrode array anteriorly, whereas the sutures and fibrous capsule that will form around the internal receiver, as well as the electrode within the trough created at the time of surgery, will stabilize this portion of the electrode array at the proximal portion of the cochlear implant. The remainder of the electrode array is coiled within the mastoid, and this air-filled space allows the uncoiling of this electrode array during development as the child's head grows. This mechanism allows

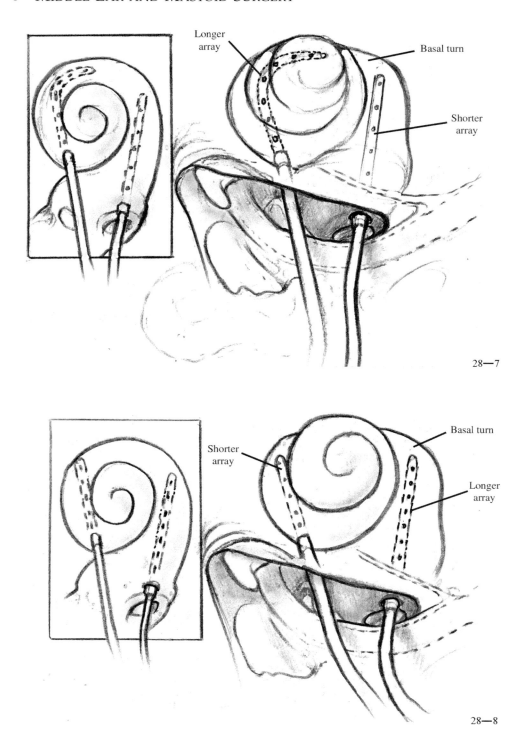

FIGURE 28–7 The Med-El C40 + GB (split electrode array) is used when there is severe cochlear ossification. If the basal turn is more ossified than the more apical turns of the cochlea, the shorter electrode array containing five pairs of electrode contacts is placed into the basal turn, whereas the longer array containing seven pairs of electrode contacts is placed more distally via a second cochleostomy. The Cochlear Corporation manufactures a similar split electrode array.

FIGURE 28–8 The Med-El C40 + GB (split electrode array) can be used when there is severe cochlear ossification. If the basal turn is less ossified than the more apical turns of the cochlea, the longer electrode array containing seven pairs of electrode contacts is placed into the basal turn, whereas the shorter array containing five pairs of electrode contacts is placed more distally via a second cochleostomy. The Cochlear Corporation manufactures a similar split electrode array.

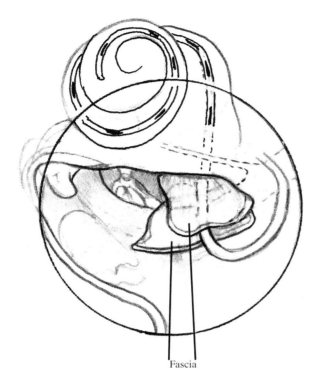

FIGURE 28–9 Fascia is placed between the electrode array and the facial nerve as well as between the electrode array and the chorda tympani/annulus. The remaining electrode array is coiled within the mastoid cavity.

Fascia

the accomplishment of natural growth and development while maintaining the integrity and position of the cochlear implant and its electrode array within the cochlea.

INTRAOPERATIVE ELECTROPHYSIOLOGIC TESTING

Intraoperative testing of the cochlear implant is a critical portion of the operation. First, impedance measurements are conducted to determine if the electrode array has been damaged during insertion and that all of the available electrodes are functional. Intraoperative neural response telemetry (NRT) is available for the Nucleus Contour device, and this allows direct recording from the eighth nerve distally following proximal stimulation. A similar system termed neural response imaging (NRI) is available for the CII Bionic Ear and HiRes 90K Bionic Ear systems. NRI and NRT function in a similar manner.

For all of our patients we perform intraoperative electrical evoked auditory brainstem response (EABR) testing. We do this with a distal intermediate and proximal electrode and determine thresholds

and maximum amplitudes of wave V. Beginning with the advent of perimodiolar electrodes, we have also been performing EABR testing both before and after placing the electrode in the perimodiolar position.[4,5] The details are provided below; however, the utility of performing EABR testing is most apparent with young children. Although behavioral thresholds can be determined in extremely young children, we have found that having objective information regarding thresholds for three of the active electrodes is extremely valuable in the initial programming of these devices. In addition, there is tremendous value to the families and to the patients receiving cochlear implants when we can state not only that the electrode array is fully inserted within the cochlea, but also that we have objective evidence of central auditory perception of the sound delivered through these electrodes. This technique has obviated the need for intraoperative radiographic studies to confirm the position of the electrode array within the cochlea.

Procedures to reliably record electrically evoked auditory potentials intraoperatively from pediatric and adult patients are described in the following paragraphs. During the surgical preparation of the patient, subdermal needle electrodes are placed on the forehead, nape of the neck, vertex, and ear contralateral to the implant. Markers that identify the electrode location are placed on the electrode leads, which are then draped under the operating table until they are needed. A subdermal needle electrode is placed on the sterile table and is inserted in the ipsilateral earlobe prior to the beginning of the surgical procedure. The electrode leads are attached to the amplifier of the evoked potential averager that is externally triggered by the stimulus output of the software for the respective implant.

After the surgeon has positioned the internal receiver stimulator and the electrode array, a sterile sheath is opened and the transmission coil is placed inside. The surgeon places the transmission coil covered by the sterile sheath over the internal device and a sterile, moistened gauze sponge separates these two structures. In this way, the external and internal devices are in communication with one another, but separated by a small space. The transmission coil is connected via a long cable to an external speech processor that is connected to a clinician's programming interface unit. When the programming interface unit is coupled to a computer, stimuli can be generated and delivered to the internal implant electrodes. Software programs provided by each of the cochlear implant manufacturers allow confirmation that the transmission coil is communicating with the internal system and that the electrodes are being activated with electrical stimuli.

From our intraoperative experience recording EABRs from patients receiving various implants (e.g., Clarion, Nucleus, Med-El), we have developed protocols for stimulation and recording that take into consideration the parameters of each device. Generally, stimulation occurs on three individual electrodes that represent apical, middle, and basal locations along the electrode array and within the cochlea. The initial stimulus levels used are those that generate a well-formed EABR. Stimulation begins on the most apical electrode, because responses from an apical position result in the best morphology, largest amplitude, and lowest EABR wave V threshold.[6] Electrical stimulation is decreased until the wave V threshold is determined. The absolute level of current varies depending on the particular cochlear implant device. The procedure is repeated for medial and basal electrodes. Waveform morphology, amplitude, and threshold are determined for all recording sets. Typically waves II, III, and V are present at higher stimulus levels, and wave V can be followed down to threshold. Wave I is never observable due to the overlap with the stimulus artifact in the early portion of the time window (less than 1 msec). We have found, as have others, that the EABR threshold represents a stimulus level that falls somewhere within the electrical dynamic range for a given electrode. This corresponds to a current level that should be audible for the patient, and can be approached from a minimum current level at the time of initial stimulation. The EABR threshold also provides prior knowledge of whether low, normal, or high current levels are expected at the initial stimulation, which can be quite helpful when presenting electrical stimuli to very young children for the first time.

EABR tracings and threshold information for each tested electrode are provided to the programming clinician prior to the initial activation of the patient. In addition, the surgical outcome and any complications (e.g., partial electrode insertion, ossified cochlea, unusual anatomy) are shared with the programming clinician. This information assists in planning for the initial activation and avoids stimulation of electrodes that could generate unpleasant sensations, such as electrodes that may be outside the cochlea. Finally, as mentioned previously, the electrophysiologic test results are shared with the patient's family and ensure that the electrode is properly placed and that electrical stimulation successfully activates the auditory system.

CLOSURE AND POSTOPERATIVE MANAGEMENT

The closure of the soft tissue varies depending on the initial soft tissue approach utilized. For young children, because the periosteum, scalp, and skin are all raised together in one layer, these are closed in two layers. The first layer is closed with inverted interrupted 4-0 Vicryl sutures (Ethicon Inc., Arlington, TX) and includes the periosteum, galea, and subcutaneous tissues. Once this layer has been closed, then the skin is closed with a running locked 5-0 plain gut fast-absorbing suture (Ethicon Inc.). The advantage of using all absorbable sutures in young children is that the skin sutures do not need to be removed.

For adult patients and children large enough to have the soft tissue approach completed in two layers, the periosteum is closed over the implant with simple interrupted 3-0 Vicryl suture (Ethicon Inc.). Another important consideration when very thick scalp or very unusually well-developed temporalis and scalp musculature is found is that debulking of the muscle can be required. Also, defatting the scalp is possible; however, the vascular supply to the scalp runs with the galea, and care should be taken to avoid compromising this. Maintaining a scalp that is thin enough to allow the magnetic attraction of the transmitter coil to the internal cochlear stimulator device magnet allows the transmitter coil to be secured to the scalp without falling off; however, if the scalp is too thick, then this is not possible. An alternate strategy is to resect the periosteum overlying the periosteum and subcutaneous connective tissue that overlies the internal device, but is medial to the galea. Surgical judgment in thinning the scalp is essential. The galea and subcutaneous layers are then closed with inverted interrupted 3-0 Vicryl pop-off sutures, and the skin is closed with a running locked 4-0 nylon for the postauricular incision and a running locked 3-0 nylon suture for the scalp incision.

For adults and children, a pressure dressing is then applied, and care is taken to protect the incision with antibiotic ointment and strips of Telfa. A small sheet of cotton is trimmed to conform to the pinna, which helps protect the pinna from pressure-induced necrosis. Fluffs are placed over the scalp and elevated flaps, and one Kerlix (Kendall Healthcare Products Co., Mansfield, MA) and one Kling (Ethicon Inc.) are wrapped around the patient's head. Umbilical tape (Ethicon Inc.) is used over the forehead to secure the dressing and to lift this dressing away from the patient's eyes. The pressure dressing is left in place for the first postoperative night and is removed the following morning.

Virtually all cochlear implant surgery is done on an outpatient basis, with children being observed for less than 23 hours in hospital, principally to control postoperative pain. Adults are typically operated in an ambulatory manner unless their surgery occurs late in the afternoon, as is the case when three cochlear implant surgeries are performed in one day.

COMPLICATIONS

The most common complications occurring after cochlear implantation are wound and flap related.[7] Wound breakdown is most often associated with placement of the internal device too close to the pinna or at the site of the skin incision. Injury to the intratemporal internal carotid artery is extremely rare; however, as discussed earlier in this chapter, in young children in whom the round window niche is not clearly seen, it is possible to follow the hypotympanic air cell tract to the carotid artery.[8] In such clinical scenarios, it is therefore important to maintain a high index of suspicion so as to identify the carotid artery prior to injury. Other risks of the cochlear implant procedure are similar to, and as rare as, those seen in chronic ear surgery: infection, facial paralysis, vertigo, cerebrospinal fluid (CSF) leakage, meningitis, and anesthesia-related risks.[9–12] Of these, the risk of meningitis most warrants further comment due to the recent heightened awareness of this complication. Early cases of meningitis are due to otitis media in the context of an unsealed cochleostomy. As discussed earlier, it is important to seal the cochleostomy with fascia. Until the subsequent fibrosis has been completed, however, the inner ear is vulnerable to the passage of bacteria into the perilymphatic space and then the CSF. Late cases of meningitis may be due to the higher risk of meningitis due to inner ear deformities[10] or inadequate sealing of the cochleostomy. In any of these scenarios, the risk of meningitis can be further reduced by preoperative immunization with Prevnar (children under 2 years of age) and Pneumovax 23 (children 2 years of age and over and all other individuals). These vaccines recognize seven serotypes and 23 serotypes of *Streptococcus pneumoniae*, respectively. Our cochlear implant program requires vaccination with the age-appropriate vaccine prior to implantation.

Facial nerve stimulation can occur after cochlear implantation due to electrical activation of the nerve by the active electrodes.[11] Placement of the fascia between the electrode array and the facial nerve as well as sealing the cochleostomy are designed to limit current spread. Certain primary bone diseases such as otosclerosis and Paget's disease increase the porosity of the bone, which may allow extracochlear current spread and activation of the facial nerve. Programming the external speech processor can deactivate specific electrodes found to be stimulating the facial nerve, thereby eliminating this problem.

The final complication that should be mentioned is device failure. Although this is extraordinarily uncommon, these failed devices are routinely removed and the cochlea reimplanted.[13] This is uncomplicated in most cases and results in comparable performance, or even enhanced performance if the failed device is replaced with a later-generation device.

SPECIAL CONSIDERATIONS REGARDING BILATERAL SIMULTANEOUS COCHLEAR IMPLANTATION

Although there are similarities between unilateral and bilateral simultaneous cochlear implantation, there are eight changes that can be made to better meet the challenges posed by bilateral simultaneous implantation and to improve performance. First, use a headlight for the soft tissue work, because the angle of the head is not as acute as is the case with a unilateral cochlear implant surgery. The draping of both the right and left side limits the ability to turn the head. Second, the side arm of the microscope is not changed between the two sides; therefore, while on the second side it requires that the resident or observer view the surgery via the video monitor. Third, in regard to draping, toweling-off the areas and using a split sheet around both sides, followed by placement of cranial incisor drapes on both sides, allows surgery to proceed in a parallel manner rather than in a serial manner. Fourth, the electromyogram (EMG) and EABR electrodes need to be individually labeled; I use all blue electrodes for the left side and all red electrodes on the right side for EMG monitoring and switch between these when skeletonizing the facial nerve on the respective side. Alternatively, a second EMG monitor can be used. Fifth, there is an aesthetic need for symmetry in placement of the internal cochlear stimulator device. Sixth, there is increased operative time, which usually requires 3.5 to 4 hours. The overall operative time includes 45 minutes of EABR testing for both the right and left sides. Seventh, close the periosteum and subcutaneous tissue as well as the skin after the first implant is placed. Eighth, use a Foley catheter because of the increased duration of surgery.

The suggested sequence is outlined here:

1. Shave and mark out incisions bilaterally.
2. Place EMG electrodes for both the right and left side (orbicularis oculi and orbicularis oris muscles).
3. Place EABR electrodes.
4. Place Foley catheter and pulsatile stockings.
5. Prepare the skin and draping.
6. Do all soft tissue work for both the right and left side.
7. Do all gross bone work for the right and left side for completing the microscope work. This includes the craniectomy or craniotomy, tie-down holes, trough, and cortical mastoidectomy.
8. Do the microscope work. Complete the mastoidectomy, facial recess, cochleostomy on the left; then repeat the above on the right.
9. Implant the right-side device.
10. Perform EABR testing for the right-side device.
11. Close the periosteum, subcutaneous tissue, and skin on the right.
12. Switch EMG electrodes.
13. Implant the left-side device.
14. Perform EABR testing for the left-side device.
15. Close the periosteum, subcutaneous tissue, and skin on the left.
16. Remove EMG and EABR electrodes.
17. Place bilateral mastoid pressure dressings.

FUTURE CONSIDERATIONS

Multiple institutions and corporations are actively pursuing the development of a fully implantable cochlear implant. Reduced power requirements, improved battery life, and the ability to recharge the internal battery via a transcutaneous route are engineering issues that are being addressed. Likewise the development of a microphone/transducer placed on the ossicular chain within the middle ear remains a technical challenge that must be resolved before a fully implantable cochlear auditory prosthesis can be created. It is anticipated that additional surgical steps will be necessary to implant this type of device. In addition, work focused on tissue engineering is targeting strategies to reduce fibrosis and neo-ossification as well as increase primary afferent dendrite growth and spiral ganglion cell survival.

REFERENCES

1. Sonnenburg RE, Wackym PA, Yoganandan N, Firszt JB, Prost RW, Pintar FA. Biophysics of cochlear implant/MRI interaction emphasizing bone biomechanical properties. *Laryngoscope* 2002; 112: 1720–1725.
2. Eby TL. Development of the facial recess: implications for cochlear implantation. *Laryngoscope* 1996;106(suppl 80):1–7.
3. Hoffman RA, Cohen NL. Surgical pitfalls in cochlear implantation. *Laryngoscope* 1993;103:741–744.
4. Firszt JB, Wackym PA, Gaggl W, Burg L, Reeder RM. Electrically evoked auditory brainstem responses for lateral and medial placement of the Clarion HiFocus electrode. *Ear Hear* 2003; 24: 184–190.
5. Wackym PA, Gaggl W, Runge-Samuelson C, Reeder RM, Raulie J, Firszt JF. Electrophysiological effects of placing cochlear implant electrodes in a perimodiolar position in young children. *Laryngoscope* 2003. In press.
6. Firszt JB, Chambers RD, Kraus N, Reeder RM. Neurophysiology of cochlear implant users I: effects of stimulus current level and electrode site on the electrical ABR, MLR and N1-P2 response. *Ear Hear* 2002;23:1–16.
7. Telian SA, El-Kashlan HK, Arts HA. Minimizing wound complications in cochlear implant surgery. *Am J Otol* 1999;20:331–334.
8. Gastman GR, Hirsch BE, Sando I, Fukui MB, Wargo ML. The potential risk of carotid injury in cochlear implant surgery. *Laryngoscope* 2002;112:262–266.
9. Luntz M, Teszler CB, Shpak T, Feiglin H, Farah-Simaan A. Cochlear implantation in healthy and otitis-prone children: a prospective study. *Laryngoscope* 2001;111:1614–1618.
10. Page EL, Eby TL. Meningitis after cochlear implantation in Mondini malformation. *Otolaryngol Head Neck Surg* 1997;116:104–106.
11. Kelsall DC, Shallop JK, Brammeier TG, Prenger EC. Facial nerve stimulation after Nucleus 22-channel cochlear implantation. *Am J Otol* 1997;18:336–341.
12. Steenerson RL, Cronin GW, Gary LB. Vertigo after cochlear implantation. *Otol Neurotol* 2001;22:842–843.
13. Alexiades G, Roland JT, Fishman AJ, Shapiro W, Waltzman SB, Cohen NL. Cochlear reimplantation: surgical techniques and functional results. *Laryngoscope* 2001;111:1608–1613.

Chapter 29

Surgical Implantable Hearing Aids

John Stewart, Trang Vo-Nuygen, Weiru Shao, and Oleg Froymovich

Implantable hearing aids, compared to conventional hearing aids, are a spectrum of prosthetic device that is wholly or partially implanted through surgery to ameliorate hearing loss.[1] To extrapolate this definition, one may consider cochlear implant and brainstem implant as close relatives, if not actual types, of implantable hearing aids. On the other end of the spectrum, a bone-anchored hearing aid (BAHA), essentially a temporal bone stimulator, also qualifies as an implantable hearing aid. Its implantation is less invasive and its method of cochlear stimulation is similar to that of conventional bone conduction hearing aid.

Recent technologic advances and innovation in digital microcircuitry have promoted the design of new implantable hearing aids. An ideal implantable hearing aid provides better sound reception and better cosmesis; is nonirritating, biocompatible, and trouble free; and has a long life expectancy. The implanted component should be easily removed or changed without incident. It should not reduce residual hearing, or limit activities such as swimming, or predispose the patient to recurrent infection. The surgical procedure should be simple and free of major complications. Finally, the cost of the device should be similar to a conventional high-power, ear-level aid.[1]

Over the past decade a number of implantable hearing devices have been introduced, but some have since been discontinued from the competitive market. With the rapid evolution of hearing aid technology, newer implantable hearing aids will soon emerge. This chapter provides a summary of implantable hearing aids: BAHA, middle ear implants, and brainstem implants. Chapter 28 discusses cochlear implantation.

BONE-ANCHORED HEARING AID

In the quest for complete hearing restoration, the cornerstone remains amplification. Many advances have been made in middle ear and chronic otomastoiditis surgery. Despite these advances, there will always remain those patients who despite aggressive surgical interventions continue to drain or begin draining once the canal is occluded with a conventional air-conduction hearing aid. Likewise, there will continue to be congenital aural atresia in which reconstructive endeavors should not or will not be undertaken by the patient or by the wishes of the family. For these patients few options exist.

Historically bone-conduction transducers are the aid of choice. Prior to 20 years ago, standard bone-conduction aids transmitted sound waves to the cochlea through the overlying soft tissues and bone. The sound quality was generally thought to be poor and the transmission inefficient. Much of the sound energy could be lost at the level of the soft tissue. The magnitude of attenuation could be as high as 15 to 20 dB in the speech frequencies. To counteract the attenuation of sound energy, the old bone conductors were driven hard, also raising the level of distortion. BAHA (Entific Medical Systems, Goteborg, Sweden) allows a direct coupling between the transducer and the skull, bypassing the soft tissues (Fig. 29–1). Energy transmission is more efficient and sound quality improved. Another advantage is the lack of discomfort from the previously required pressure of the transducers to the soft tissues by the headbands, metal springs, or heavy frames. It should not be disputed that this is the simplest hearing aid implant with respect to both functional concept and implantation.[2]

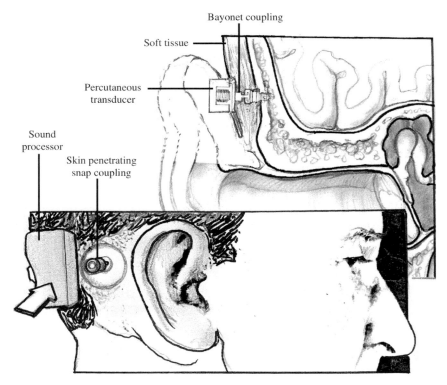

FIGURE 29–1 Schematic drawing of the bone-anchored hearing aid (BAHA) in bone.

A surgically implanted titanium screw is allowed to osseointegrate into the skull to reduce extrusion and to improve acoustic transmission. The timing of applying a load to the screw after surgery ranges from 1 to 3 months to allow for osseointegration and to reduce irritation of the surrounding soft tissues in the operated field. The BAHA vibrates the screw and skull, which in turn vibrates the cochlear fluids directly. Patient selection involves two main groups of patients: patients with chronically draining ears and a conductive, sensorineural, or mixed hearing loss; and patients with bilateral ear canal atresia whose reconstruction is not advisable, such as those with a Jahrsdoefer rating of 7 or less,[3] or in pediatric patients whose reconstructive surgery will be delayed until adulthood so that they can then contemplate the risks of facial nerve injury and hearing loss themselves.[4]

Acceptable hearing loss for BAHA depends on the use of the ear-level transducer such as the BAHA HC 300 Classic or the body aid transducer BAHA Cordelle, which is more powerful and allows for greater hearing loss. Patients with better cochlear function, such as discrimination scores better than 60% and bone conduction less than 45 dB, have better outcomes with the HC 300 Classic style. Many patients demonstrate a mixed loss. Those with a mean bone conduction loss of 45 dB and an air–bone gap of 60 dB (with a total of 105 dB speech threshold) through the speech ranges may consider the Cordelle. Those with a mean bone conduction loss of 60 dB and a maximal air–bone gap of 60 dB (with a total of 120 dB speech threshold) are more likely to require the Cordelle.[4–7]

Preoperative evaluation is limited to audiometric testing and imaging studies. A high-resolution computed tomography (CT) imaging study of the temporal bone is performed in anyone whose sigmoid sinus, middle fossa plate, or facial nerve position is in question as in congenital ear cases. Informed consent should include local infection, subcutaneous tissue reduction in the area, alopecia in the operative site, bleeding from violated sigmoid sinus, and possible dural disruption if a shallow bone plate or low-lying middle fossa is present. In addition reasonable hygiene is expected because the implant penetrates the skin. The surgical steps are relatively simple and are easily learned. Most adults can have this performed under local anesthesia, whereas children usually have a general anesthetic for practical purposes only.

The proposed site is marked 55 mm posterior to the external meatus and superiorly in the linea temporalis. The transducer should not contact the pinna when attached to the screw (Fig. 29–2). The following are the operative procedures[4]:

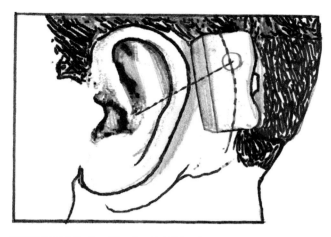

FIGURE 29–2 Site for BAHA placement.

1. A 30-mm radius shave and sterile prep and drape.
2. A 20-mm anteriorly based ∪-shaped incision is carried down through skin and soft tissues and the flap is reflected forward.
3. The flap is thinned of subcutaneous tissue and sometimes hair follicles.
4. The underlying bone is cleaned of muscle and periosteum in a 6-mm radius in the proposed drilling site.
5. A low-speed (1500 to 2000 rpm) drill, saline irrigation, and a 3-mm drill guide is chosen to allow a 1.8-mm diameter bit.
6. A countersink hole is created with a 4-mm drill guide always remaining at the same initial perpendicular angle of entry to the bone surface.
7. A 3- to 4-mm titanium tap is loaded onto the stainless steel drill hand piece with touching of gloves and will be tapped at an ultralow drill speed of 8 to 15 rpm and at a torque setting of 20 to 40 N · cm depending on bone softness.
8. The tap is removed by slowly reversing the drill.
9. The fixture flange is implanted by screwing the internal screw and holding the fixture mound with the organizer.
10. A skin punch is utilized directly over the area of the fixture device.
11. If fixture device is stable, the skin abutment is connected immediately. If it is unstable, the connection is delayed 3 to 4 months to allow for osseous integration.
12. The skin flap edges are approximated with 6-0 nylon monofilament.
13. A healing cap is affixed to the abutment cap; gauze and a light mastoid dressing are utilized. Mastoid dressing is removed on the following day.
14. Gauze and cap are maintained until suture removal in one week.
15. Gauze and cap are reapplied for another week.

Postoperative complications include local skin reactions treated with topical antibiotic ointments and good hygiene, granulation tissue formation, and loose screws that can usually be tightened without anesthesia with the screwdriver and wrench supplied. Granulation tissue is removed by standard techniques, and the device is not used until the wound is well healed.

Overall, the BAHA has specific indications; the technique for implantation is easily learned and the minor complications easily dealt with, making this a worthwhile device that is likely to stand the test of time.

MIDDLE EAR IMPLANTS

Implantable middle ear hearing aids directly drive the ossicular chain or its attachment by means of the implanted components. They are intended for use in patients with residual cochlear function who could benefit from amplification. Based on the different transducers used in the design, current technology offers two types of middle ear implants: piezoelectric and electromagnetic. *Piezoelectric* implants use ceramic structures that are capable of temporary bending if electric current is applied. The implants may be single layered or bilayered, that is, monomorph or biomorph, respectively. When attached to the ossicles, the implants create vibrations with alternating current. The amount of the structural bending is proportional to the overall length of the implants that are attached to the ossicles, a limiting factor for amplification power in piezoelectric implants. *Electromagnetic* implants convert electromagnetic signals into ossicular vibrations via a nearby coil without physical contact. A magnet is implanted onto the ossicle and vibrates according to the electromagnetic signals that are transmitted to the coil from the sound processor. A major limitation of the device is the distance between the coil, usually in the external auditory canal, and the magnet. Its power output is inversely proportional to the cube of the distance.[8]

There are a number of middle ear implantable devices currently available: Direct Drive Hearing System (DDHS, SOUNDTEC, Oklahoma City, OK), Envoy (St. Croix Medical, Minneapolis, MN), Middle Ear Transducer (MET, Otologics, Boulder, CO), and Rion (Rion Company, Tokyo, Japan). The Totally Integrated Cochlear Amplifier (TICA, Implex, Munich, Germany) and Vibrant Soundbridge (Symphonix, San Jose, CA) have been discontinued in the United States. Table 29–1 provides a summary of the devices.

DIRECT DRIVE HEARING SYSTEM

The SOUNDTEC DDHS design consists of an external and an internal unit. The external part includes a processor that is worn behind the ear and an electromagnetic coil in the ear canal in a conventional ear mold. To minimize the distance between the coil and magnet, the magnet is placed at the incudo-stapedial joint (Fig. 29–3). The magnet is coated with Parylene C and sealed in a laser-welded titanium cylinder. A titanium alloy ring is used to secure the implant around the incudo-stapedial joint.[9]

The audiologic indications are bilateral mild-moderate to moderately severe sensorineural hearing loss (SNHL), bone thresholds within 10 dB of air thresholds, high-frequency pure tone average of 1000, 2000, and 4000 Hz between 35 and 70 dB hearing level, and discrimination scores greater than 60%. A recently completed phase II clinical trial demonstrates that the SOUNDTEC system provides statistically significant reduction in feedback and occlusive effect as well as a statistically significant improvement in the following categories: functional gain, articulation index scores, speech discrimination in a quiet environment, perceived aided benefit, patient satisfaction, and device preference over the patient's optimally fit hearing aid.[10]

The surgical technique is a transcanal stapedectomy approach. A standard stapedectomy-type tympanomeatal flap is elevated to expose the tympanic cavity. The incudo-stapedial joint is then separated in a careful manner so as not to disrupt the stapes superstructure. The long process of the incus is then separated enough to allow for placement of an attachment ring. A 4-0 silk suture is placed and advanced beneath the long process of the incus. This sling then allows the surgeon to use his or her nondominant hand to elevate the incus during implant insertion. The implant is then inserted using the suction-operated SOUNDTEC insertion instrument or the SOUNDTEC open-mouthed cylinder-holding forceps. Only special nonmagnetic instruments and specula are used during the implant process to allow for exact positioning of the implant. The lenticular process is then allowed to rejoin with the capitulum of the stapes through the ring. The magnet cylinder is axially aligned with the ear canal. A cast made from absorbable Gelfoam is used to stabilize the implant. Care is taken to ensure that the promontory, the posterior canal wall, and the under-surface of the tympanic membrane do not come into contact with each other to prevent synechia formation. The tympanomeatal flap can then be returned to its original position. If the magnet comes into close apposition with the undersurface of the tympanic membrane, then a cartilage cap obtained from the tragus should be placed in the undersurface of the tympanic membrane to minimize the risk of implant extrusion. Following implantation, a 10-week period is allowed for healing to take place. Then the SOUNDTEC search coil is used to locate the optimal area for placement of the electromagnetic coil within the external auditory canal (ECA). Once the ECA is fitted, the device is activated.[10]

ENVOY

The Envoy is a totally implantable hearing system developed by St. Croix Medical Products of Minnesota. The Envoy hearing aid consists of a sensor, a driver, and a sound processor. The sensor is placed in the mastoid cavity in such a way that the transducer tip can be adhesively attached to the

TABLE 29–1 IMPLANTABLE HEARING DEVICES

Device	Manufacturer	Transduction Mechanism	FDA status	Implantability
Direct Drive Hearing System (DDHS)	SOUNDTEC	EM	Phase II completed	Partial
Envoy	St. Croix Medical	PE	Phase I	Total
Middle ear transducer (MET)	Otologics	EM	Phase II	Partial
Rion	Rion Co	PE	NA	Partial
*Totally Integrated Cochlear Amplifier (TICA)	Implex	PE	NA	Total
*Vibrant Soundbridge	Symphonix	PE	Phase III completed	Partial

*Product discontinued.
EM, electromagnetic; NA, not approved; PE, piezoelectric.

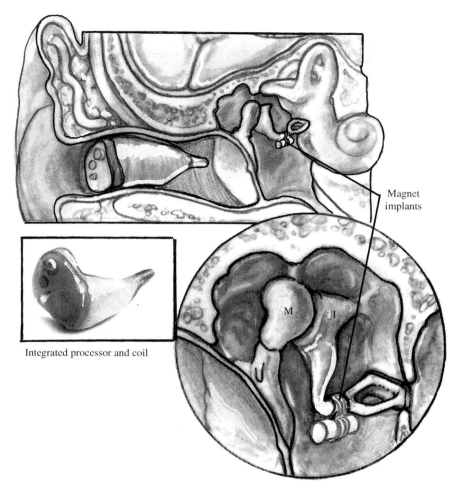

Integrated processor and coil

Magnet implants

M   I

FIGURE 29–3 The Direct Drive Hearing System.

stapes. The body of the sensor is secured to the mastoid cavity using bone cement. The driver is also positioned within the mastoid cavity (Fig. 29–4). The sound processor is typically implanted in a bony cavity created behind the ear, in a similar fashion as cochlear implant. The sensor acts as a microphone. It converts sound vibrations into electrical signals. The electrical signals are then amplified by the sound processor. The driver converts the electrical signals into mechanical vibration to drive the stapes.[8,11] The Envoy system is currently undergoing phase I clinical trial in the United States.

MIDDLE EAR TRANSDUCER

The MET is produced by Otologics, LLC, of Boulder, Colorado. It is approved in both the United States and Europe for implantation. It has an implantable part and an external part in a behind-the-ear case. A probe is placed in the body of the incus and generates vibration in the ossicles (Fig. 29–5). The

audiologic indication is moderately severe to severe SNHL.[12] A postauricular approach is typically used for implantation. Currently, a phase II clinical trial is being conducted in the United States.

RION

The Rion is manufactured by Rion Company in Japan. It is approved for implantation in Japan and is not available in the United States. Indications for the device include patients with conductive deafness and mild to moderate mixed hearing losses due to chronic otitis media, tympanosclerosis, or total loss of the sound conductive mechanism. The device's usage has been limited to patients with bilateral deafness. It is implanted in the ear with greater hearing loss (Fig. 29–6). The audiologic criteria for selecting candidates are (1) an average bone-conduction hearing threshold for speech frequencies not exceeding 50 dB; (2) speech discrimination score better than 70%; and (3) intraoperative hearing testing that demonstrates the effectiveness of the implant. The device is implanted via a mastoidectomy, canal wall up or down.[13]

TOTALLY INTEGRATED COCHLEAR AMPLIFIER

The TICA has been developed by Implex Corporation, Munich, Germany, and approved in Europe for moderate to severe high-frequency SNHL. The device is implanted through a mastoidectomy and has a small remote control to adjust the device. The battery is charged transcutaneously with a portable charger within approximately 90 minutes. The running time is about 50 hours, and the battery may require replacement every 3 to 5 years. The indications for the new model TICA LZ0331 include lack of benefits from conventional hearing aids, normal

pneumatization of mastoid, and SNHL from 50 to 90 dB above 3 kHz.[8]

VIBRANT SOUNDBRIDGE

The Vibrant Soundbridge system was developed by Symphonix Devices, Inc., of San Jose, California. In November 2002 the company was dissolved by its board and the system withdrawn from the market. Prior to its withdrawal, the device was approved by the Food and Drug Administration (FDA) and the European Union for implantation. A phase III study demonstrated effectiveness for moderate to severe SNHL in adults.[14] The device consists of two parts: the external speech processor and the implanted vibrating ossicular prosthesis. The surgery includes a mastoidectomy, similar to cochlear implantation.

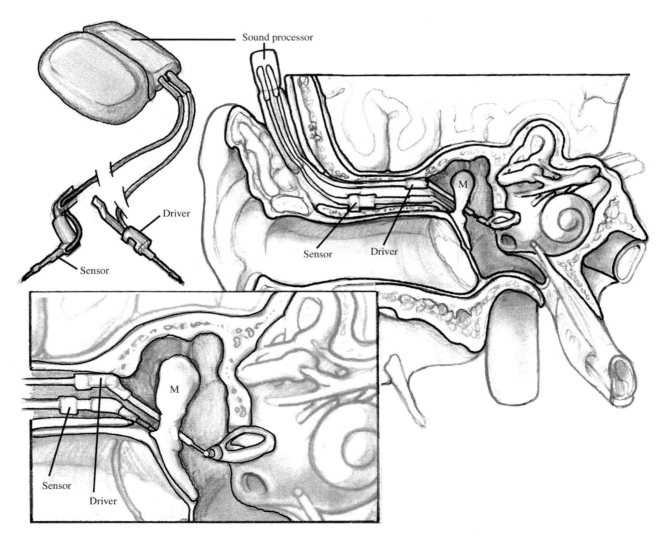

FIGURE 29–4 The Envoy.

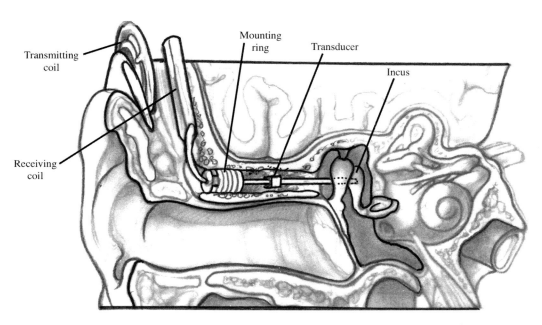

FIGURE 29–5   The middle ear transducer system.

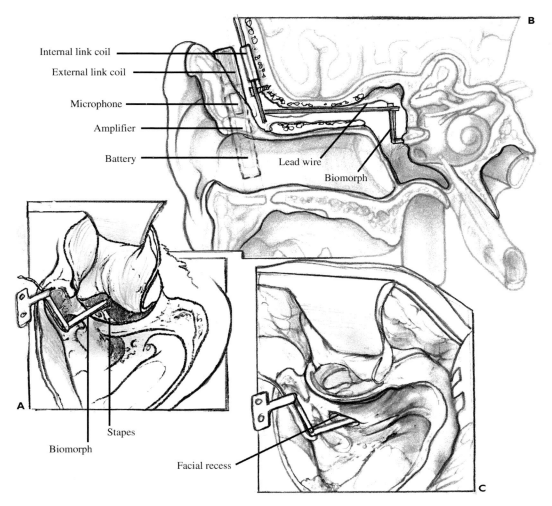

FIGURE 29–6   The Rion system. (A) Canal-wall-down mastoidectomy. (B) Canal-wall-up mastoidectomy. (C) Coronal cross section, canal-wall-up mastoidectomy. (Adapted from Slattery and Soli,[8] with permission.)

AUDITORY BRAINSTEM IMPLANTS

The first report of direct stimulation of human auditory cortex is attributed to Penfield in the 1950s, which was done under local anesthesia. In 1964 Simmons and his group described their experience with electrical excitation of the cochlear nerve and inferior colliculus. William House implanted the first auditory brainstem implant (ABI) with single-channel electrode array in 1979 after removal of an acoustic tumor.[15] Since 1992, advanced multichannel ABIs have been implanted.

At the present ABI has a narrow set of indications related to bilateral retrocochlear deafness. The leading cause is loss of bilateral auditory nerve function after vestibular schwannomas removal in neurofibromatosis type 2 (NF-2) followed by other rare bilateral auditory nerve pathologies. Approximately 90% of NF-2 patients exhibit bilateral acoustic neuromas.[16] In the United States patients undergoing ABI are under strict protocols including a comprehensive battery of psychophysical and speech perception tests.

In deciding on a patient's candidacy for cochlear implantation versus ABI, the surgeon must have a clear distinction between cochlear and retrocochlear deafness. Pre- and postoperative topodiagnosis of deafness after bilateral tumor resection in NF-2 may be crucial in determining hearing rehabilitation

strategies. Transtympanic extracochlear monopolar electrical stimulation on the promontory or round window in conjunction with transtympanic electrocochleography is a well-accepted method of distinguishing cochlear from retrocochlear deafness. It has been postulated that in patients with acoustic neuromas, cochlear deafness, either before or after tumor resection, is of vascular etiology when the auditory nerves are preserved. Only very large acoustic tumors are thought to affect auditory nerve

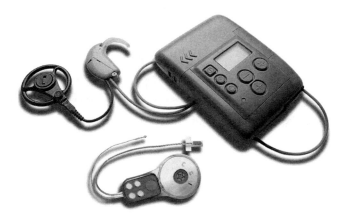

FIGURE 29–7 Auditory brainstem implant receiver/stimulator (bottom), and auditory brainstem implant speech processor, postauricular microphone, and transmitter coil. (Courtesy of Cochlear Corp., Englewood, CO.)

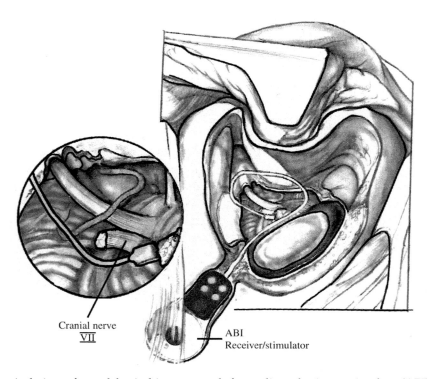

Cranial nerve
VII

ABI
Receiver/stimulator

FIGURE 29–8 Surgical view of translabyrinthine approach for auditory brainstem implant (ABI).

directly. Therefore, preserving the integrity of auditory nerve is a major surgical consideration so that cochlear implantation can be performed in the future. If surgical preservation of auditory nerve cannot be accomplished, however, subsequent hearing rehabilitation with ABI should be considered. Topodiagnostic studies are of great value in these situations.

Thorough knowledge of anatomic landmarks is essential in the localization of cochlear nucleus. Finding the lateral recess depends on identifying a 5- by 6-mm triangle formed by the exiting nerves of VII, VIII, and IX as well as the foramen of Luschka.[15] The design of Nucleus 22 and the more current model, Nucleus 24, ABIs takes into account the structural nuances of the lateral recess and the surface of cochlear nucleus (Fig. 29–7). As essential as anatomic landmarks are, the optimal placement of ABI electrode array largely depends on intraoperative monitoring via evoked auditory brainstem responses.[17]

In terms of surgical approaches there are certainly multitude routes to the internal auditory canal (IAC) such as translabyrinthine, transcochlear, middle fossa, retrolabyrinthine, retrosigmoid, and suboccipital approaches. Translabyrinthine approach was originally advocated by House and Hitselberger et al[15] as the most direct access to the foramen of Luschka (Fig. 29–8). The retrosigmoid approach in combination with the transmastoid approach appears to offer several advantages in situations where either cochlear nerve preservation or simultaneous ABI implantation is performed.[18] Significant features of this route are the ease of intraoperative monitoring of cochlear nerve action potentials, excellent visualization of the lateral recess of the fourth ventricle, and greater room to manipulate skull base endoscopes as means of improving three-dimensional orientation.

From 1992 to 1999, 58 patients were implanted with ABIs at 18 centers in Europe and Asia.[19] Most patients were noted to use their ABI daily. Some reported perception of different sounds and frequencies, enhancement of lip-reading ability, and even the use of telephones. Patients in multiple electrode array studies demonstrated different pitch perception and the use of tonotopic organization of cochlear nucleus complex. Similar results were also reported by the House Institute in Los Angeles.[20]

Surgical application of ABIs and postoperative rehabilitation have demonstrated effectiveness and safety in helping patients improve their communicative skills, acoustic orientation, and overall quality of life.

CONCLUSION

Implantable hearing aid technology has evolved over the past several decades. With the recent advancement in the semiconductor industry, its development has accelerated. Cosmesis, comfort, safety, and effectiveness are important factors in their design. During the rapid growth in their use some devices will stand the test of the time and be widely accepted. It would be exciting to witness their development as the paradigm of the fusion between medicine and modern technology.

REFERENCES

1. Goode RL, Rosenbaum ML, Maniglia AJ. The history and development of the implantable hearing aid. *Otolaryngol Clin North Am* 1995;28:1–16.
2. Snik AFM, Mylanus EAM, Cremers CWRJ. The bone-anchored hearing aid. *Otolaryngol Clin North Am* 2001;34:365–372.
3. Jahrsdoerfer RA, Yeakley JW, Aguilar EA, et al. Grading system for the selection of patients with congenital aural atresia. *Am J Otol* 1992;13:6–12.
4. Tjellstrom A. The bone-anchored hearing aid. In: Brackmann DE, Shelton C, Arriaga MA, eds. *Otologic Surgery.* 2nd ed. Philadelphia: WB Saunders; 2001:360–370.
5. Hakansson B, Liden G, Tjellstrom A, et al. Ten years of experience with the Swedish bone anchored hearing system. *Ann Otol Rhinol Layngol Suppl* 1990;99:1–16.
6. Tjellstrom A, Hakansson B, Granstrom G. Bone-anchored hearing aids: current status in adults and children. *Otolaryngol Clin North Am* 2001;34:337–363.
7. Abramson M, Fay TH, Kelly JP, et al. Clinical results with a percutaneous bone-anchored hearing aid. *Laryngoscope* 1989;99:707–710.
8. Slattery WH, Soli SD. Implantable hearing devices. In: Brackmann DE, Shelton C, Arriaga MA, eds. *Otologic Surgery.* 2nd ed. Philadelphia: WB Saunders; 2001:350–359.
9. Food and Drug Administration. Summary of safety and effectiveness data on SOUNDTEC Direct Drive Hearing System (DDHS), September 2001.
10. Hough JV, Matthews P, Wood MW, Dyer RK Jr. Middle ear electromagnetic semi-implantable hearing device: results of the phase II SOUNDTEC direct system clinical trial. *Otol Neurotol* 2002;23:895–903.
11. First Chronic Implant Performed, Envoy-Voices, St. Croix Medical, Minneapolis, MN, March 2000.
12. Kasic JF, Fredrickson JM. The Otologics MET ossicular stimulator. *Otolaryngol Clin North Am* 2001;34:501–513.
13. Yanagihara N, Sato H, Hinohira Y, Kiyohumi G, Hori K. Long-term results using a piezoelectric semi-implantable middle ear hearing device. *Otolaryngol Clin North Am* 2001;34:389–400.
14. Luetje CM, Brackman D, Balkany TJ, et al. Phase III clinical trial results with the Vibrant Soundbridge

implantable middle ear hearing device: a prospective controlled multicenter study. *Otolaryngol Head Neck Surg* 2002;126:97–107.

15. Hitselberger N, House WF, Edgerton BS, Whitaker S. Cochlear nucleus implant. *Otolaryngol Head Neck Surg* 1984;92:52–54.

16. Ricardi VM. Neurofibromatosis. *Neurol Clin North Am* 1987;5:337–349.

17. Niparko JK, Kileny PR, Kemink JL, et al. Neurophysiologic intraoperative monitoring. II: facial nerve function. *Am J Otol* 1989;10:55–61.

18. Colletti V, Sacchetto L, Giarbini N, Fiorino F, Carner M. Retrosigmoid approach for auditory brainstem implant. *J Laryngol Otol Suppl* 2000;(suppl 27):37–40.

19. Sollman WP, Laszig R, Marangos N. Surgical experiences in 58 cases using the nucleus 22 multichannel auditory brainstem implant. *J Laryngol Otol Suppl* 2000;(suppl 27):23–26.

20. Otto SR, Brackmann DE, Hitselberger WE, Shannon RV, Kuchta J. Multichannel auditory brainstem implant: update on performance in 61 patients. *J Neurosurg* 2002;96:1063–1071.

AFTERWORD

In 1938 Julius Lempert boldly developed a one-stage operation for otosclerosis, the lateral semicircular canal fenestration procedure. Because of his success, medical school professors began to encourage students to enter the field of otolaryngology, and subsequently John Shea, Jr. performed the first stapedectomy on May 1, 1956. Thousands of stapedectomies are now routinely performed throughout the world each year, many by general otolaryngologists who learned the technique in residency and maintain a high level of otologic prowess in their practices. This book has presented surgical approaches to the treatment of otosclerosis as well as other ear diseases in a way that should encourage the general otolaryngologist to continue to practice the procedures they were trained to perform. Each chapter has covered a surgical procedure or set of procedures in a way that is clear, concise, and with illustrations to clarify the technique. From an editorial point of view, the reader is offered a chance in one book to read about techniques in ear surgery written by recognized international experts with an emphasis on presentation to the general otolaryngologist. Clearly, we did not want to write a book to serve as a teaching tool for the experts who wrote the chapters. Instead, we decided to offer the vast majority of practitioners in our specialty, that is, the general otolaryngologists, a textbook that should be easily decipherable, applicable to their practices, and up to date in terms of recent operative innovation.

The book was organized by procedure rather than by diseases or anatomy. That way, a practitioner can easily make reference to a specific chapter to prepare for an upcoming case. If one is about to perform a canal-wall-down mastoidectomy, what better way to prepare than to read and review the chapter by Thomas McDonald, chairman at the Mayo Clinic

and an expert in the canal-wall-down technique. If one is to prepare for a tympanoplasty, there is not anyone better to read than Edwin Monsell, professor at Wayne State University and a renowned authority in otologic surgery. If your approach requires a lateral graft technique, then one must assume that a writer from the House Ear Clinic would be the author, and indeed that is the case. Rick Friedman presents an excellent review of the technique that should be easily appreciated by the otolaryngologic practitioner. The intact bridge mastoidectomy, presented by Hamed Sajjadi, provides an alternative approach to mastoid and chronic ear disease that has broad applicability. The textbook covers most of the otologic operations that a general otolaryngologist would perform, and even goes beyond that, as in the case of posterior semicircular canal occlusion or implantable hearing aids, procedures that may not be readily performed by many otolaryngologists, but could be if the surgeon prepared adequately. That brings us to the question of who should perform otologic surgery. Should procedures be relegated to neurotologists or subspecialists in otology? Should stapes surgery be limited to specific otologists? Should those at universities perform only mastoidectomies? I think that most general otolaryngologists are excellent otologic surgeons and should perform the procedures that they feel comfortable doing, and that includes stapedectomy and mastoid surgery as well as most middle ear and mastoid surgery. Thus, there seems to be no better time than now to publish a textbook like this one, complete and operationally sound, and part of the library of practicing otolaryngologists.

This is the first edition of *Middle Ear and Mastoid Surgery*, but it should not be the last. Over time, techniques will become more refined and today's operations may soon be part of tomorrow's otolaryngologic history. New innovations will arise and technology will advance, and that puts the emphasis on the surgeon to keep up with the times and stay current with novel and groundbreaking developments. In the next edition, changes will no doubt occur and the presentation may be different or slightly altered to reflect changes in the ever-changing field of otologic surgery. There may be different authors or an expanded number of authors, depending on the number of chapters written or if new technologies and techniques become more commonplace. What is assured is that the world of modern middle ear and mastoid surgery will be presented in a format that is easily usable by the general otolaryngologist.

I would like to thank the many authors who contributed to this project. They were asked to contribute to the current state of hard-bound text literature by spending hours of extra time on chapters about which they are recognized experts. It is a thankless job and requires many hours of diligence to achieve the high degree of excellence that is required to be acknowledged as an expert or authority. They did it without remuneration. Instead they present a commitment to excellence that makes my job as editor easier, knowing that the information presented is the best the world can see.

I would like to thank the publisher, Thieme Medical Publishers Inc., for soliciting my involvement in this project. I wasn't sure at first how it would play out, but now I'm convinced that this book is a necessary addition to the current literature. I look forward to the next edition!

Rex S. Haberman II, M.D.